R. BROBY-JOHANSEN

BODY AND CLOTHES

An illustrated History af Costume

R.BROBY-JOHANSEN

BODY

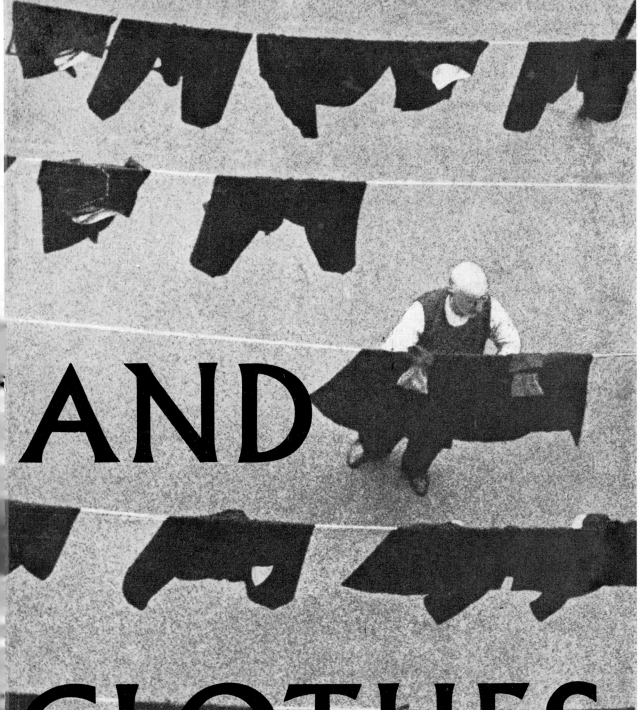

AND

CLOTHES

FABER & FABER LTD

Published in Great Britain, 1968 by
Faber and Faber Limited
24 Russell Square London W C 1

Translated from the Danish by Karen Rush
and Erik I. Friis
Drawings by Ebbe Sunesen
All rights reserved
Printed in Denmark by Krohns Bogtrykkeri,
Copenhagen

S.B.N. 571 08731 0

Published in Copenhagen by Gyldendal
under the title Krop og Klær
© 1966 by R. Broby-Johansen, Copenhagen
Translation © 1968 by Faber and Faber Limited,
London

Acknowledgement
We would like to thank Penguin Books Limited for
permission to reproduce an excerpt from
Nevill Coghill's translation of The Canterbury Tales
by Geoffrey Chaucer.

Title page, left   Cave-painting of naked Bushwomen, South Africa
Title page, right The modern man's wardrobe

CONTENTS

Foreword 5

Primitive Peoples 6

Classical Dress 33
  The Wrapped Garment 33
  The Egyptian Loin-Cloth 35
  The Mesopotamian Wrap 41
  The Greek Chiton 46
  The Roman Toga 52
  The Arab Haik 59
  The Indian Sari 62

Workaday Clothes 67
  The Armour of Antiquity 67
  The Goat-Skin Skirt of the Aegean 73
  Persian Leather Trousers 77
  The Indian Feather Poncho 83
  The Mongolian Silk Kimono 89
  The Eskimo Skin Clothes 98

Clothes and Status 101
  Historical Costumes 101
  Robes of Byzantium 300—1100 102
  Romanesque Shift and
    Monk's Cowl 800—1350 111
  Gothic Armour and
    Pointed Shoes 1350—1490 121
  Renaissance Fashion 1490—1625 133
  Baroque Lace and Footwear 1625—1710 . . 147
  Rococo Fashion and
    Powdered Wigs 1710—1790 163

Changing Fashions 175
  Fashion During and After the French
    Revolution 1790—1830 176
  Crinolines and Stovepipes 1830—1870 . . 185
  Jackets and Bustles 1870—1890 195
  Corsetted Waist and
    Wing Collar 1890—1920 201
  Functional Design 1920—1950 215
  Today's Fashions —
    and What the Future May Bring 226
  Expanded Table of Contents 235

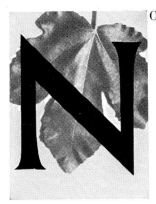

NO REASON exists for feeling that one's body is a forbidden topic. What might make it seem so are the associations of fear it has come to carry. After all, it is only in very recent times that the body, after being assiduously concealed for hundreds of years, has been revealed. This process, once begun, seems almost to be escalating. The increasing manifestation of the body has caused a measure of surprise, and the phenomenon is still regarded with deep suspicion.

It must, nevertheless, be acknowledged that we relate many of our concepts of nature to the human body. We refer, for example, to 'the foot' of a mountain and 'the neck' of a river isthmus, and we say that a tree 'stands'. Michelangelo extended this parallel when he stated, 'The man who cannot master the human body, and particularly its anatomy, will never understand the meaning of architecture.'

All our ideas of proportion are related to the body. Our movements arise out of our sight and our instinctive muscular reactions. Whether we are sleeping or waking, our feeling for rhythm is closely connected with our regular heartbeats and the rise and fall of our breathing.

Clothes assume significance only when they are on the body. When they are hung up in a wardrobe they look pathetically helpless; they seem to be voicelessly denouncing the cruelty of the tailor who forced them into their state of sad dependence. To really understand clothes it is necessary first to see the reasoning behind them and then to see them, as it were, in action. Clothes are more than just products of a textile factory or exhibits in a museum; they are artefacts, used by people in all activities of dayly life — standing, sitting, dancing, working or dying. Their true significance only becomes apparent when we consider how they are related and adapted to the body. So many different human types exist: thin people, fat people, people with large heads, pin-headed people. But human nature being perverse, styles do not always echo the body framework. If the body does not suit a certain style of dress then it is the clothes and not the body which should be modified.

But the determining factor is really neither the body nor the clothes. It is Fashion. Fashion extends far beyond mere clothes; it is affected by how we stand, sit, smile and cry, how we love and how we hate. It is nothing less than an attempt to unify all the expressive capacities of language, gesture and physiognomy in a given society.

Clothes represent an art form rising out of a period and environment and as such are no less valid than other artistic creations. Dress design is a craft comparable with architecture, but lacking the latter's permanence. It is an art which, like music, is in constant movement but, unlike music, it cannot express direct emotion. As are both these arts, dress design is also non-figurative. It seeks not to pretend, but rather to display. It is at one and the same time fettered and free, as is all genuine art. There is the simple type of dress which innocently declares its purpose, like a ball-dress, and then there are carefully constructed complex compositions like the armour of the Middle Ages.

As do all other works of art, clothes reflect the times in which they were created. People reveal themselves unconsciously both in the art forms they accept, and those they reject. No form of art is more subtle than the variations that dress design creates upon that most fascinating of all themes — the human body.

When we consider the subject of dress through the centuries, it is not details of the dressmaker's skill which concern us most, but rather a gradual awareness of fashion as a camouflage, as a long series of devices for hiding the true nature of men and women, created by God in his own image. The value of such duplicity is surely negative, on a par with the conjuror who draws attention to his empty hand which does not do the trick.

The history of dress is full of deception and self-delusion, deliberate mistakes and unconscious mistakes, the calculated and uncalculated in a long and illogical record of human folly. In short, it is simply the history of mankind. The interplay between the two sexes, with the whole range of shifting emotions that it encompasses, forms a mirror in which is reflected the ever-changing world of fashion. Dress does not merely show how men and women wish to appear; it provides answers to many questions and also a criticism of the people who ask them. Women's fashions through the ages can provide a mass of silent evidence against the tyranny of the male at various times, and men's fashions can make out an equally strong case against the female sex. These situations occur because each sex reacts in accordance with the demands of the opposite sex. In a subtle way, the nature of one sex is revealed in the concealments of the other.

The history of dress cannot be treated as a conducted tour in which wheels revolve and carry both author and reader to a predetermined destination. The reader must be a pedestrian and use his legs; he must halt continually to adjust his bearings and change his point of view, sometimes to regard woman from the man's angle and at other times vice versa. It is necessary to observe and study all aspects of the history of dress from both these standpoints before we can hope to gain a real understanding of fashion.

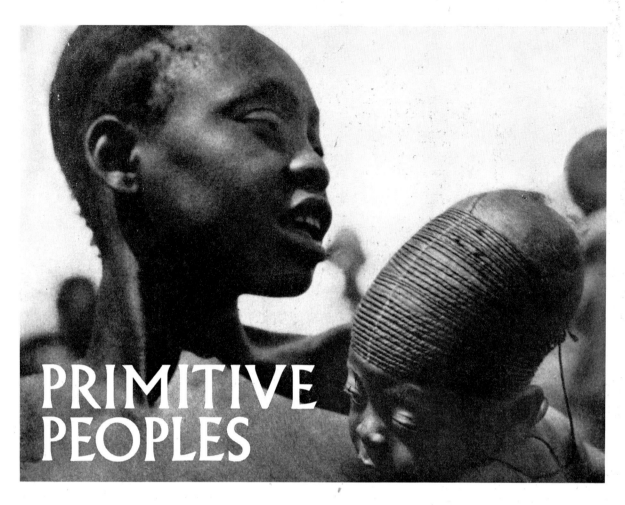

PRIMITIVE PEOPLES

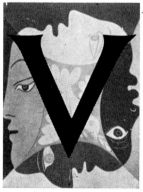

VALUES and attitudes influencing the way we clothe ourselves have changed over the centuries. Nowadays we are so accustomed to clothes that we regard them as an integral part of ourselves and of our personalities.

All over the world, peoples of every race and nationality have gradually accepted clothes, in icy climates because of the cold and in hot climates because of the heat. It goes without saying that clothing can serve as protection. One has only to cite the foundry worker's asbestos apron which insulates him from the blast of the furnace or the Arab's turban which shields him from the sun.

On the other hand we find clothing which is worn for reasons other than protection, for example bathing suits. It is noteworthy that we do not cover extremely sensitive organs such as the eyes, nose and ears, as Montaigne pointed out in the sixteenth century.

The sparseness of hair on the human body is often used as an argument for the necessity of clothes. Wearing fur is one way of insulating the body against the cold, but it is wrong to think that all warm-blooded animals are provided with fur. The whale, a warm-blooded mammal who lives in the Arctic and Antarctic Oceans, has a smooth skin, and so does the porpoise. These animals rely on the same principle of insulation as we do, namely, a layer of fat under the skin.

Smooth-skinned human beings have lived on the earth for hundreds of thousands of years without ever knowing about clothes. In cave-paintings dating from the Ice Age mammoth and reindeer and naked hunters run side by side. The truth is that the very wearing of clothes has made the human body more sensitive to cold. We know, for instance, that the Patagonians, who lived near the southernmost tip of South America where the climate is severe, used to go about completely naked. When white missionaries came they insisted that the natives be decently dressed, and the race died out.

Another misguided belief is the conviction that the human body must be heated from without. Our internal metabolic processes make it essential that heat is shed continually. A substantial rise in body temperature above 98.6° Fahrenheit would result in certain death.

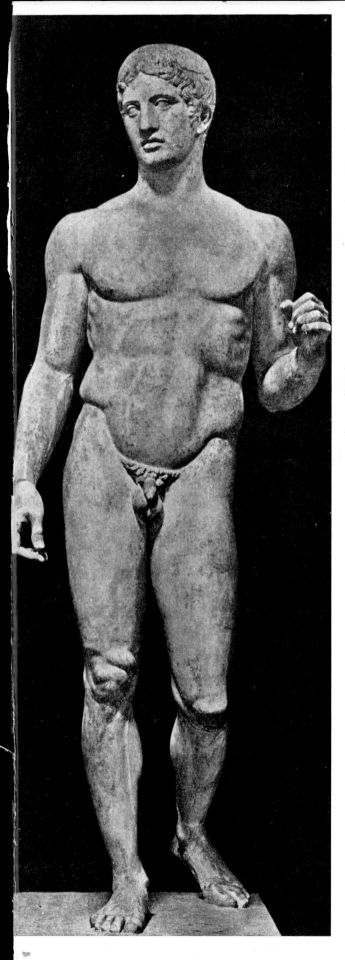

The Price of Nakedness

The human body can, to some extent, be trained to produce heat in order to adjust to the temperature of its surroundings. The Finns, for example, jump from hot Sauna baths into the snow, and Eskimo women take their children, stark naked, out of their carrying-bags in the middle of a snow-storm when the temperature is 30 degrees below freezing-point.

The human skin is almost certainly man's greatest advantage over the animal world. Compared to the human skin with its capacity to react to and adjust itself to changes of temperature, the fur or hair covering of the animal is an extremely primitive form of protection. Yet instead of conditioning and training this organism to perform its natural function, we seem to do our utmost to put it out of order. The 'normal' temperature for the air surrounding the human body is a question of habit. Many doctors maintain that children should get used to running about naked in normal indoor temperatures from an early age. It is worth noting that the average woman wears between a half and one tenth of the amount of the clothes worn by men. One explanation given is that women have a thicker layer of fat under the skin and therefore need less protection. In fact, the exact opposite might well be the case. It is a question of habit surely. Boys become accustomed to wearing thicker clothes from babyhood. Compare a photograph of a beach fifty years ago with one of today and you will see how emaciated men's legs and thighs then were since they were covered up all the year round; they probably wore long woollen underwear as well. Sheer stockings not only show of a girl's shapely legs, but they actually encourage those curves. In his book, *Woman's Beauty*, the Renaissance writer, Firenzuola, says, 'A woman's leg should be like the contours of an antique vase, with the outlines rising and falling gently.'

Cold Shoulders and Empty Stomachs

The normal process of heat regulation has had to be supplemented by artificial means and one saves on food, or body fuel, by being clothed. Another thing to be taken into account is that man is made to work, which entails activity and keeps him warm. But our civilized schools make children sit stock still. Mechanized transport also demands little movement and the motorist actually wraps himself up in the same way as primitive people used to do when they went to sleep.

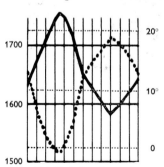

The thick black line shows the metabolism in the human body throughout the twelve months of the year. The dotted line indicates the average temperatures during the same twelve months. During the cold months the consumption of calories – the numbers on the left – is heavy while it is light in the warmer months

The words 'cold' and 'warm' are also associated with the feelings. We speak of a cold ex-

The Spear Carrier, Polycleitus (about 450 B.C.)
The statue embodies the Greek conception of the ideal male body

7

pression and a warm smile, of warm and cold colours. When we are miserable or depressed, we feel we need more clothes than when we are happy. Clothes are portable houses which have grown around us like the shell of a snail. But the fetish for encasing ourselves in layer upon layer of clothing is gradually breaking down and we have now discovered that we can come out of our shells and move freely in the sun, the air and the water. This, and not the television or the atom bomb, is the greatest step forward of our time.

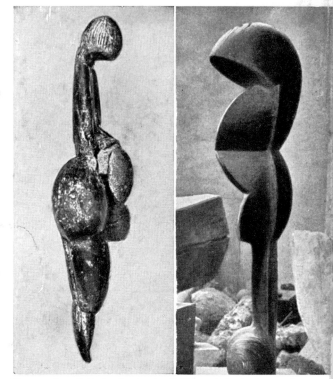

The rear view of this Ice Age figurine (left) was obviously the one that mattered. The sculpture of a woman by the contemporary sculptor, Brancusi (right) emphasizes the front view.

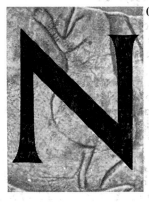

NO SIGN of clothing has been found in Southern Europe before the end of the so-called Reindeer Period, which came after the Ice Age fifteen to thirty thousand years ago. A number of small figurines from that era, worked in stone or bone, give a clear impression of the feeling which men of that time had for the unchanging female shape. They are small statuettes, without any feet, whose gentle curves could be stroked or caressed by rough hands.

In our times naked girls are no less objects of appreciation; magazine covers, films and paintings give ample evidence of this. Today's cult of the female nude has, however, an abstract character about it which is quite different from the rough realism of the Ice Age figurines. Among the latter, the female forms swelled in exaggerated pregnancy similar to the style in which animals were painted on the cave walls.

The only piece of clothing found on a few of these figurines is a kind of small apron secured at the back by a belt. This apron could have been made of thongs or twine. Its use cannot, however, be related to civilized conceptions of modesty. The intention was indeed not to obscure, but rather to emphasize sexual characteristics. For example, some male pygmies wore nothing but a yellow calabash or gourd two inches in diameter and sixteen inches

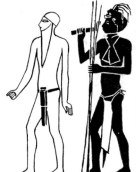

Penis cases from Egypt and New Caledonia

long between their legs; penis cases adorned with precious stones were worn by certain tribes of South American Indians.

The extraordinary thing about the apron shown here is that it covered the buttocks. Most of these figurines appear to have been designed to be looked at from behind, and many have enormous posteriors. These over-developed buttocks are still fashionable; present-day African Hottentots achieve them by binding the body tightly from early childhood. In the Ice Age they were a result of its being a man's world. Hunting wild animals demanded courage and a strong physique. (The justification for referring to man as the stronger sex possibly lies in his ability to produce a concentrated amount of strength when necessary.) At that time woman was a prey to be hunted and run to ground by the male pursuer who sank his teeth into her neck. The woman's rear apron was there to attract the male; and this was the first and basic purpose of dress.

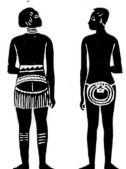

Rear aprons worn by Kaffirs and Congolese Negroes

A figurine from the Ice Age wearing the rear apron

8

Opposite A relief from the Ice Age showing a woman with a drinking-horn. The work still carries traces of red paint. Actual height is about eighteen inches

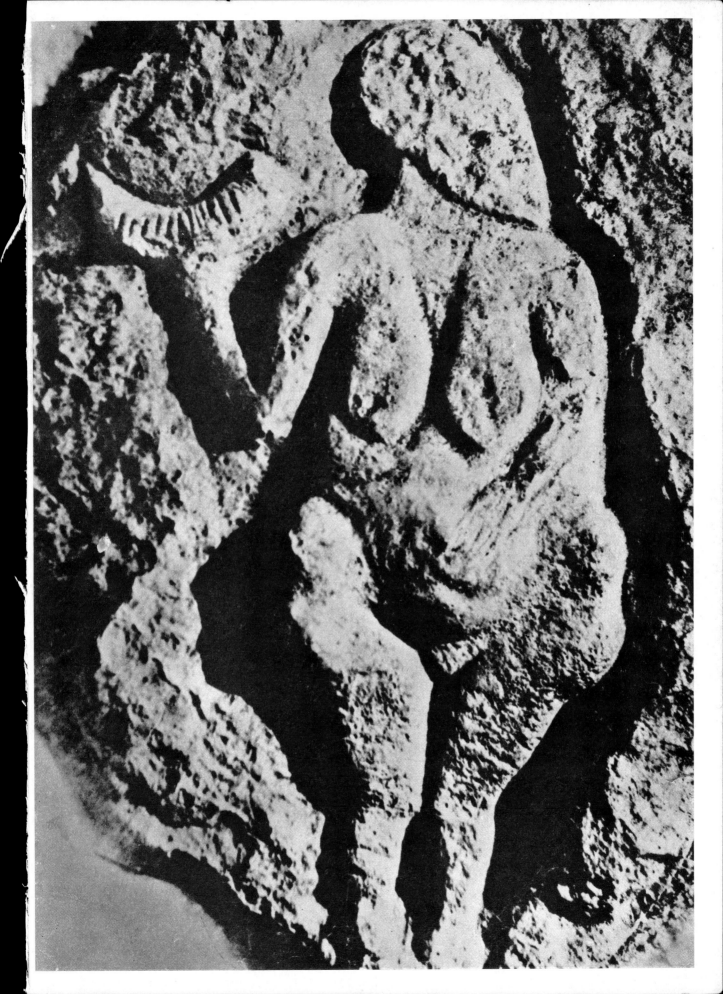

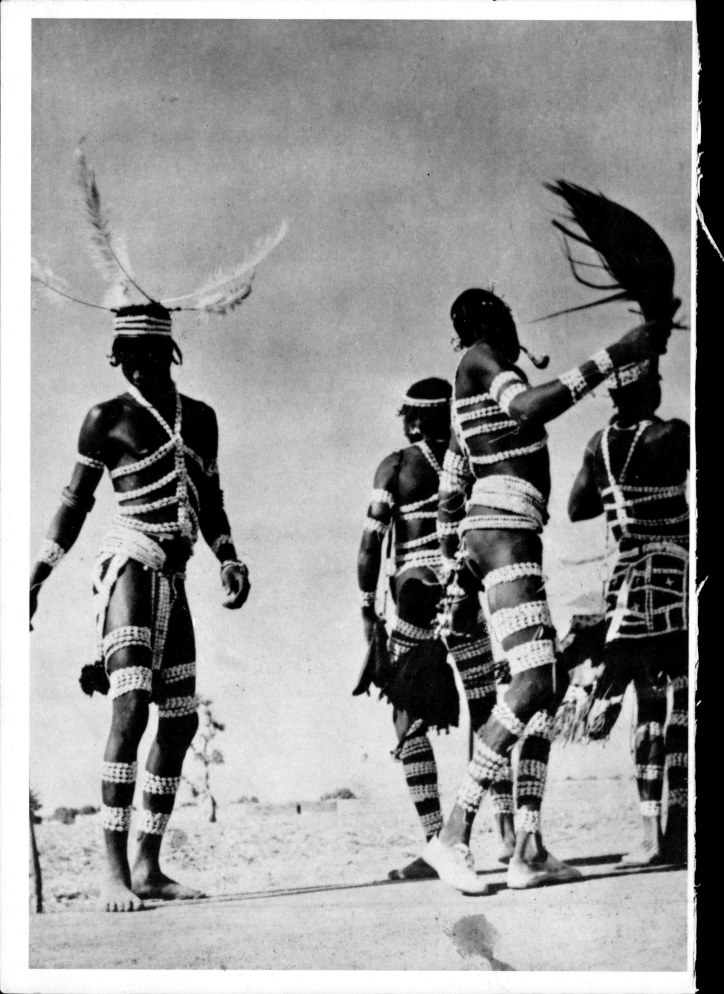

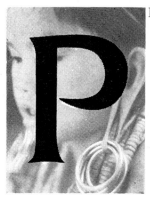

PEOPLE began to till the soil in the agricultural era, no longer roaming the country in small nomadic groups as the primitive hunters had done. They joined together in communities and could thus co-operate in agricultural activities. As they cultivated their fields they became more cultivated themselves. Well-nourished girls came to be prized, and it was regarded as an indication of prosperity to be fat and to have a fat wife. The Indian moralist, Manu, said that one ought to choose a wife with the walk of an elephant. Some African tribes pay for their brides according to weight. Arms and legs were thickened by the application of tight bandages. The first American Indians to be encountered by European explorers had their knees and ankles bound, causing the calves to swell up like balloons. The Papuans in New Guinea wore tight metal rings around their upper arms so that their arms grew thicker and the muscles swelled on either side of the ring.

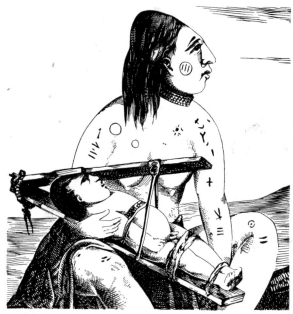

Leg bandages used by the Caribe Indians and an arm ring from Melanesia

Flat Foreheads. The shape of the head was altered by tying tight bandages around the head of a new-

The method employed in Central America to flatten the foreheads of children

born child. The American Indians changed the shape of the child's head by pressing it between wooden boards, a custom which still persists in certain parts of Africa. Portraits of the ruling classes in Egypt of a certain period show that the back of the head was greatly enlarged, almost like a balloon. The common people in all these ancient races had to carry water pitchers and other heavy burdens on their heads. By having an elongated head, a person clearly indicated that he belonged to a higher social class and that his head was not utilitarian but solely an object of beauty.

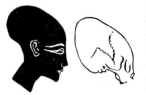

An Egyptian head and a cranium from Peru

Plate-Shaped Lips and Elongated Ears. In some African Negro tribes, the women insert pieces of wood as large as plates behind their lips. An interest-

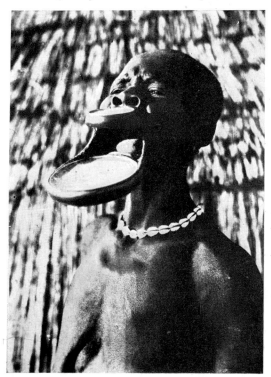

An African Negro with plate-shaped lips

ing theory is that these deformities were perpetrated for very practical reasons. When marauding Arabs carried off African girls to be slaves in their harems, they did not look at girls with misshapen or deformed lips. This was because the Arabs kiss like Europeans, whereas, among the tribes concerned, kissing is quite unknown. Another

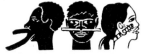

An East African Negro with plate-shaped lips; an adornment for the nose from Australia; and a decoration for the ear from Formosa

custom is piercing the cartilage of the nose and inserting pieces of wood, metal or shell.

It is the ear, however, on which primitive peoples lavish the greatest artistic energy, and it would seem that its very toughness has encouraged experiments in decoration. There are practically no primitive people who have not reshaped the ear. In places such as South India and among the Papuan tribes, ear-pierc-

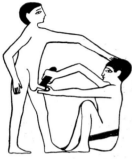

Circumcision in an Egyptian relief

ing is a religious ceremony on a par with our christening. Among the Kaffirs, the reshaped ear is reserved for 'men only'. Some Zambesi Negroes' ears hang down over their shoulders with a hole in the lobe large enough for an arm to pass through. The New Caledonians sometimes carry small objects inside the ear, as if it were a case.

Self-Mutilation and the Gods. Circumcision is another simple incision, whose hygienic significance in hot climates is indisputable. In Europe it is regarded as being mostly a Jewish custom, but it is observed in all Islamic countries, by many African Negroes, Australian Aborigines and by Indians of both North and South America. Primitive peasant communities believe in spirits and gods who resemble human beings. In these societies, circumcision is based not on practical value, but forms part of religious ritual. In another puberty ceremony, the front teeth

Front teeth that have been filed down. From West Africa

are extracted or filed down, so that an exit may be provided for the free passage of the soul. Mutilation causes blood to flow, and to see blood — or even to read about it — stimulates excitement. (Newspapers today make capital out of the same instinct in reporting violence and murder.) Blood is a vital and precious thing, an offering of which a man can be proud. Therefore there is good reason to preserve and even enlarge the scar, so that it constitutes a continual reminder to everyone that a worthy offering has been made.

Civilized Body Culture. When hair is pulled out, shaved off or cut, a part of the body is removed. Hair

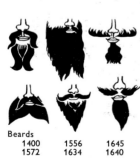

Beards
1400 1556 1645
1572 1634 1640

styles, therefore, are really a deformation based on fashion. Some of the Crow Indians grow long hair, while the women wear their hair short. Curiously enough, straight-haired people do their utmost to make their hair curl, whereas naturally curly-haired people do just the opposite. Racial groups

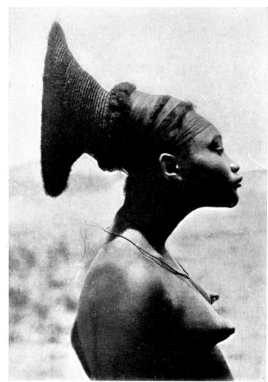

Coiffure from the Congo. It shows a striking resemblance to hair styles seen in Spanish cave-paintings dating from the Ice Age (see illustration below)

with short, thin hair make it solid and stiff by applying clay, tallow or cow manure, and then decorate their heads with animal hair and feathers.

Among civilized peoples, mutilation is largely confined to ear-piercing. In India, one side of the nose is still pierced for the insertion of a piece of gold, silver or a precious stone.

Even down to present times, the heads of children in Europe have been reshaped by tight bandages. Deformed skulls dating from the thirteenth century have been found in the Riddarholm Church in Stockholm. During the National Socialist Regime in Germany in the 1930's and

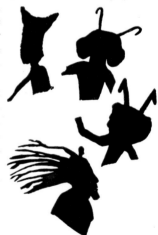

Hair styles of the Ice Age

1940's, the delichocephalic 'Aryan' head was greatly valued and many parents tried to improve their children's cranial index. Generally speaking, however, the white man has confined his attention to the more central parts of the body. Piercing the ear or the nose is a comparatively harmless adornment which affects neither the sense of hearing nor of smell; and altering the shape of head or limbs likewise causes no harmful effect on the general health. But, on the other hand, the white man's maltreatment of the waist and feet has given rise to serious physical consequences.

The tightly laced stays and bindings worn by Europeans and Indians, from the Bronze Age right up to the present day have resulted in deformities even more shocking than those known among primitive cultures. Throughout the centuries stays and corsets have been connected with all kinds of female diseases and infirmities. It is true that some

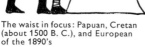

The waist in focus: Papuan, Cretan (about 1500 B. C.), and European of the 1890's

tribes, such as the Mehuans in Papua, have worn tight belts, but no primitive peoples have ever tried forcibly to reshape the entire human torso.

Cinderella's Glass Slipper. Only the tiny feet of the Chinese women of the past can compete with the average Western European feet of our time. One of the principal differences between the human skeleton and that of other vertebrates lies in the bone structure

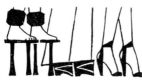

Lofty people: shoes for Syrian, Chinese, and European ladies

of the foot. In the human frame twenty-six bones combine to form a resilient arch. High-heeled shoes or boots destroy the elasticity of the foot, while low heels tend to do much the same. High heels also cause bent knees, a protruding posterior and a zig-zag posture. Under these conditions, no single organ retains its natural position. Laced-up shoes enclose the foot like a box and press down on arch and instep.

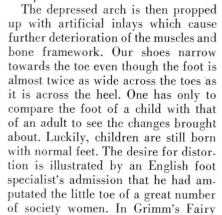

The depressed arch is then propped up with artificial inlays which cause further deterioration of the muscles and bone framework. Our shoes narrow towards the toe even though the foot is almost twice as wide across the toes as it is across the heel. One has only to compare the foot of a child with that of an adult to see the changes brought about. Luckily, children are still born with normal feet. The desire for distortion is illustrated by an English foot specialist's admission that he had amputated the little toe of a great number of society women. In Grimm's Fairy Tale the prince's bride had to have a foot small enough to fit a glass slipper. In order to make the shoe fit, Cinderella's elder sister cut off her

Four degress of elevation: European shoes of the 17th, 18th, 19th and 20th centuries

big toe. 'After all,' said her mother, 'Once she is queen she won't need to walk any more.' Cinderella's younger sister then cut off the back of her heel. But both sisters were given away by the blood that filled the shoe. Physical deformity can be an indication of social status: a small foot is regarded as the foot of a true queen.

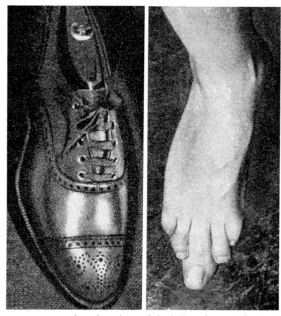

A modern shoe and the foot, as shoe manufacturers evidently imagine it to be

Nature provides a normal body free of change, but we go to great expense to achieve small feet and unnaturally slender waists through methods possible for only the privileged few in our society.

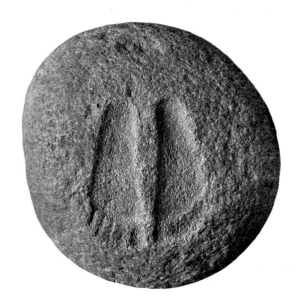

A Dane's feet. A Bronze Age rock-carving of 1000 B.C.

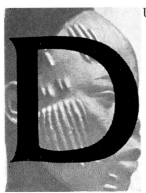

DURING THE ICE AGE it appears that corpses of important people were painted with a red colouring. It is possible that colour was also used as adornment during life. The same colours used in cave-paintings may have been used on the human skin, thus making them the forerunners of powder, lipstick and rouge.

We know that the types of hunting weapons used by primitive people, such as the Bushmen of South Africa, made it necessary for them to get within a very close range of their prey. Consequently, they found it advantageous to paint themselves with red and yellow stripes and thus camouflaged they blended into the landscape. The Ona Indians of the snowy Tierra del Fuego paint themselves white in winter for the same reasons. Similarly, the army of the Swedish king, Charles Gustavus X, who besieged Copenhagen during the winter, wore white shirts on top of their uniforms, as did the Finns in the Winter War of 1939-40.

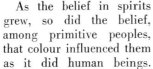

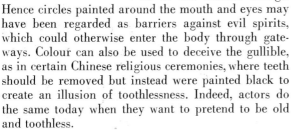

Terracotta figures of the Neolithic Age showing patterns of painted or tattooed lines

As the belief in spirits grew, so did the belief, among primitive peoples, that colour influenced them as it did human beings. Hence circles painted around the mouth and eyes may have been regarded as barriers against evil spirits, which could otherwise enter the body through gateways. Colour can also be used to deceive the gullible, as in certain Chinese religious ceremonies, where teeth should be removed but instead were painted black to create an illusion of toothlessness. Indeed, actors do the same today when they want to pretend to be old and toothless.

Colours for Identification. Colour may be used to indicate order in a stratified society. In many tribes, the men are painted red-brown to signify outdoor life and being bronzed by the sun, while the women paint themselves a pale yellow as a sign of innocent womanhood. Different colouring makes it easier for a tribal chief to identify his men in battle — as is still the case in football games, for instance, today. The tribal colour serves much the same purpose as the military uniform of later ages. The warrior identifies himself with the totem of his tribe or state, and he fights or dies for his national colours.

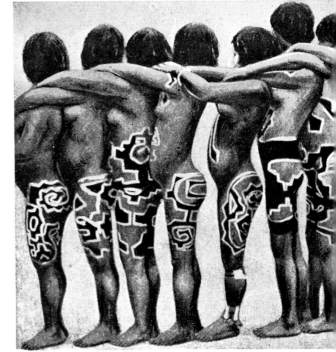

Painted Indian girls of the Amazon region performing a snake dance. This dance symbolizes the unity of the tribe under the leadership of the chief, "the snake's head"

Fear-Inspiring. Festive and Mourning Make-up.

The Indians in our childhood stories were called Redskins. The name was derived not from the natural yellow-brown of their skin, but from their warpaint. Red warpaint was a symbol of the enemy's blood. In Ancient Rome, victorious leaders were carried in triumph to the Capitol, their faces and chests painted with red lead. The purpose of brightly coloured uniforms was to strike terror into the heart of the enemy. The white design sewn onto the Hussar tunic suggested the ribs of a skeleton supplemented by the skull and crossbones of the cap.

The women of the ancient Celts painted themselves blue on special festivals. The Caledonians paint their bodies black for certain occasions to provide a flattering background for the garlands of flowers which they hang around their necks. Javanese women colour the upper part of the body with saffron yellow powder. In certain North American Indian tribes the widow paints her face black for her husband's funeral, and even nowadays it is customary for a widow to cover her face with a black veil in many countries.

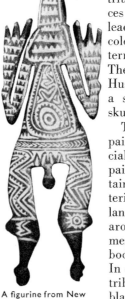

A figurine from New Guinea, indicating how the men painted and decorated themselves

Whatever may have been the original reason for

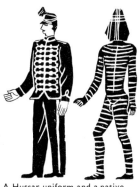

A Hussar uniform and a native of Tierra del Fuego whose body is painted with white stripes

applying colour to the face or body, it is clear that the principal object was to make the men look ferocious and the women attractive. The colours used evolved into cosmetics applied for the same purpose. Young Jibaro South American Indians applied rouge to their cheeks. French explorers recorded in the seventeenth century that just as Frenchwomen rouged their cheeks, so did Tahitian women paint their bottoms blue!

Decorative Scars. Tattooing is a versatile method of permanent body decoration. Dark races, such as African Negroes, boast scars which stand out white or

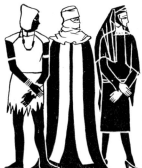

Tattooed legs from the Marquesas Islands and a decorated embalmed head from New Guinea

pink against their skin. Fair-skinned Polynesians and Europeans apply colour to wounds in order to produce striking and vivid scars. In general, scars and tattoos signify courage. German university students used to prize the facial scars acquired in fencing duels, but these could also be produced artificially for decorative purposes. In the South Sea Islands tattoo marks are the privilege of the well-to-do, while the Haida Indians

Widows' weeds: in New Guinea, Europe in the 16th century, and Europe today

in North America are tattooed in order to convey family and rank. Darwin regarded tattoos as artificially

Ainu woman from Japan

created secondary sex characteristics, since their design and use always differed between male and female. A curious example of how far people will go in stressing natural differences, is the custom among Japanese Ainu women of having moustaches tattooed on their upper lip, and Aleut men who carefully pluck all hair from their faces.

Moving Pictures. Lombroso, with his famous theory that criminals are born and not made, maintains that tattoo marks indicate a moral deficiency. Splendid, you might say, so potential criminals supply the police with ready-made identification marks. It may, however, be more reasonable to assume that tattooed people are comparatively less complicated in their attitudes and relationships.

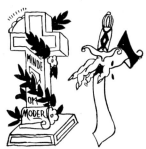

Modern tattoo patterns. The one on the right shows Asian influence

Primitive designs were geometric, whereas designs nowadays are usually naturalistic. Examples of old unsophisticated humour, in which the arms and legs of tattooed figures can be manipulated, with incongruous effect, may still be found beneath many a sailor's uniform. As far back as the Ice Age this form of humour caused hilarity. Some of these older patterns were undoubtedly intended as magic symbols. In the Far East, the body may be so completely covered with a tattooed pattern that it looks almost like a garment; the work of tattooists the world over is based on Japanese and Chinese designs. This oldest form of art, painting the human body, has, like much of modern art, renewed itself from oriental sources, without, however, losing its primitive closeness to nature. Perhaps this is worth remembering by people who fear that man may be losing his contact with nature in the machine age.

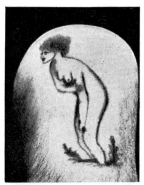

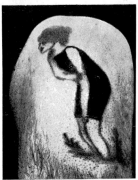

A tattoo on a sailor's knee. The original (above) and as completed (below) after the owner reached maturity

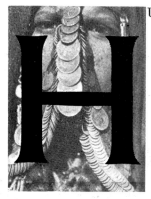

HUMAN BEINGS' delight in decoration has its counterpart in the animal world. Apes sometimes adorn themselves with fruit and foliage and entwine vines and lianas around their necks. An ape can comport himself with the dignity of a man wearing insignia and decorations. Darwin once gave a piece of red cloth to a member of a tribe in Tierra del Fuego because it was cold and the man wore no clothes. The man immediately tore the cloth into strips and handed them out to his friends who tied them round their arms and legs as adornment.

Naked people obviously have no pockets in which to carry valuables, or clothes on which to attach jewellery. They therefore display their valuables and jewellery on their bodies, and become almost a travel-

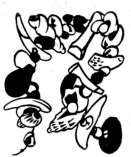

A necklace from the Ice Age

ling exhibition. Since jewellery is often made from precious metals, although non-precious metals might be just as beautiful, its use must obviously indicate wealth, calling and status.

The ornaments worn by the hunters of the Ice Age signify their social position and their renown in hunting. Such ornaments, nearly always found in graves beside male skeletons, include diadems, necklaces, bracelets, belts and anklets made from bone and shell. Some of these may have been hunting trophies worn as evidence of strength and courage.

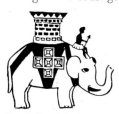

The Order of the Elephant

Whenever spirits are thought to be present the ornament becomes an amulet, acting as a protective charm against evil. Evil spirits fear the amulet, while good spirits are attracted. The ear-ring may serve as a warning, meaning 'keep away!' But ornaments, first and last, are for decoration; they are a means of creating or enhancing physical attractions. The American Indians provide many salient examples of this, with their proud and warlike feathers, their epaulettes that broaden the shoulders, necklaces that rest with contrasting grace on the broad powerful chest, and ear-rings that emphasize the gentle curve of the cheek and ear.

The recent fashion in the West of using sunflower seeds, apple pips, brown beans and shells to make necklaces and bracelets is one of the many signs of today's revolt against dress and jewellery that imply class distinction.

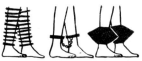

African anklets

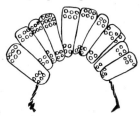 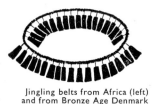

Jingling belts from Africa (left) and from Bronze Age Denmark

Heavy jewellery is most often worn by slender races who have fine limbs and slim necks. More delicate less massive jewellery is worn by races who are more heavily built. Silver is a favourite of dark-skinned peoples, gold of brown races, jade of yellow-skinned people and amber of fair, blonde-headed girls. The jingle of metal and sound of shells make delightful music which can be produced by the slightest movement. In modern society jewellery does not play such an important part. Necklaces, bracelets and rings are now much more modest in size, and their jingle would not be generally considered as consonant with respectability.

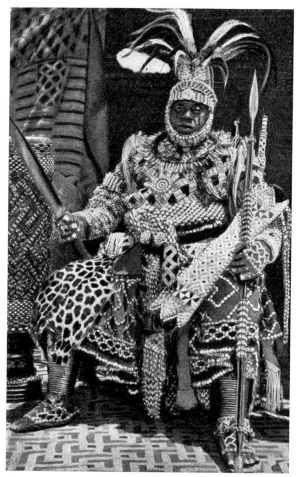

West African chief in full regalia, so weighty that without help he is unable to move

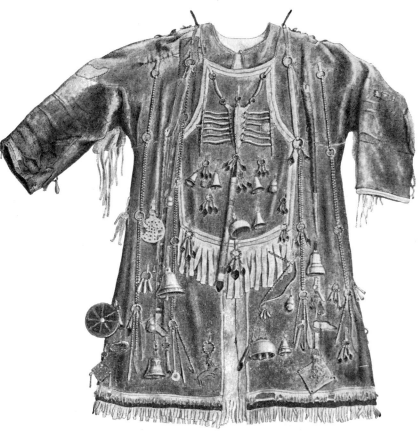

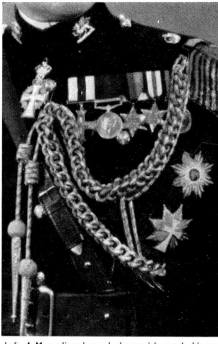

Left, A Mongolian shaman's dress with metal objects, bells and chains attached. Right, Modern military decorations
Below, Stone face from Easter Island with an 'ear-ring'. This large round piece of metal piercing the lobe is still worn among the Indians of Central and South America

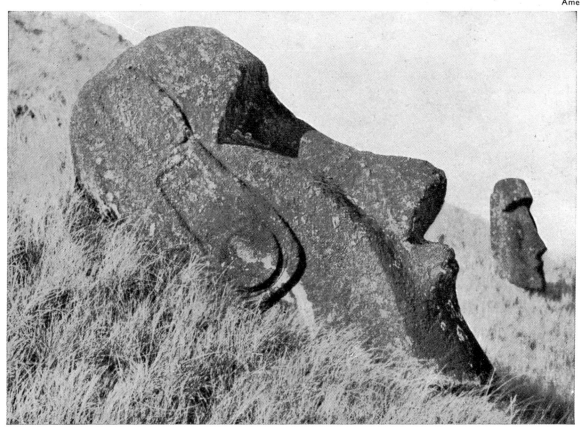

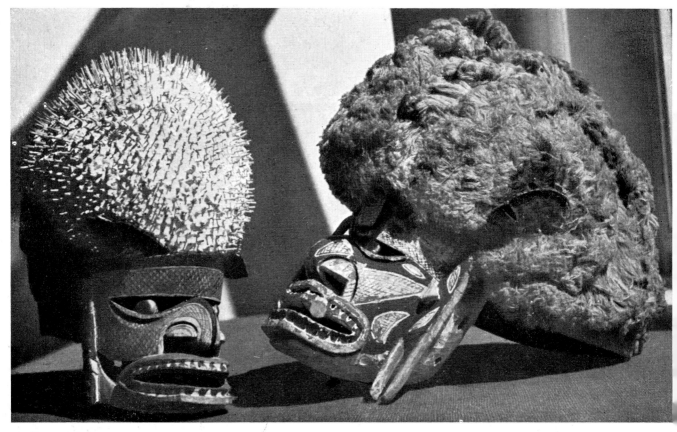

ISCOVERIES of Ice Age paintings have included few pictures of human beings. Those few, however, often show men with animals' heads; some are partly covered with skins. Primitive hunters who still live in a culture no higher than that of the Stone Age, cover themselves with animal skins and put masks over their faces so that they can creep up undetected on their prey. It is not a very big step for such disguises to be worn on other occasions and to be regarded as magical. After all, if magic can bring luck to the hunt, why not to life in general? The mask forms a central part of religious ceremony and helps man to identify with the powers of the spirit world. His normal self then ceases to exist, he transcends it in a burst of ecstasy. The barriers of human existence are broken down by these fantastic disguises and human beings are invested with supernatural powers far exceeding their ordinary limitations. The hunted animal will move closer to the hunter's spear, fish will muster in his net, the rain will fall and the corn will sprout — when the exorcism has been properly carried out. Evil spirits turn to stone confronted by the ritual movements of the masked dancers.

Masked ceremonies were restricted by the Roman Catholic Church to Mardi Gras. Putting on masks came thereby to signify only the abandoning of restraint, since contact with the spirit world had become the function of the Church. Fashions as well as customs underwent certain changes and the

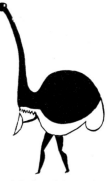

A Bushman's impression of an ostrich hunter

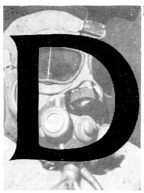

Animal masks as pictured in Ice Age cave-paintings

Man with bird mask holding an egg. From Easter Island

Top, Dance masks from New Guinea   Opposite   African dance mask

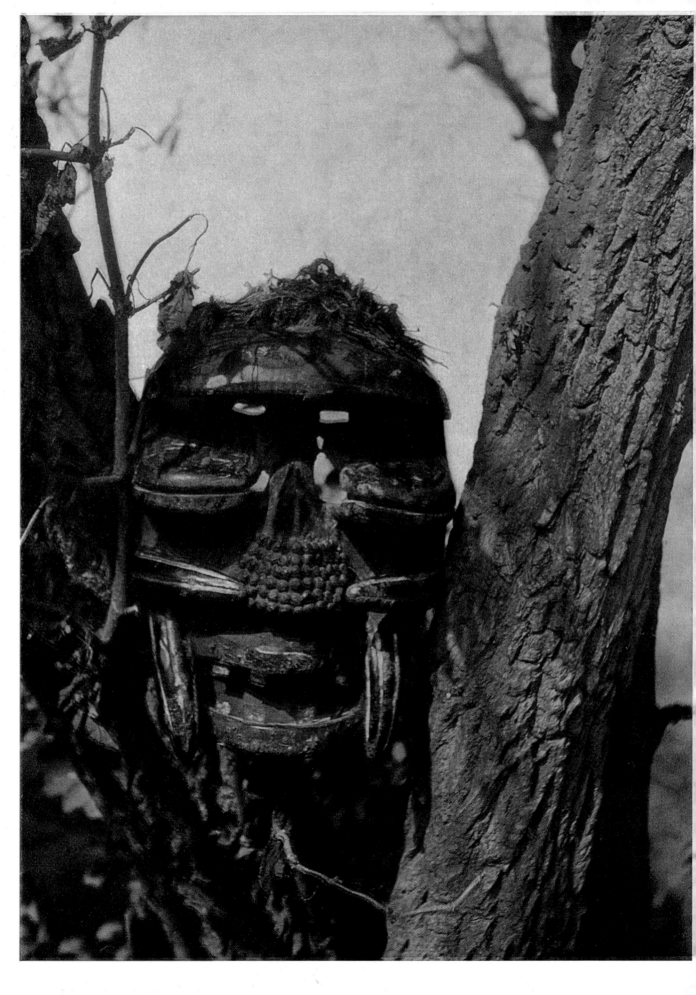

parties. It has, however, reappeared with the demonic shroud of the Ku Klux Klan, and the utilitarian gas-mask of the war years.

The Magic of Clothes. The conception of magic which primitive people associated with amulets and masks was later transferred to dress. Carlyle made the following colourful observation on the English legal scene:

'We see two individuals, one arrayed in sumptuous velvet and the other in coarse worn blue clothing. Red says to Blue: You are about to be hanged and your corpse will be dissected. Blue hears this with a shudder and, miracle of miracles, walks quietly to the gallows. He kicks about a bit as people do when they are hanged, after which the doctors dissect his body and re-assemble his skeleton for the benefit of science.

'How can such a thing happen? Red lays no hand on Blue nor has any direct contact with him. The people who are in contact with him: the prison governor, the warders and the hangman have no personal grudge against him, but they are so much in the power of Red that they do whatever he tells them to do. Each of these people is an individual personality, yet as soon as Red has spoken all become active and eventually the rope and the trap door function in the way it is supposed to do.

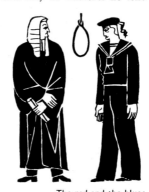

'It seems to me, intelligent reader, that two forces are at work. Firstly, man is a spirit tied by invisible ties to his fellow men. Secondly, he wears clothes which are the visible expression of this fact. The man in the velvet robe and the horse-hair wig, with power to condemn another to death, has surely demonstrated to all men that he is in fact a Judge?'

The red and the blue: an English judge and a British sailor

Carlyle concludes by saying, 'The more I think of it, the more it appears to me that dress is the foundation of society.'

The surprising thing is that the magic of dress influences not only others but also the wearer himself. A red scarf makes cheeks look rosier and a fur coat creates an illusion of animal strength. The blind man's stick becomes an extension of his hand, while the man in a top hat grows in his own imagination as high as the crown of his hat. Square shoulders indicate strength, even though they be made of buckram and cotton wool. The woman with a sweeping train pervades the whole atmosphere with the dignity of her presence. Clothes become one with the body. If, for example, something is thrown into the lap of a man, he will instinctively bring his legs together. A woman on the other hand will spread her legs to catch the object in her skirt. It feels good to be well-dressed, our self-confidence increases and our personality expands. Could anyone imagine Hitler making an oration dressed only in a pair of socks, or with bare feet and sandals? Or could one imagine Members of Parliament conducting affairs of state completely naked?

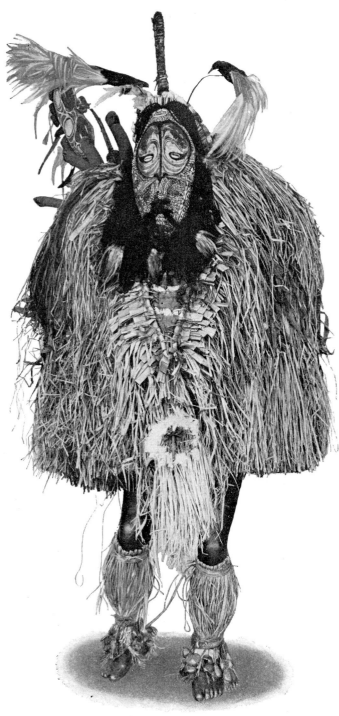

Ritual dancer from New Guinea

significance of the mask changed accordingly. The mask, originally used only for hunting, had gradually assumed magical powers until it became a visual expression of the deity. We may recall that Moses wore a mask when he came down from the mountain with the Ten Commandments. Eventually the use of the mask became limited to carnivals and to children's

But it would be wrong, on the other hand, to think that the intellectual life can only be lived with a collar and tie. Socrates always preferred to lecture in the nude. In some countries, people have to remove their clothes before entering holy places; Hindus should be naked above the waist in their temples. Covering the head before entering a church is a vestige of this connection between clothes and religion.

The Mask Changes — But the Mask Remains.

The origins of dress are to be found in a combination of decoration, disguise and magical power. The principal charm of all methods of covering the body lies in the variety of contrasts possible, when compared with the unchanging nature of the human frame. The human body will always remain the same

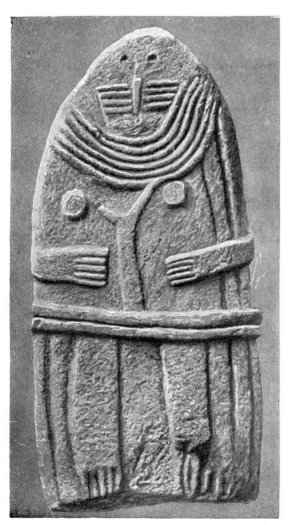

Stone figure from the Neolithic Age. A woman with a tattooed face wearing cape, belt and necklaces

but its covering can be infinitely varied. And with changing fashions, the outward appearance of the body varies accordingly. Human nature has a weakness

for novelty. We hardly notice what is always there; on the contrary, the slightest hint of something exceptional attracts our attention and is also an integral part of the whole concept of beauty. Undoubtedly the way to gain attention is to be different. But dress, like the mask or artificial colouring, carries a measure of sleight-of-hand. We want to be noticed, but we must somehow do it unobtrusively within recognised customs and conventions. No one must suspect we are striving for attention.

Herbert Spencer has claimed that no religion can give us the peace of mind that comes from knowing that we are well-dressed. It can be nothing less than a nightmare to arrive at a party incorrectly dressed, to be wearing, for example, flannel trousers and sports jacket when everyone else is immaculately turned out in evening dress. Nothing can do more to undermine one's self-confidence and even one's self-respect. One of the causes of merriment connected with a clown is that his clothes never fit him.

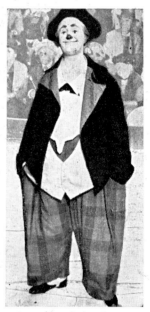

A clown's costume

There is no need to try to look like everyone else; the important thing is to look natural, to look as one really is or as one wishes to be. The housewife who has a lot of work to do around the house dresses up when she goes out shopping, so as to give the impression that she has a retinue of maids. Again, dress is a mask.

Clothes have taken over the task of denoting people's place in society, a function which in primitive times was fulfilled by jewellery and coloured decoration. Instead of the African chieftain's lionskin, there is the postman's uniform, the bellboy's jacket with its row of shining buttons, the prisoner's drab garb or the patch of scarlet cloth on the leper's tunic.

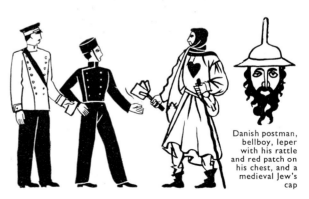

Danish postman, bellboy, leper with his rattle and red patch on his chest, and a medieval Jew's cap

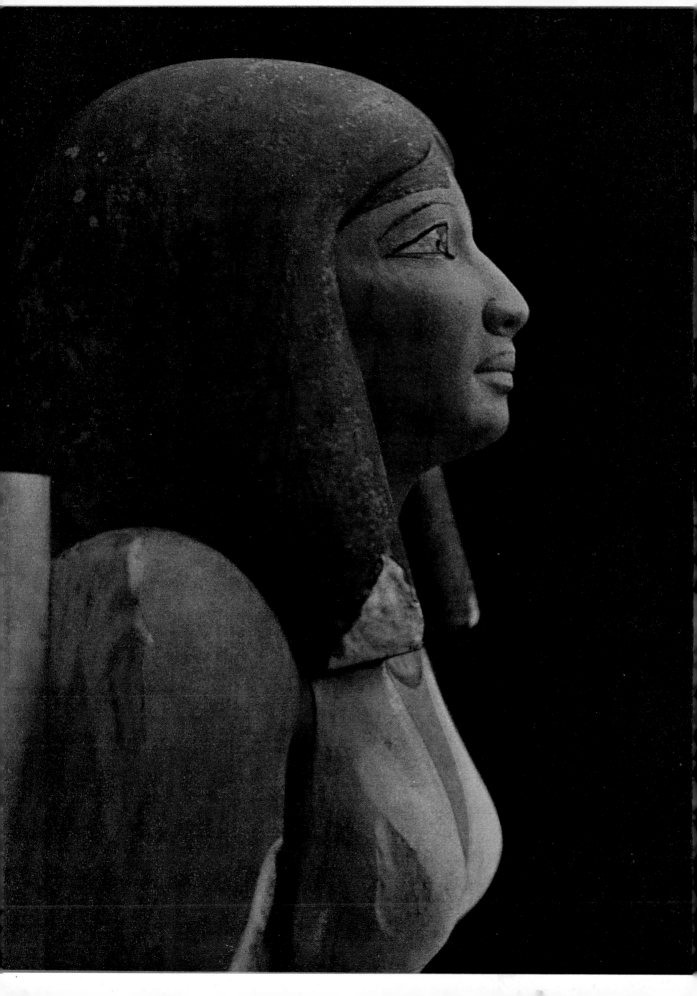

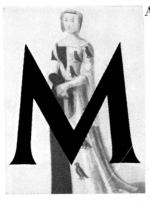

MASK OR CLOWN'S COS-
TUME, both — like all
clothes — indicate social
and economic standing. In
much the same way, mili-
tary uniform designates
country, rank and regi-
ment.

Clothes also reveal a
continuous clash between
younger and older gene-
rations; the former always
anxious to prove its ma-
ture strength and virility,
while the latter tries to hide its loss of such qualities.
While the old endeavour to keep the young in check,
the example of the young also forces them to try and
keep up to scratch. So we see a constant battle waged
between the two age groups. One is best served by
clothes which reveal, and the other by clothes which
hide. Clothes are fundamental weapons in the war
between the sexes also, a war which is even more
varied and extensive than the war between generations, social classes or nations.

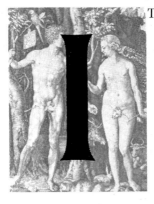

IT WAS our premise that
women in prehistoric times
were the ill-treated slaves
of the great male hunters.
The early origins of agriculture may be sought in
the fact that the women
began to gather roots and
seeds to supplement the
meat which the men
brought back from hunt-
ing. Tilling the soil in
those early days was al-
ways regarded as women's
work. Man ceased to be master of the cave if he came
home empty-handed, while his woman had brought
back the fruits of her garden or cornfield. Our conception of man as the active force and woman as the
obedient passive mate has been superseded by the
idea of competition between the two sexes.

Tools made of stone and bone were used and fire
was known before the age of agriculture, whereas
basketmaking and pottery did not develop until later.
When hides were too scarce to satisfy the demand
other materials had to be found as substitutes, and
spinning and weaving sprang up.

An even greater discovery was made when man's
interest was diverted from the beloved's hair, back
and buttocks and became focused on her face, bosom
and lap. Woman became man's equal and a new world
was born in the human embrace.

A society emerged in which the communal ownership of land eliminated the need to hunt and in which
the woman took her place with the man in tilling the
soil, making laws and governing their community.

Society now became peaceful, and men had no longer
to concentrate their energies on fighting and killing.
The agricultural activities of women had already
made them used to the idea of cautious progress. The
normal function of a woman — producing, educating
and feeding her young — had extended to include
sowing, tending and harvesting the crops. The care of
her children developed into a care for the whole community, of which she felt herself an integral and useful part.

The Submission of Man to Woman. All the world
over, both in the past and present, we can find traces
of the original matriarchal society still existing in
laws, customs, religion and dress. The law of inheritance through the female line is still observed in
many countries. This type of *jus familias* is interested
in mainly the rights and responsibilities of the mother,
and not of the father. Customs continue to be observed
which are fathomable only if we understand the kind
of man-woman relationship in which the man is help-
mate to the woman, and not vice versa. For example,
there is the custom of 'couvade', in which the father
takes to his bed on the birth of a child and remains
there long after his wife has gone back to work. The
anthropologist, Margaret Mead, describes the matriarchal society of the Tchambuli in New Guinea in
terms of 'mutual help'.

'They live on fish of which there is an abundance. Fishing
is woman's duty and the women make their own netting. It is
the women who take the initiative in marriage. It is the man
who must make himself attractive. He learns for instance to
play the flute, imitates the sounds of the rhinoceros bird and
the barking of dogs, and on the flute with many pipes to
make sounds like the roaring of a waterfall. Woman's attitude
towards man is characterised as friendly tolerance. They appreciate the efforts of the man to entertain them as, for example, when they dance before them in masks which are decorated with flowers.
'The men live by themselves in the "men's houses" where
they do the cooking and in all respects look after themselves.
The same atmosphere of work does not exist in the "women's
houses" where the children are brought up.'

Mother-Worship. In later times the old worship of
a female goddess occasionally survives side by side
with newer patriarchal religions and their dynasties of
male gods. This has occurred, for instance, in the
adoration of the Virgin Mary in the Roman Catholic
Church. The whole life-principle in a matriarchal society was conceived as embodied in the female; woman represented earth, all was brought forth through
her, all would return again to the great mother earth.
In contrast to matriarchal societies, patriarchal societies have one or more 'father gods' who created the
world.

The female monthly cycle was considered a holy
occurence under a matriarchal regime, but a token
of uncleanliness and sin in male-oriented societies.

Ruth Benedict, the American ethnologist, states that
she has herself seen old Apache medicine-men crawling solemnly on their knees to bless a group of young
girls who were having their first monthly periods;

afterwards old people and sick children were brought to the girls to be healed. This is indeed a striking example of the homage paid to the miracle of creation.

The Amazons. There was certainly a period during which female rule was accepted. But for thousands of years after this, male rule has been predominant. A

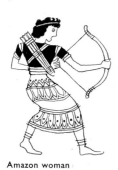

great deal of our knowledge of this early time is derived from accounts by the Greeks of their wars with matriarchal tribes. Robert Graves gives a vivid picture, based on the material collected by Bachofen, of the matriarchal woman. He writes about the reactions of the priestess of Majorca who was told by a Greek refugee how the male-oriented society in his country operated. She asks,

Amazon woman

'Who can this father god be? A father is a man who is used by a woman either because she wants him or else because she wants to become a mother!'

She laughs contemptuously and exclaims,

'By heaven, this is the worst I have ever heard. This is the height of all nonsense, father indeed! I suppose that in Greece the fathers suckle their children, sow the corn, pollinate the fig-tree, make the laws and carry out all the other female prerogatives.'

She stamps her foot impatiently and her face grows dark with anger.

'Is it not the woman who decides and not the man, ... She is the hand and he is the tool. She gives the orders and he obeys. Is it not so that the woman chooses her man and conquers him with her perfume and her charm? She orders him to lie on his back, rides him like a wild horse to get her pleasure, and leaves him as dead when she has finished. Is it not the woman who rules the cave and banishes her lovers to the men's cave if they are lazy or ill-tempered after a thrice repeated warning?'

Warrior versus Housewife. The militant Amazon regime resulted from a clash between matriarchal societies and male rulers. Primitive forms of agriculture called for the female understanding of peace, their ability to care for children, for flowers and all growing things, to nurture them and bring them to fruition. In many primitive societies, the women were regarded as sacred and inviolate, and kept separate from war and bloodshed. They were frequently employed on diplomatic missions for this very reason. Men have always been the superior in fighting and women the superior in rearing children. The effect of each on politics have corresponding results.

Women in matriarchal societies must have worn clothes which were comfortable and in harmony with the body. The appearance of uncomfortable dress, as for example armour, has always been precipitated by men. Throughout the entire history of dress, women have struggled to have easy loose-fitting clothes. Men, on the other hand, have dressed themselves in clothes that are close-fitting. They have always been ready to fight, and weapons, tools and fighting techniques

have interested them above all else. The central male concern is with how things should be done, whereas the female concern is with what should be done. This underlines, to some degree, the egocentric nature of the male, but also suggests the extent to which vast technical advances have had no effect on women. Until quite recently, relatively old-fashioned domestic appliances and utensils were retained, and indeed in many households are still retained.

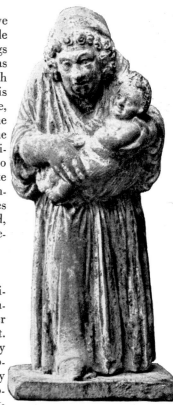

Greek terracotta figure of a woman and child

The Fight for Freedom. Although they have ostensibly accepted male domination, women have never fundamentally accepted it. The civilized world of today is like a model pioneer society, in which the primary duty of the man is to protect the weaker sex, permitting the latter to drag their lives out in this type of security with as much contentment as they can discover. But all suppressed people hide a dagger in the folds of their festive garments, and are reduced to methods of underground sabotage and guerrilla warfare. The unwritten law for both sexes is never to show its true colours. All the absurdities in the history of dress are explained by the fact that dress, as we know it, is first and foremost a secret weapon. It is employed in both attack and defence, in provocation and ambush, for blatant propaganda in hidden psychological warfare, lightning attacks and prolonged wars of attrition.

The Struggle for the Trousers. Clothes, unlike the deer's antlers or the peacock's tail, are not secondary sex characteristics. They are an artificial form of sexual attraction and can be used by either sex. In the Ice Age, the necklace was a male ornament, but now it forms a part of female embellishment.

The war over trousers has gone on for hundreds of years and has always been a favourite subject for western satirists. Trousers, for them, are always a symbol of masculinity (though it can hardly be said that the women in Persian harems or Eskimo igloos were lacking in feminine charm). Skirts are regarded as feminine and it is held contrary to human and moral law that men, apart from Greek soldiers and Scottish Highlanders, should wear them. The opposite would really be more understandable because, when all is said and done, the cut of a pair of trousers is

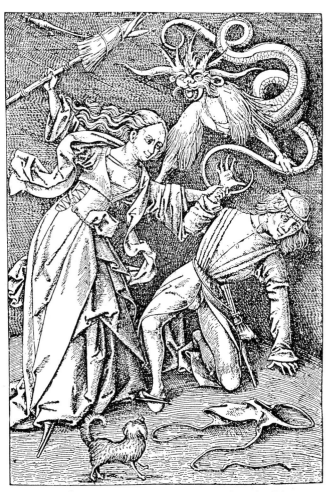

The struggle for the trousers. Satirical woodcut from the 15th century. The trousers, on the ground here, are hardly more than a strap and were worn with wide stocking hose

appeared *in puris naturalibus*, but wearing slippers and top hat. Australian aboriginal women, who normally go about naked, don feather skirts for certain indecent dances. The Indians from the Shingu Springs on similar occasions paint sex symbols on their palm skirts.

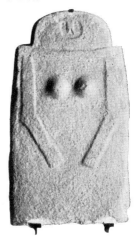

The dress of a modest Neolithic Age woman

We ourselves do much the same. The dress of today is designed to emphasize the differences between the sexes when fully dressed. Men and women seem to be totally different creatures, although they differ in only a few details when naked. Even without knowing an individual, we can at least tell whether that person is male or female. There is no pronoun to denote a human being; we cannot say 'it said' or 'it did'. Before we can take any interest in a person, we want to establish the potential role of that person in the reproductive process. Even the gods are given genders.

not in accord with the male anatomy. But trousers show off a strong leg — or create the impression of one. A skirt, on the other hand, can with a sufficiently vivid imagination, be regarded as an invitation. Icelandic sagas tell us that men divorced their wives simply because they wore trousers. In the Laxdale Saga, Aud burns down her former husband's house and wounds him with a sword, 'And then she surely wore breeches,' exclaims the narrator.

From Feast Hall to Prison. Dress, like any secret weapon, can be used with hypocrisy and deceit. Its basic logical purpose in the sex war is to cover up the sexual difference. Nudity is penalized by law in all civilized countries; everything below the neck and above the knee is regarded as a danger to society. Exposure of much more than face and hands is taken as a violation of modesty, except in such places as the ballroom or the beach. It is even claimed that the injunction to cover the body springs from natural modesty and a desire to conceal one's sex.

When an African Negro observed Dr. Livingstone's scrupulous attire in the presence of the female sex, he

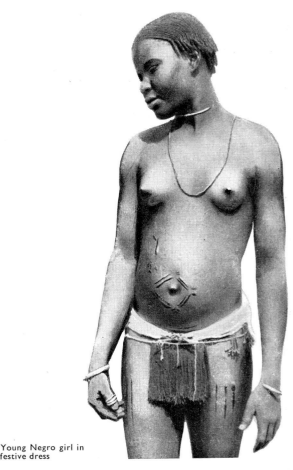

Young Negro girl in festive dress

25

The clothes of primitive people were more simple and loose-fitting than those of civilized societies, and more open in expressing their purpose. If clothes were intended merely to protect, then that was obvious; if they were meant to be seductive, there was no doubt in anyone's mind. Civilized man seldom shows his true colours. Love-making, for instance, is inhibited by talk of decency. Modesty has its basis and origin in dress. If we look closely we can begin to see the true nature of prudery. We think we are better than those ignorant souls who do not know that one is not supposed to express one's true feelings. Hypocrisy has gone so far that certain parts of the body are no longer mentionable. Prudery is also another form of social snobbery: a foreign word, for instance, may pass where the same word in our own language would just not do. The point is made that one does not belong to the common herd, leaving the latter no choice but to use the basic word or else keep quiet. What a disgrace it is to dress in coarse homespun and to speak vulgarly! But in the midst of this tailor dictated modesty, is the unhappy human body. Innocent as Adam and Eve, it writhes, cringes and wails. Behind its enforced armour it screams like the victims in Falarie's 'bull of copper', the throat of which was shaped in such a way that cries of pain were turned into beguiling music.

The people depicted in the large animal paintings of those early times were naked apart from their animal masks. Later rock paintings, dating from the end of the Ice Age and found in the eastern part of Spain, show many human figures including women dressed in skirts and a kind of shawl. These pictures are not sufficiently clear to give us a proper impression of design or style, but it can be taken for granted that the hides had to be cut and sewn together in order to produce a comfortable garment. The oldest representations of human beings

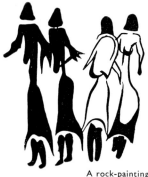
A rock-painting from the east of Spain

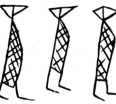
Three figures dressed in capes. Stone Age drawings from Denmark

made in Denmark in particular were carved on aurochs' bones about seven or eight thousand years ago; these people, too, appear to be dressed in hides.

The masculine dress of today, based as it is on the cut and sewn suit, probably derives from the dress of the ancient hunter in a period when man was the dominant sex; female clothes, where the material was draped easily on the body, probably developed when women were in the ascendency. By this time, the art of weaving had been developed and made draped garments possible (which may explain, to some extent, the origin of trousers and skirts). Bridging the gap between hides and woven fabric, are clothes fashioned from material made from bark, generally

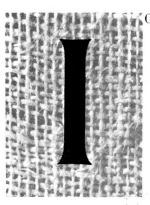

CE AGE CAVES have revealed a large number of beautifully made bone needles complete with eyes. Animal bones found in the same places show that the sinews have been cut out and evidently used as thread. Thus crafts calling for the use of hides were obviously practised in those days, just as they are among the Eskimos today. Piercers of bone, used to make holes, are strikingly similar to those still in use among the Eskimos. One implement frequently discovered, which archaeologists at first called a 'command stick' and long found difficult to explain, is identical with the tool used by the Eskimos to stretch and dry their hides. It is likely that the primitive hunters first of all sewed hides so that they would hold liquids. Pottery-making had not yet been developed; when it was, the first vessels were intended not to stand but to hang, hence suggesting that their forerunners had been sacks or bags.

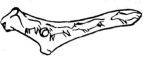
A 'command stick'

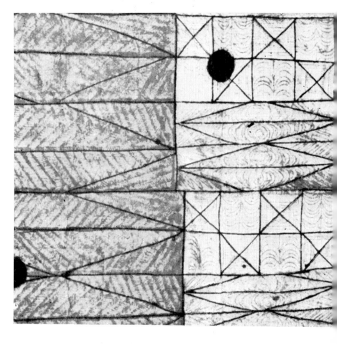
Painted tapa from Polynesia

referred to by its Polynesian name, tapa. This was made from bast soaked in water to make it soft, and then beaten with wooden clubs to a paper-like material. It was then varnished to render it waterproof with a concoction made from plants, and decorated with painted or printed patterns. A similar process was employed using hair and wool which were beaten and pressed into felt.

The Spun Thread. The development of agriculture resulted in thread made from coconut fibre, cotton and flax being introduced, and this became the essential element in making cloth. These fibres when spun, were twisted into a continuous thread. The same result was achieved by the simpler process of rubbing the fibres between the palms of the hands, but this was extremely slow since the spinner had to stop every

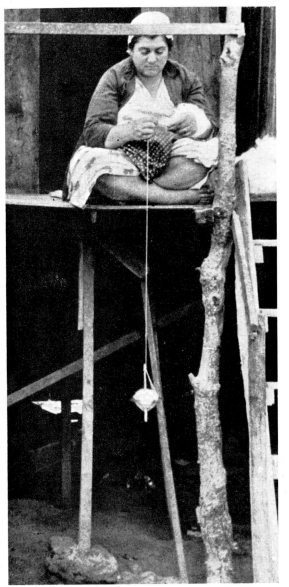

Syrian woman spinning with the help of a spindle identical to those used in the Stone Age

few minutes to take up more fibre. If, however, the fibre was rubbed against the cheek or the thigh, one hand could be continuously employed while the other was left free to add new fibres from the nearby heap. It was discovered that even longer thread could be produced if the fibres were allowed to hang free; in the Stone Age in Europe earthenware weights were

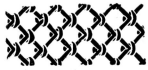

Plaiting

used to keep the thread taut and impart a rotary movement to the spindle.

The knot is one of the greatest inventions in the history of man, comparable in importance with the discovery of fire or the invention of the wheel. The most simple method of joining threads together is plaiting and the oldest materials from the Ice Age were made this way. The art of knotting was a further development. In lace and in fishermen's nets, the threads are not only intertwined but also knotted together.

Knotting

Weaving is a method of plaiting using two sets of thread, the warp and the

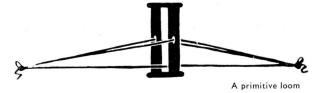

Weaving

weft. A wattle hurdle gives an idea of the principle of weaving: its upright poles represent the warp and the horizontal wattles which are laced through form the weft. The genius of the loom lies in the fact that mechanism raises and lowers the warp in various combinations. For example, threads 1—3—5 are lifted together, followed by threads 2—4—6 and so on, each move enabling the weft to go through the opening or shed thus formed to create the pattern. The weft is secured firmly as the warp changes position. The material is pushed down and packed tightly by a beater.

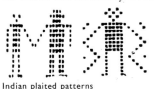

A primitive loom

Female Occupations. Plaiting and weaving were no doubt the discovery of women, whose patience and skill were obtained from their work in the fields. All the tools and implements from the latter part of the Stone Age and the beginning of the agricultural era show the influence of women. The decorations on ancient earthenware pots give evidence of the systematic, graceful

Indian plaited patterns

and patient work done by women, in contrast to the rapidly executed drawings made in the Ice Age by men.

Dyeing material was also carried on by women. It was often felt that the work would turn out badly if men were allowed to glimpse the process. The

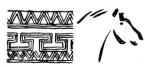
A pattern representing a row of jugs from the Neolithic Age and a picture from the Paleolithic Age

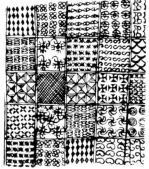
Printed fabric from the Sudan

use of templates and cartoons is known the world over. In Java and the East Indies the dyeing process is known as batik. The parts to be left without colour are coated with wax. In India, Indonesia and Peru, the dyeing process is called ikat: here the parts not to be dyed are tightly bound with bast.

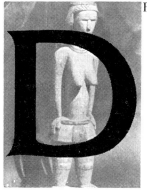

DRESS of every kind, whether simple or elaborate, must be made to fit the human frame in some way. There are three principal focal points around which clothes can be fitted: the waist, the shoulders and the neck. Another way is to envelop the whole body in a sort of cloak. Arms, legs, hands and feet offer additional opportunities for attaching clothes to the body.

During ancient times, when Asia and the Americas formed one continent, it was discovered that if a hole were cut in a piece of hide the head could be inserted and the hide would then hang comfortably from the shoulders. This is called the poncho in South America, and from it developed the tunic, the skirt and the

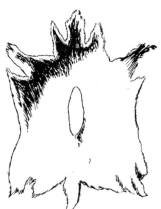
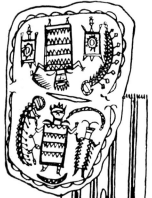
Ponchos used by North and South American Indians

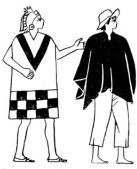
An Aztec poncho and one used in present-day Mexico

ordinary female dress. The poncho is worn from Colombia to Chile in South America, in Tibet, throughout Indo-China and the Polynesian Islands, Egypt, Lapland and in northern Siberia. And, of course, the skirt is an important part of everyday dress in all Western countries. So a simple hole cut in a piece of material probably somewhere in Central Asia became a pattern for the rest of the world.

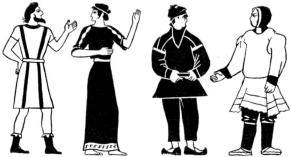
Tunics worn by ancient Greeks, Lapp and Samoyed

It was also discovered that instead of cutting a hole for the head, the garment could be placed over the shoulders and fastened in front like a mantle or a cloak. Eventually sleeves were added and this form of dress became known as the caftan. This type of garment is worn open in Japan as the kimono, tied with a scarf in Turkey, fastened by a belt in the Caucasus and with buttons or cords in China. It travelled to Europe via Russia, and buttons and buttonholes were added to transform it into the overcoat, jacket and waistcoat.

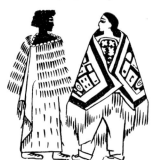
Capes worn by a Maori, and an Indian from North-West America

Another form of clothing developed from various types of loin-cloth. Australian aborigine men wear a

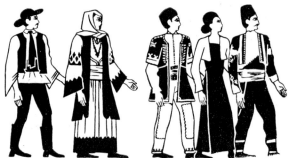
Waistcoats and jackets from Rumania, contemporary Greece, Bulgaria, Burma and Turkey

28

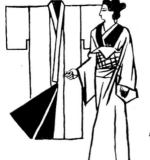

A Japanese kimono

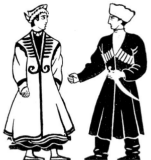

A Siberian and a Cossack caftan

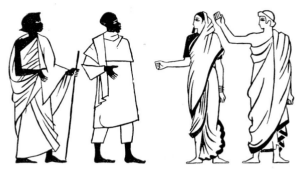

Wrapped garments from Somalia, Ethiopia, India and Ancient Rome

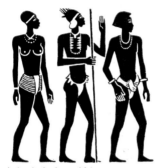

Loin-cloths from Africa,
Central America and Micronesia

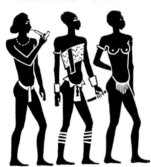

Aprons from Indonesia, Africa
and South America

narrow belt of raffia or human hair. South African Bushmen slip a piece of hide between their legs and fasten it front and back to a belt. Loin-cloths of this kind are commonly worn in the Pacific islands to the east of Australia, in the eastern and southern parts of Asia, in Africa and in North and South America.

Loin-cloths are worn in the front like a small apron. Over the whole of the Far East, Indonesia and Africa the shape is square; in the regions round the Amazon it is triangular. The primitive skirt is a development of the loin-cloth. This can be made of raffia, grass or even leaves. In a more developed form it covers the entire lower half of the body, as for instance in Africa and Melanesia.

In Mediterranean countries, South Asia and North Africa, wrapped garments cover the upper part of the body too. The type of dress used by the Eskimos and Persians encases more or less the whole body. This

garment was originally made from a whole animal skin, its front legs being made into sleeves and its rear legs being used to cover the legs of the wearer.

Covering for the hands seldom developed beyond simple adornment, in the form of rings and other ornaments, or protection against the cold, in the form of gloves and mittens. Covering for the feet however, is a long and varied chapter in the history of dress. Moccasins were made from deerskin folded and laced together. There were two basic designs of sandals: one with thongs to fit between the toes, and one with loops and holes along the edge for tying them. Snow-shoes, ice-skates and skis are actually sandals designed for special purposes. Sandals and stockings made from hide were the forerunners of boots and shoes, while the clog developed as a variation.

The use of headgear dates from the time of the first hunters. The cap of muskox skin worn by the Eskimos and the reindeer skin cap of the Tungus both developed into the hooded cap used as protection against the cold. The Arabian turban of twisted material gave protection from the sun, while the helmet gave protection in battle.

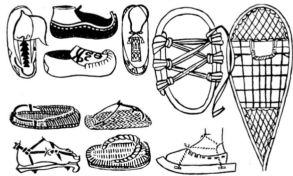

Above left, A Lapp and a Siberian shoe between two Indian moccasins. Below left, sandals from Korea, Arizona, South Africa, Japan. Above right, snowshoes used by Japanese Ainus and by Indians in Alaska. Below right, an ice-skate from Central Europe

The tiara or diadem took the form of a circle surmounted by decorative feathers, notches or spikes to

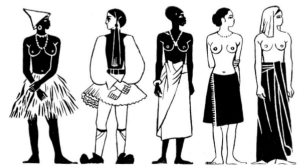

Skirts from Melanesia, contemporary Greece, Central Africa, Indo-China and Indonesia

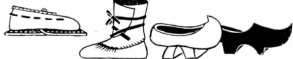

Leather shoes from Egypt and Alaska, and wooden shoes from Korea and Denmark

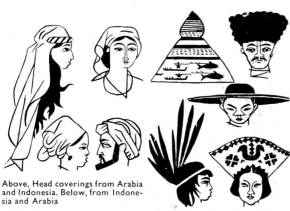

Above, Head coverings from Arabia and Indonesia. Below, from Indonesia and Arabia

Headwear from Colombia, the Caucasus, China, North America and Estonia

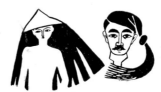

Headgear with tassels as worn in Indonesia and in Albania

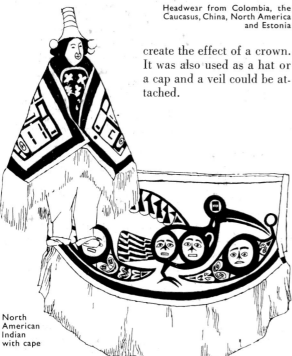

create the effect of a crown. It was also used as a hat or a cap and a veil could be attached.

North American Indian with cape

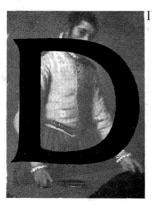

The types of clothes they choose sometimes leave unsaid what they wish to say, sometimes reveal what they dare not put into words.

The history of dress changed through the ages with the influence of powerful rulers since they could not only decide what they would wear, but also dictate what their subjects should not wear. The lower classes inevitably adopt a cheaper, simplified version of upper class style. This may often take the form of an outdated style, as, for instance, the elaborate livery of the footman, the tailcoat of the waiter, or the Baroque costumes adopted by folk-dancers of various countries. Little, however, is known about the dress of the lower classes and its development. Descriptions and illustrations are few and far between.

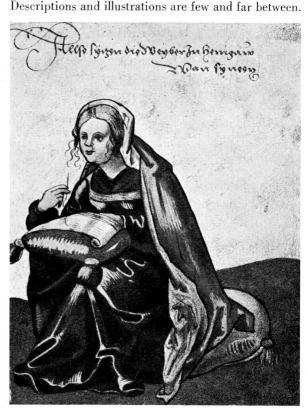

German seamstress sitting on a cushion on the floor. Drawing by Christoph Weiditz, ca. 1530

DIVERSITY is the most striking element in the history of clothes, as varied and complex in type as languages themselves; the abundance of materials, shapes and colours equate with a large vocabulary. Ways and means of covering and adorning the body constantly alter their accent and stress, much as the voice is modulated to introduce music and expression. The language of dress, like any other collective art, has its own principles of beauty that are independent of simple reasoning. An effect is produced, an idea is expressed. People are given away by dress — more often than they themselves might realise.

Although we have an intimate knowledge of the pyramids and mediaeval cathedrals we know next to nothing about the houses in which their builders lived. Similarly, all we know about humble weavers and lace-makers are the materials and brocades which they created. When all is said and done, however, the history of dress has been made by the creators and not the wearers. To discuss the style of clothing worn by the tailor or seamstress is as irrelevant as describing a great artist's house. It is, above all, the work produced by such people that in the chapters to come will be our concern.

Opposite   Women in the tropics work naked from the waist up; Eskimo women wear reindeer-skin trousers indoors

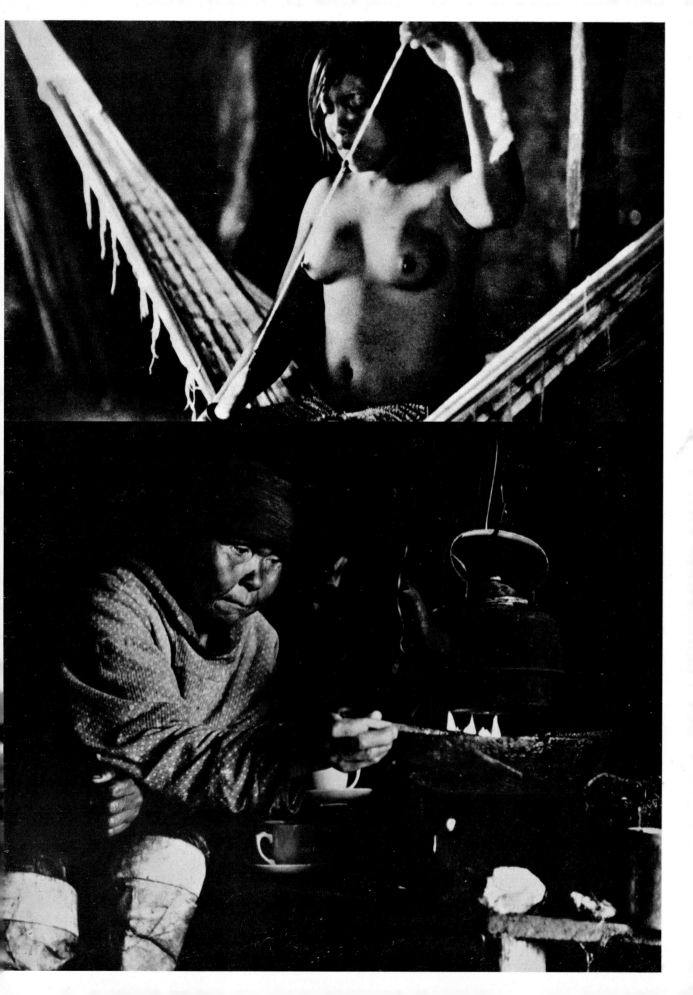

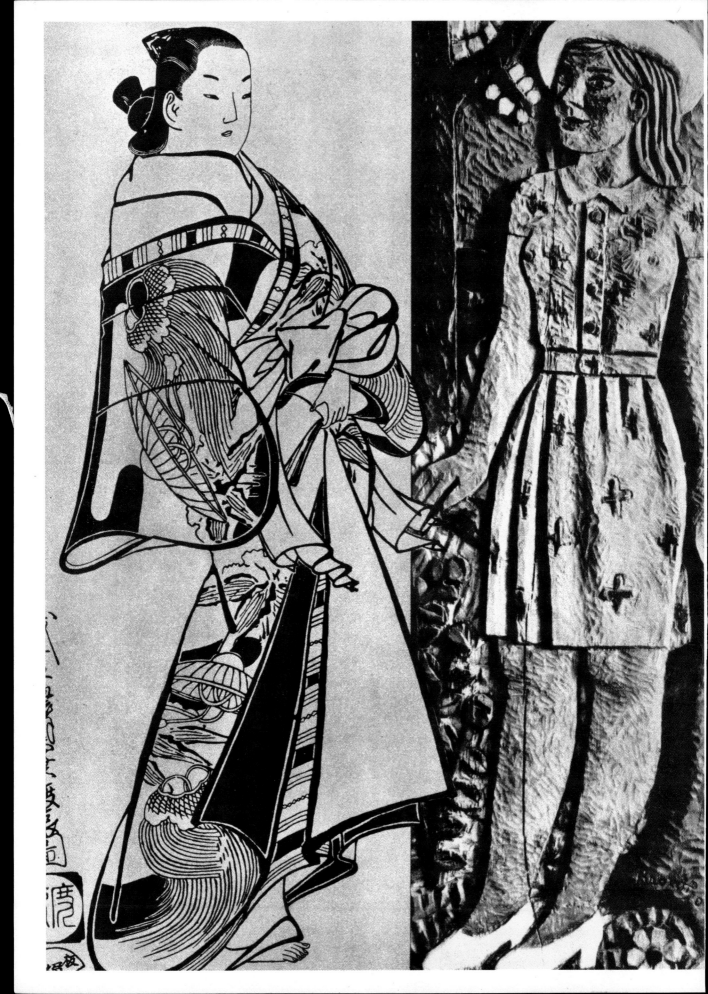

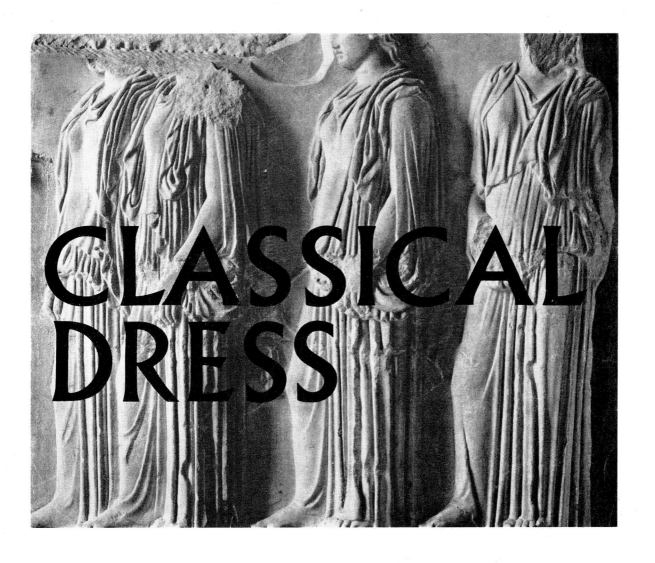

CLASSICAL DRESS

THE WRAPPED GARMENT

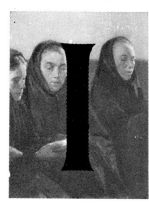

I T WAS in the very earliest stages of civilization that weaving first developed. At that point, agriculture was the principal means of livelihood and the substances for clothing came from the soil. So great was the respect for the art of weaving, that people could not bring themselves even to cut the piece of fabric which was the produce of the loom. The material was therefore wrapped, folded or knotted. Such garments are the only form of clothing not fastened in any way to a particular part of the body.

The draped material and wrapped garment clearly speak of their feminine origin. Masculine interest is concentrated on place, period, temperament and detail, whereas feminine interest centres around the overall effect.

Jewellery played an important part in all early civilizations, but transcending even the beauty of precious stones and gleaming still brighter than silver or gold, were the beautiful white linen draperies. No element in nature could compare with the delicacy, fineness and exquisite folds of the draped woven cloth, that contained every nuance of light and shade. The wrapped garment is usually white; in hot climates it deflects the sun's rays. Its loose folds provide cool for the body and allow the skin to breathe. Nowadays, however, the main concern of the tailor is to eliminate loose folds. The great distinction of woven material

Opposite   Japanese kimono and modern Swedish tunic-style dress.
Bas-relief carved in wood by Brør Hjorth

lies in its infinite capacity to catch in its drapery, every variation of light or shadow — to the endless delight of artists throughout the ages.

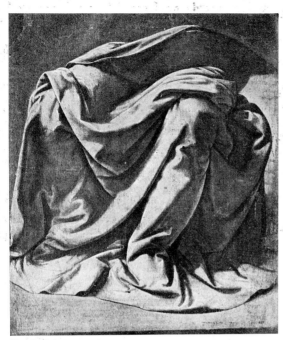

Sketch of drapery by Leonardo da Vinci

It is significant that the wrapped garment, originating in those southern countries where temperaments tend to be fiery, is unsympathetic to sudden or violent movement. Such garments educate the wearer to preserve at all times an outer calm and dignity. One is

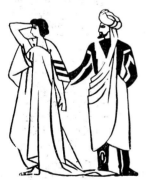

Arabian haiks as worn by women and men

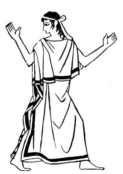

Open chiton fastened with two clasps

inclined to think that the toga played its part in creating the dignified manners and attitudes of Ancient Romans.

An account by a European dating from 1729 describes the Arabic haik as a loose vestment, and claims that it is impractical because of its tendency to come undone; the wearer is thus constantly concerned with keeping it properly tied. That particular observer may

not have considered that this feature might have been an advantage for the person who always liked something to do, rather like today's cigarette smoker.

Another advantage of the draped garment lies in the fact that it can be folded after wearing and stowed away in a minimum amount of space, in contrast with modern clothes which involve wardrobes, drawers, clothes brushes, hangers, irons and ironing boards to keep them in a good state. All that now remains in Western civilization of the wrapped garment is the kilt, the shawl and old-fashioned swaddling clothes, unless we count robes of office, such as the priest's cassock, the monk's cowl and the king's coronation robes.

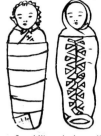

Swaddling clothes still used in southern Italy

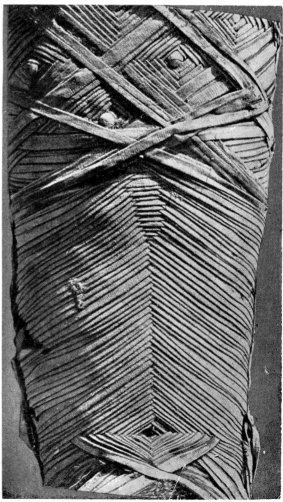

Cloth in which an Egyptian mummy was wrapped

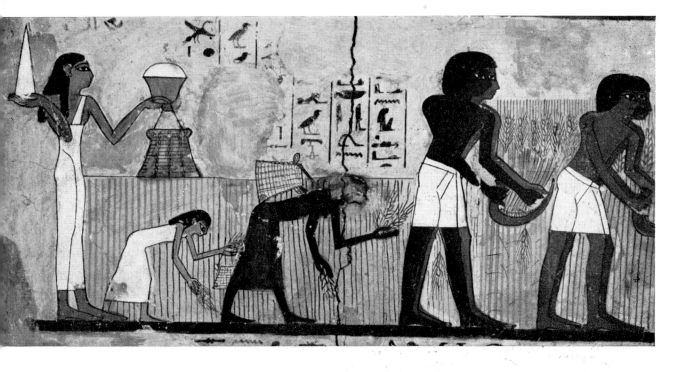

THE EGYPTIAN LOIN-CLOTH

FAR OLDER than any other article of Egyptian dress was the wolf's tail, which formed part of the Pharaoh's ceremonial dress. This remains with us, to some extent, in hunters' trophies, first worn attached to their caps by Canadian trappers, flying rabbit tails on children's bicycles and similar adornments on the aerials of scooters and cars.

Before weaving was developed, the Egyptians covered themselves with fur like everybody else. The leopard skin was used as a priestly robe until the rise of Western civilization. When the Egyptians learned to weave, the loin-cloth came into being and remained the most important part of male dress for thousands of years.

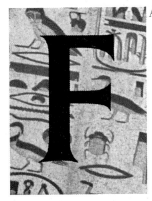

Leopard skin and loin-cloth worn over tunics

Everything in Egypt had to go from left to right, so the loin-cloth was also put on in this way. Statues stand with the left foot forward; similarly, when one faces south, towards the source of the Nile whence all good comes, the sun rises on the left.

As the art of weaving developed, the loin-cloth became broader and more elaborate, gaining coloured borders and pearl embroidery. From around 2000 B.C., men of high rank wore a double loin-cloth, the outer one being longer and made of thin, transparent, stiffened linen. Sometimes a short cape was worn over the shoulders, one side of which was passed beneath one arm and fastened on the opposite side with a buckle.

After 1500 B.C., the upper part of the body was covered by a tunic. It resembled a sack worn upside down, with holes for the head and arms. The double loin-cloth was worn below. This form of dress gradually lengthened, and with a belt at the waist, became normal dress for upper class society. Egyptian society was divided into classes, and these were denoted by the clothes they wore. Civil servants, for example, wore variously coloured ribbons on their shoulders, much as stars or stripes indicate rank in armies today. Manual workers, peasants and shepherds continued to wear the

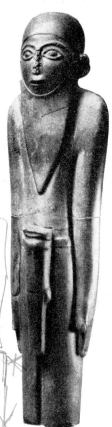

Male figure with false beard and penis case, ca. 3500 B.C.

Top Egyptian harvesters from a painting in a burial vault

35

3*

original loin-cloth, not so much from a sense of decency, since the loin-cloth hid nothing, as to indicate their position in society.

The Long Dress. Women have always used much more material for their clothes than men have. This may have been because they were the weavers of the cloth and may also have felt a great deal of material enhanced their appearance. (And perhaps the men, on the other hand, demanded greater freedom of movement.) Their dress was suspended by two shoulder straps and reached from below the armpits to mid calf. About the year 1500 B.C., we find this insubstantial slip covered by a loose sleeveless cloak, twice as long as the wearer was tall. This was knotted over the chest or shoulders, or simply wrapped around the body, like the Greeks' clothing later on or as in Spain today.

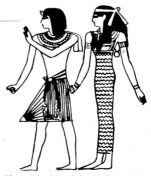

Man with pleated double loin-cloth and a woman's dress

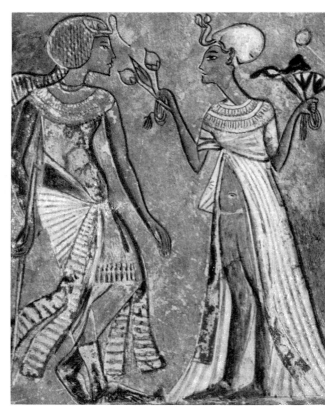

The Pharaoh Akhnaten and his queen, Nefretiti, ca. 1380 B.C.

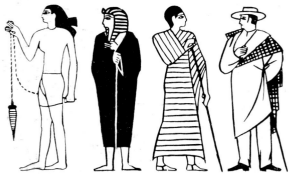

Female spinner with spindle, two Egyptian cloaks and a modern Spanish cape

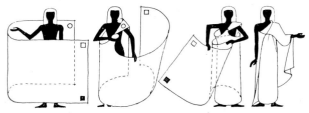

Egyptian woman wrapping her dress around her body

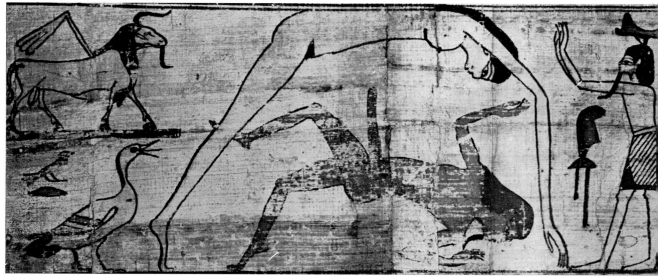

The heavens represented as a woman arched over the earth which is symbolized by a man. Drawing in *The Book of the Dead*

Opposite   Servant girls, ca. 2000 B.C.

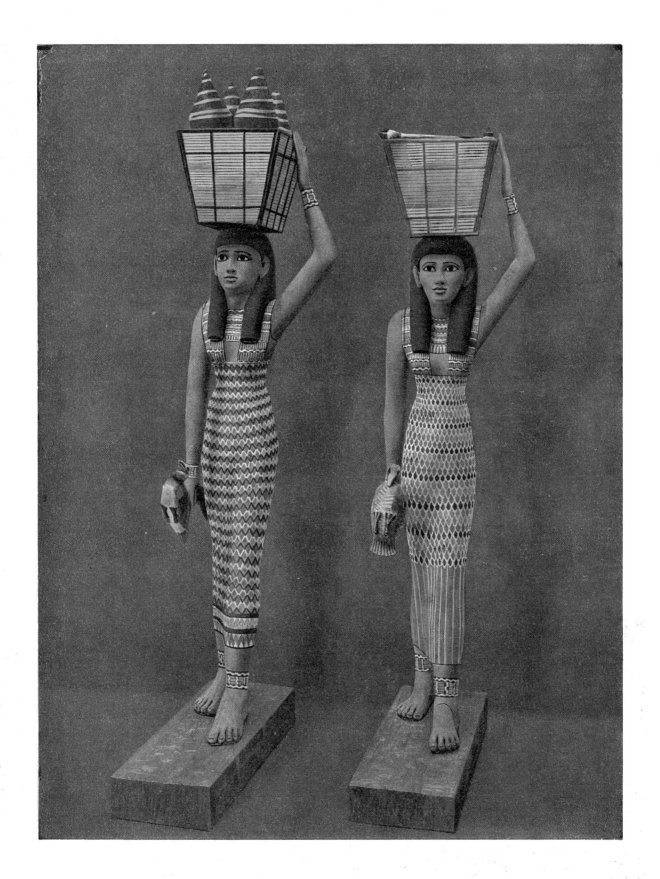

Light Clothing. Cotton, made from flax, came to be used as well as the usual linen. It was woven as finely as some handkerchiefs today, sometimes of even near transparent thinness. The colour was normally white, but singing girls wore yellow and mourners were dressed in blue. Egyptian garments always produced a light airy effect, and never became the straitjackets other civilizations would have made of them. The human body was treated in Egypt as a living and breathing thing. The Pharaoh went about in private with bare head and feet, though as time went by he adopted elabor-

ate headgears and wore various decorative signs and tokens of his high office. Boys and girls went naked and workmen removed their clothes when engaged in strenuous work.

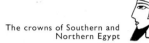

Greek and Egyptian versions of the same dress, the latter having added a transparent 'shawl' tied in front

The crowns of Southern and Northern Egypt

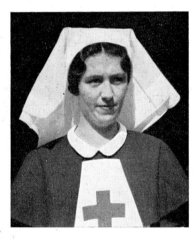

Pharaoh, his headgear similar to that nurses wear today (right). (Tutankhamun's coffin of gold)

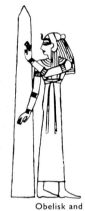

Obelisk and woman's dress

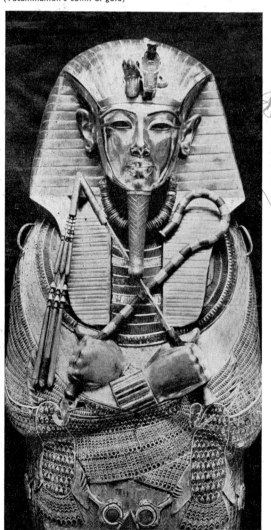

The Slender Line. The ideal Egyptian figure was tall and graceful with narrow hands and slim hips. Both men and women had broad, straight shoulders (sloping shoulders are never found in Egyptian painting). Beauty in body and limb was developed by physical exercises, dancing and swimming. Their carriage was erect, calm and composed. Their feet were of ample size and beautifully shaped, never having been compressed into close-fitting 'boxes'. Sandals were worn only if the going was rough, for which event people of high rank had slaves to walk behind them carrying their sandals. The Egyptian was evidently never tempted by a fashion for small feet; Egyptian sculptors appear always to have made the feet as large as possible. Our own attitude seems to be based on the basic principle that feet are something to be covered up and, as far as possible, hidden.

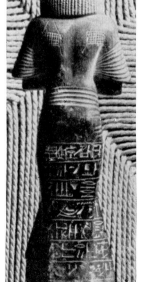

Woman with long wig

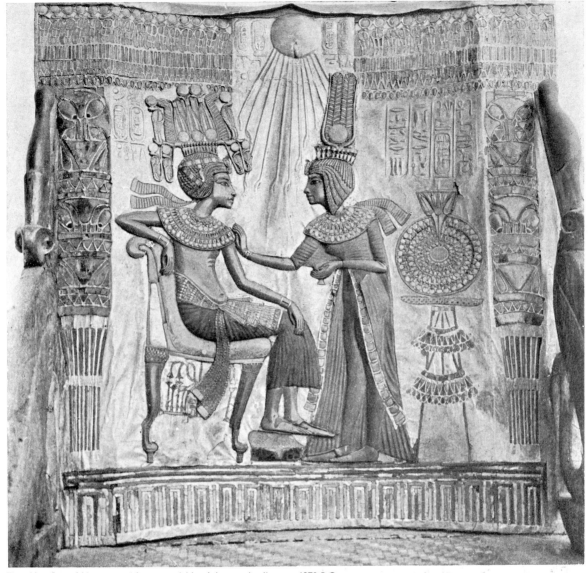

Tutankhamun and his queen with ceremonial head-dress and collars, ca. 1370 B.C.
He is naked above the waist; she wears a transparent draped garment.

Pharaoh's Throne. It is somewhat ironical that the chair which derived from the throne of the Pharaohs has done more than anything else to develop large posteriors among white races. The throne, originally designed for state occasions, was copied by the Egyptian aristocracy and gradually deteriorated into the ordinary chair of today. The average chair is neither comfortable nor restful. We therefore instinctively adopt positions when seated, such as putting our feet up or sitting on our legs, which restricts the blood circulation and is neither healthy nor restful. Squatting eases the pressure on the heart by halving the natural height, but the only time our hearts get a real rest is when we lie asleep flat on our backs.

Sitting positions in Ancient Egypt

Cosmetics and Wigs. Cosmetics were used by both sexes in Ancient Egypt, and various ointments and pigments were also known. Eye-shadow, which was made from a green mineral known as malachite, was painted on the eyelids. Galena or lead sulphide was applied to eyebrows and eye-lashes, as Arabian women still do today. The lips and finger-nails were painted with a dye known as henna, made from Egyptian privet. The first recorded strike in history was caused during the building of the Pyramids by a shortage of make-up when supplies of ointment and dye had failed to come through.

Affluent men and women wore tightly-curled wigs made from sheep's wool or human

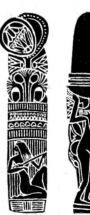

Make-up jar and spoon

39

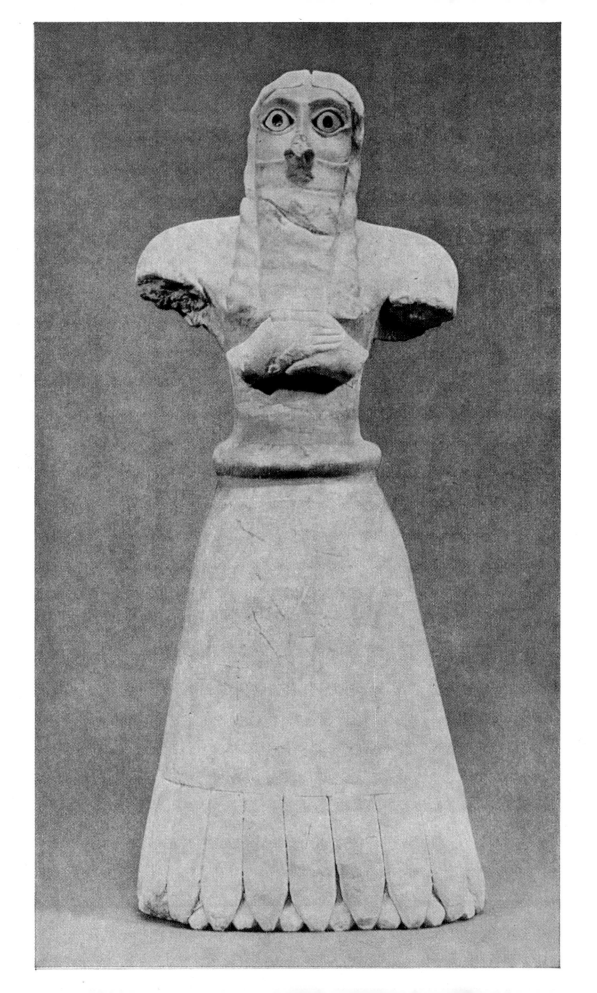

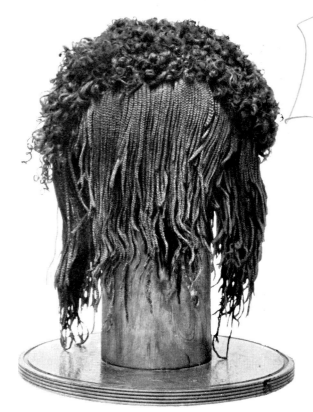

A wig made from wool and human hair found in an Egyptian tomb

Peaceful Coexistence. Life in Ancient Egypt was reasonably tolerable even for the slaves, even though the form of government was essentially despotic. In the first place, peace had been maintained for thousands of years because of the protection against invasion provided by the surrounding desert. So long as the water supply from the Nile was controlled, the necessities of life were secure.

People concentrated on peaceful occupations. Throughout that period, women were given the respect which they deserved, as they had also been in the most primitive agricultural societies. The kings of Ancient Egypt were portrayed beside their consorts, and the queens were given equal stature. For a considerable time after the year 2000 B.C., inheritance went not to the son but to the eldest daughter. Women joined in all festivities, worshipped with the men and attended ceremonies for the dead. When the men went out hunting their wives accompanied them and they ate their meals together. In the language of Ancient Egypt the wife is simply called 'the ruler of the house'.

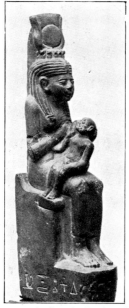

An Egyptian 'madonna' from about 600 B.C.

hair as protection against the sun. In the case of priests and professional men, the head under the wig was shaved. But on the other hand, various prescriptions for baldness surviving show that people were interested in keeping their own hair.

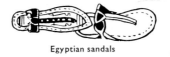

Egyptian sandals

THE MESOPOTAMIAN WRAP

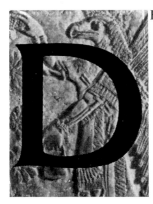

DEVELOPING side by side with the civilization of Egypt was Mesopotamia's civilization. The development of agriculture followed a similar pattern in both societies. The oldest and most interesting discovery was made at Ur in Mesopotamia: this was the grave of a queen dating from about 3500 B.C. The body and the casket had turned to dust as well as the clothing, but it was evident that the clothes had been made from a red woollen material. Articles such as jewellery and weapons of metal and precious stones were, however, uncovered more or less intact. Also found was a

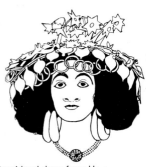

Regal head-dress from Ur, about 3500 B.C.

royal tiara in the form of a broad golden circlet, to be placed like a garland around the head and the wig. The wig was also encircled by three wreaths, one of linked gold rings, one of beech leaves and one of small willow leaves. The willow leaves were in groups of three, with white and blue enamel set between. On top of this tiara was placed a comb, its points surmounted by golden flowers with calyxes of lapis lazuli. On either side of the head heavy spiral rings were attached to the wig, and large crescent-shaped ear-rings reached down to the shoulders.

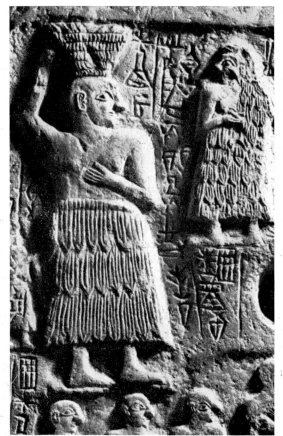

Laying the foundation stone for a house, about 3000 B.C. The king carries a basket with building materials on his head; his eldest daughter, wearing a wrapped fur garment, looks on

The history of dress in Mesopotamia begins with this unique find. Subsequent records speak only of male clothing, which was much the same as women's. The ancient queen, Semiramis, was described by a Greek historian as wearing male dress.

The place of women in Mesopotamian society changed considerably in later times. Early reliefs depict the eldest daughter of the family twice the size of the eldest son.

Draped Clothing. In earliest times, people went about naked, except for a belt or a strip of fur they wound spirally like a soldier's puttee round the lower part of the body. The top end of the strip was secured by a belt or thrown over the left shoulder. Presumably

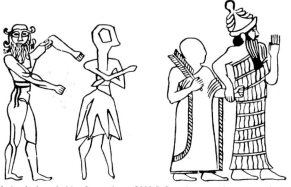

Loin-cloth and skirt from about 3000 B.C. and wrapped garments from about 2000 B.C.

some kind of woven fabric was used as a backing for the fur which was usually from small animals like the weasel. If it was, then it must have played some part in determining the shape of the garment it lined.

In later times, clothing was fashioned from rectangular pieces of fabric with fringes at the edge; these fringes were made by combing out the ends of the warp and weft threads. Men wrapped the cloth round their bodies and fastened it over the left shoulder, thus leaving the right arm free and unencumbered.

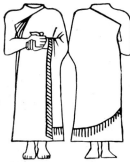

Statue from about 2400 B.C.

In the case of women, the cloth usually crossed over the chest to cover the bosom, then went under the armpits and came over the shoulders. This was a practical form of drapery and was capable of many variations.

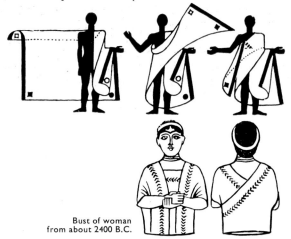

Bust of woman from about 2400 B.C.

Heavy Wool. Wave upon wave of nomads descended on Mesopotamia's old centres of culture. They depended ultimately on their animals for survival and maintenance, a source of supply to which they frequently resorted. Unlike sun-baked Egypt, where linen provided an ideal protection against the desert sun, Mesopotamia had copious mists and rain. Against these natural greasy wool was good protection and, above all, a good tough covering.

Notwithstanding constant foreign infiltration, the Mesopotamians remained a sturdy people with thick necks, arms and legs. The norm was

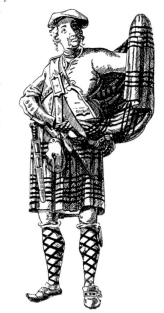

European wrapped garment: Scottish kilt

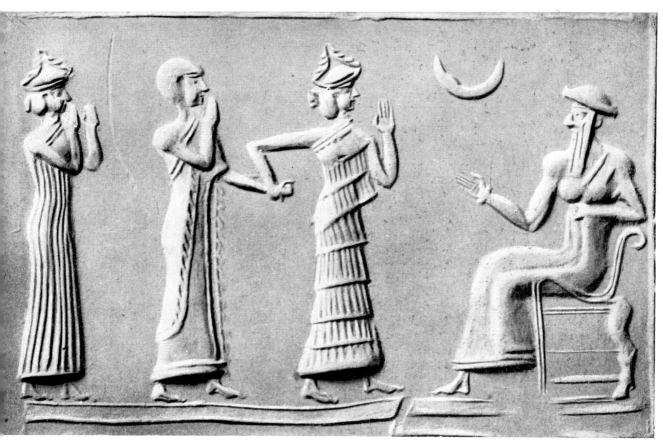

Moonlight scene, 2300 B.C. All the garments are draped over the left shoulder. The scene depicts a judge, the husband, unfaithful wife and a witness

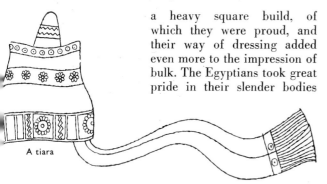

A tiara

Mesopotamian handbag and fly-whisk

a heavy square build, of which they were proud, and their way of dressing added even more to the impression of bulk. The Egyptians took great pride in their slender bodies and brought up their children to adopt elegant poses, with those graceful and artistic arm and leg positions seen in their temple pictures. The Mesopotamians, on the other hand, hold their arms close to the body in illustrations, and at most show their legs only to the knee.

Perhaps this impression of bulk is due to the scarcity of stone in this land of rivers, a situation which may have influenced the sculptor to limit his chipping and thus produce these block-like figures.

This tendency to bulk extended to articles which were in everyday use. The women's fly-whisks were something like Russian knouts and their handbags looked like flour sacks. Heavy rounded folds of woollen material were

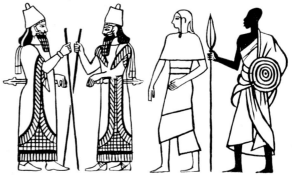

An Assyrian pictured from right and left, a Syrian from an Egyptian relief and a Somali warrior

considered more attractive than delicate sharp linen pleats. Vertical pleats, of course, lengthen the general appearance, whereas horizontal pleats or folds broaden it. The way the Mesopotamians wrapped themselves made them look like pillars with spiralling horizontal folds.

The buildings in their towns were made of sunbaked clay, not wood or

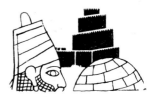

A Mesopotamian spiral-shaped tiara, a step-temple and an Eskimo snow hut

stone. Their temples, with banked up spiral walks, had the shape of a twisted turban. The Greenlander builds

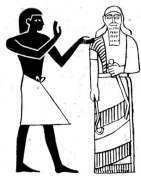

Egyptian and Mesopotamian

his snow hut in a spiral fashion to avoid it collapsing during construction; perhaps the soft Babylonian clay may have necessitated a similar building technique. The spiral may also have been regarded as a symbol of strength.

The Egyptian was smooth-skinned; he had a thin growth of hair on his chin which was usually shaved off. The Mesopotamian, on the contrary, was hairy and although in earliest times the hair on his chin was removed, it was later allowed to flourish luxuriantly.

Rich Colours. A shift-like shirt with sleeves was worn as an undergarment from the year 1000 B.C.

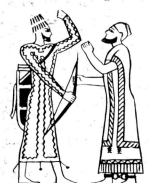

Syrian warrior of about 1600 B.C. and a captured ruler, probably a Hebrew, of about 700 B.C.

But the outer clothing remained the rectangular cloth with the weft ending in tassels and the warp threads combed out and tied to make a fringe. Colours were bright red, saffron yellow, violet, indigo, blue or deep olive green. The most popular patterns took the shape of squares or circles. Ornaments were attached, such as precious stones, rosettes made from metal or leather, and bells. The garment

was edged with broad borders embroidered with figures. The main effect came from the weave, the weight of the material, the colours and the decoration.

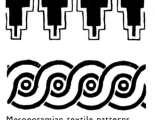

Mesopotamian textile patterns

The Mesopotamian love of heavy, thick material and rich, full-bodied colours contrasts sharply with the Egyptian reverence for white linen, pure lines and unconfining drapery.

The Babylonian reliefs depict the vestments of the priests, so colourfully described in the Old Testament. Evidently the Jews were not blind to all of this during their captivity in Babylon. A procession in Mesopotamia must have comprised great masses of people in richly coloured robes which were decorated with glittering gems, wearing gilded tiaras and carrying burnished weapons. The noise must have been equally intoxicating, with the loud clash of cymbals, rolling drums, tinkling bells and the sensuous sound of flutes; and enveloping the whole procession would have been the smell of heady, strong perfumes.

Ointments and perfumes were valued by the Mesopotamians. Soldiers and artisans received a considerable portion of their wages in the form of sweet-smelling ointments.

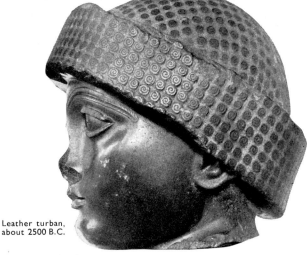

Leather turban, about 2500 B.C.

Exposed Borders – Concealing Dress. Unlike Egypt, Mesopotamia was a country whose borders were unprotected by nature and its history tells of little but continuous warfare. As its civilization developed, the neighbouring countries grew envious and launched attacks. After several generations, the invaders themselves developed a related form of culture. This, in turn, attracted their neighbouring countries and precipitated further invasions; so history repeated itself continuously. In Egypt, a state of war was quite

Assyrian sandals

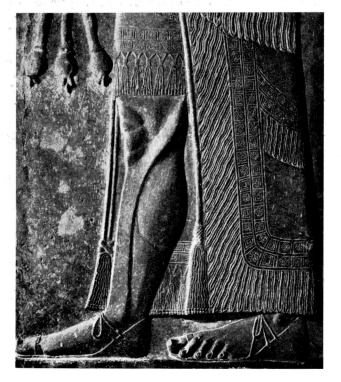

An Assyrian garment from about 700 B.C. Our modern dressing-gowns are tied with similar tasselled cords

exceptional, whereas in Mesopotamia it was almost an everyday occurrence.

The Mesopotamians did a great deal of marching, and their sandals therefore had thick soles, solid heels and heavy thongs. Life under this male regime was hard and tough. The barracks life gave rise to an atmosphere of virile sensuality, characterized by a crude enjoyment of power and opulent display, and by pride in physical strength. Extravagance in dress was tempered by military discipline. For example, only two of the three principal colours could be used together in any one piece of decoration; one colour always had to be omitted. Their clothes were designed to cover and obscure. They were thick and heavy, forming a shield against the outside world. To expose the body was considered shameful. Of the girls, only those in the slave market were naked, while the only naked men were prisoners of war, stripped of their uniforms and decorations. Sex was an unmentionable subject. To obtain pleasure from gazing on the beauty of the human body, however tender, gay and innocent it might be, was equally forbidden.

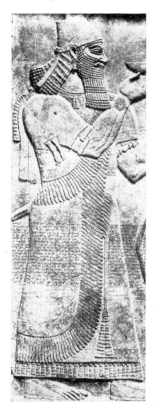

Assyrian, 800 B.C.

Female Duties. In the period during which Mesopotamia was ruled by warrior kings, the central figure among the deities continued to be female, but the attitude changed. The old worship of fertility began to lay more stress on the satisfaction of man's physical desire and the Ishtar temples degenerated into brothels. The temple girls performed their usual duties, but in addition they also did the work of clerks. Hundreds and thousands of clay tablets have been discovered, mainly business letters and undoubtedly the work of women. Women did the spinning and weaving, dyed the yarn and made the embroidery. Well-preserved tablets record the names of weavers, the amount of wool used, hours worked and food consumed.

Male attire was magnificent and male hair styles elaborate and complicated. Male rulers and warriors wore heavy, valuable jewellery which covered head, neck, arms and chest. Female jewellery, such as the elaborate tiara discussed above, was not worn in later times.

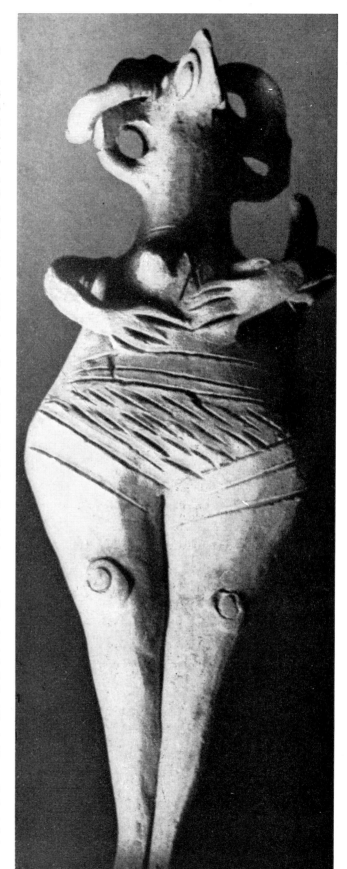

The warrior's ideal woman. Ishtar figurine found in Cyprus, from about 1500 B.C. The idol has in the course of time lost three of her four enormous ear-rings

45

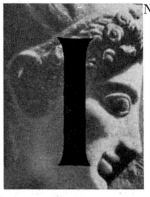

I N the period between 700 B.C. and the beginning of the Christian Era, the beauty of the human body was revered in Greece, to an extent difficult for us to comprehend. There is, for example, an anecdote about Phryne, a famous courtesan and the model for Praxiteles' Aphrodite of Cnidas. She was apparently on trial at one time and her defending lawyer, seeing that her case was going badly, removed her clothes, revealing her beautiful naked body to the judges. They promptly brought in a verdict of not guilty. In the eyes of the Greeks, a perfect body was indicative of spotless character.

The Naked Athlete. In Greece, complete exposure of the body was not a remnant of primitive times. It was, in fact, usual practice for Greek youths of the Classical period to disport themselves quite naked on the athletics field. Orsippos is remembered for divesting himself of his loin-cloth in the middle of a race (in 720 B.C.) and going on to win first prize. Plato writes, 'It is not so long since the Hellenes — as did most Barbarians — appeared to regard the naked man as something shocking and ludicrous.' An unexpected aspect of Greek fashion is the narrow waist of early times. This can be attributed to tightly-laced garments similar to those later adopted by other primitive peoples. But in Classical Greece, the waist was not pulled in but was, on the contrary, broad and well-developed. The Greek physique was characterized by broad shoulders, a strong neck, a navel that sat high above slender hips. The lower part of the back was tapered, thighs were long and straight and women's breasts were rounded and set far apart.

Head and Feet. The Greeks were always barefoot at home; out of doors, however, they occasionally wore

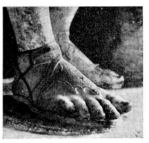
Greek sandals

leather sandals with a thong that went between the big toe and the second toe. The Grecian foot therefore retained its natural shape. They usually went bareheaded and adopted a broad-brimmed hat only for travel.

They were a clean-shaven race like the Egyptians, but for a different reason. Although a naturally hairy people, they did not prize a hirsute appearance. In very early times, the men plaited their hair; later it was worn long and kept in place by a head-band. Later still, the hair was cropped and curled. Long hair was impractical in battle because it could be seized by an adversary.

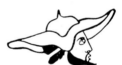
The Greek rain-hat, which looked rather like an umbrella

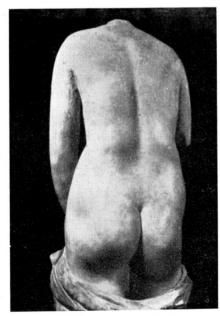

Wasp-waisted Greeks from a vase-painting of about 900 B.C.

The back of the ideal woman, Aphrodite from Syracuse

Women too wore plaits in very early times, which came down over their shoulders and breasts. In the fifth century, a bun at the nape of the neck took the place of the plaits. This was neatly secured by a ribbon or a net, and a wreath of leaves was sometimes worn for feasts. A loose veil was used to keep the hair in place when out of doors, or a fold of the cape was thrown over the head for the same purpose.

Greek Stances. The Greek figure differs from the figure of the statuesque Egyptian and the ponderous Mesopotamian. Rather, it is functional and well suited to work and athletics. We can observe the various positions of hands in the statues. The worthy matron stands with her hands on her hips like a washerwoman. The young girls, like those in the Parthenon frieze, have hands hanging loosely at their sides, almost like idle labourers. The old Greek sculptures show very relaxed figures, and if seen away from their pedestals (for instance in the store-room of a museum) they appear often as if resting before entering a sports arena.

They rarely sat upright except in the theatre. They ate their meals in a reclining position. There was no need for them to learn to relax. Their example could well be followed by some of our athletes today.

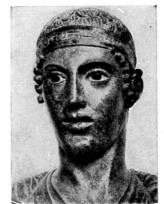
Athlete with short cropped hair and a head-band.   About 470 B.C.

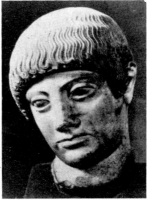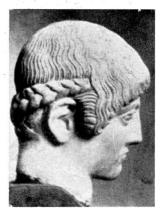
Young man with braids underneath his forelocks.   About 470 B.C.

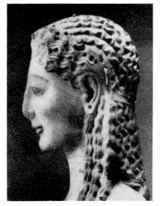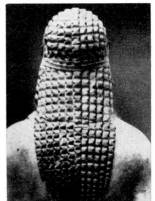
Young woman with long hair falling over her shoulders and breasts.
About 550 B.C.

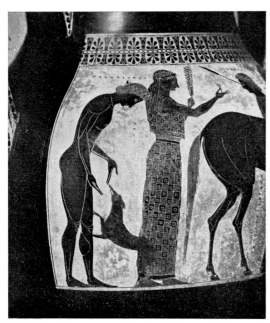
Figures in motion on a vase from the 6th century B.C.

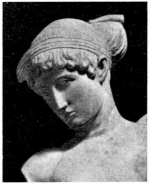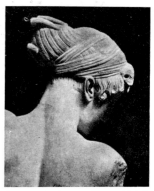
Young woman's hair style with bun held in place by bands. About 470 B.C.

The Significance of Folds. The Greek garment was loosely draped, its shape being derived from the figure which it covered. Dignity was achieved not by embellishment, but rather by the very simplicity of the folds. The character of the wearer was revealed by the way the garment was carried and not by the garment itself. It might express charm and intelligence, not neces-

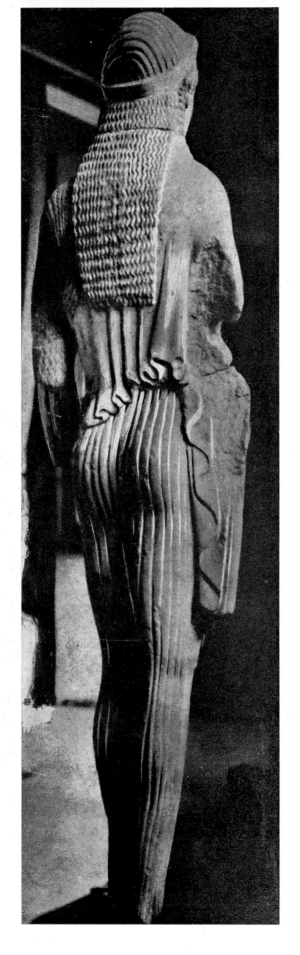

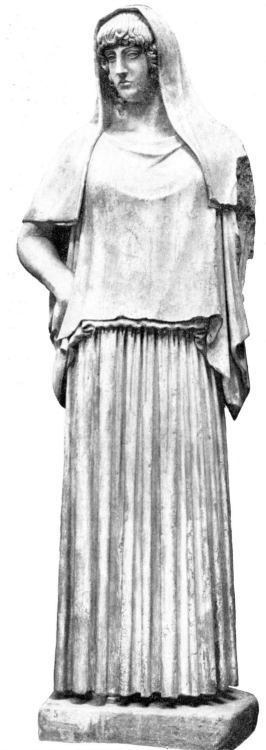

Doric peplos from about 460 B.C.

sarily wealth and prosperity. Materials were hand-
woven. The various articles of clothing were made up
from rectangular shapes produced in a number of
standard sizes laid down by tradition. This form of
dress was worn by all free citizens. But ancient statues
indicate that, in spite of its democratic nature, great
variation could be achieved in the way the garment

Young girl dressed in long Ionian chiton with a cape over her shoulders.
About 550 B.C.

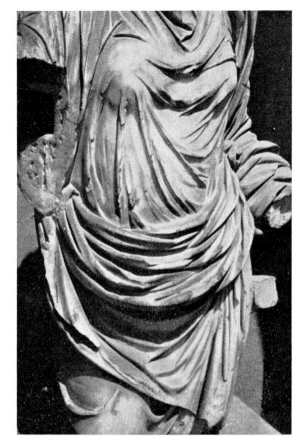
The beautiful draped effect of the chiton of antiquity

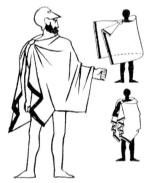
Putting on the chlaina

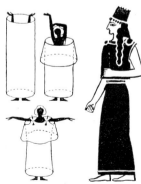
Putting on the peplos

was draped and carried. By comparison, current fashions look uniform and dull.

In the earliest times, Greek men and women wore a kind of light blanket known as the himation. This hung over the shoulders and was fastened by a buckle in the day; at night this garment acted as a coverlet for its owner when he slept. The chlaina was worn by men and was just long enough to reach the knee. The peplos was the women's garment; the material for it was wide enough for it to be doubled over as the diploidon which came over the shoulders and breast. The edges were sometimes stitched together to form a sheath which enveloped the whole body. An undergarment called a chiton was added later, the combination becoming standard women's wear, also occasionally worn by men.

The material for this outfit was usually sewn together, but sometimes appears to have been entirely draped and secured round the waist by a belt. It was sometimes accompanied by ribbons crossed over the chest and shoulders.

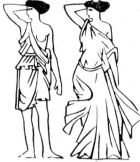
Doric and Ionian chiton

The Amazons are shown wearing the knee-length Doric chiton. Peasants and artisans wore the Doric chiton and the exomis, which was fastened with a buckle on the left shoulder and had no belt. Town-dwellers wore the chiton fastened

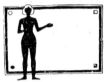 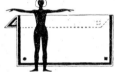

with a buckle on each shoulder and one or two belts with overlapping folds. About 600 B.C., the long Ionian chiton from Greek Asia Minor replaced the short Doric chiton. It was worn in Athens and most of the other Greek city-states, with the exception of Sparta. When young Spartan girls came to Athens wearing the short Doric chiton, they were laughed at, teased and referred to as 'hip displayers'.

The Ionian chiton was looser and had more voluminous folds. It was cut so wide that something like sleeves could be formed by fastening it on the shoulders and around the upper arms. Double buttons were used for this,

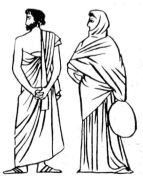
Man wearing a himation and woman wearing a peplos over a chiton

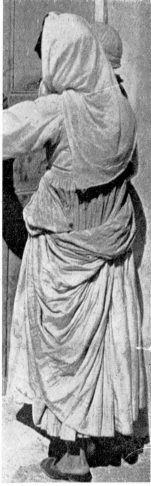
Greek peasant-woman of today

49

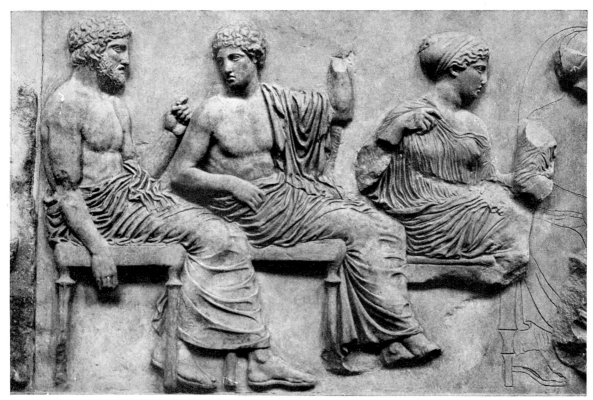

Greek deities: Poseidon, Apollo and Artemis. The gods have short hair and are naked from the waist up. From the Parthenon frieze, about 400 B.C.

very much like modern cuff-links. After 450 B.C., the man's chiton reached only to the knee. They often used only the himation as their sole piece of clothing.

Wool and Linen. The Greeks were descended from many different peoples, some of whom were nomads in Southern Russia before they invaded Greece and settled there. Their clothes at that time were made of wool, and the peasants continued to use this material for their rough peplos and exomis. When they established themselves as farmers in Greece, where flax was an important product, linen became popular. From then on, the chiton was made from either linen or cotton. Vegetable dyes were used for wool; colours recorded are: frog green, apple green, olive, amethyst and hyacinth. Mention is also made of a purple which varied from poppy red to deep violet. Linen garments were usually white, with gold, silver or coloured borders for women. Printed and embroidered patterns were also used, with designs of animals and flowers; printed patterns were never woven into the material.

Greek ornamental patterns: maeander, running dogs, wavy-leaf pattern, palmetto border

Dress and Body. When describing Greek temples, one is almost tempted to refer to the 'linen effect', in the same way as we can speak of the 'silk effect' of China. The fluted columns of Greek temples resemble heavily draped material. Indeed the Greek form of dress itself has an architectural quality, which does not mean that it alters the shape of the body at all but rather that it has its own existence although in such close contact with the body.

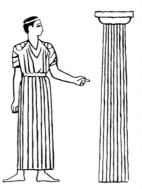

Man wearing a chiton, about 475 B.C.

The inherent sense of clarity and order which underlies all things Greek permeates the whole existence and culture of that people. Fringes, for example, were too indefinite, too fussy to be admired. An edge must be an edge. Body and dress are not confused or mixed, which is unavoidable in a dress shaped with shoulders, sleeves, waist or trousers. Dress should be an entity in itself, just as the body should stand on its own, each possessing perfect harmony and together forming a balanced unified whole. This type of dress is not designed as a set of separate units nor is its object to conceal the body. This does not mean that the Greeks always went about naked. It is true that clothes were not worn at home or in athletic clubs, but a free-born citizen would always wear his mantle in the town square and at gatherings. At

50

the theatre also, it was felt that a certain separateness from one's fellow should be observed, so the mantle was obviously regarded as a kind of formal limit or boundary between persons.

For a woman, dress became a covering that was gently flattering, its soft folds moving rhythmically with the body like the ripple of music. Greek dress gave full scope to the natural allure of the body and achieved this frankly with no coquettry or deception.

Ceremonies in the Greek temples which were connected with education were followed by music and dancing. The harmonious lines and movement of Greek dress were influenced by the flowing rhythms of these ritualistic dances, still to be found in Caucasian folk-dances. The natural calm and dignity of the Greek people were balanced by the controlled passion which gripped the dancers during the festivals of Dionysos; obviously there was latent fire burning beneath the snow of their raiments!

Democracy. The draped garment was impractical for slaves and other labourers, who wore either a shirt

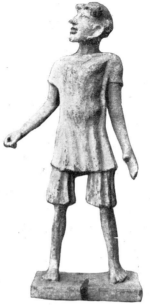

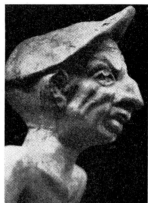

and trousers like the Barbarians, or the plain exomis. A voluminous garment was obviously unsuitable for physical work.

It must be borne in mind, when speaking of Greek democracy, that the states were ruled by the patrician classes on whom the remaining three quarters of the population had no influence whatsoever. However, especially after iron became the basis of technical development, a higher form of civilization did develop. The wealth of Greece came to benefit all people to a higher degree and culture became more generally suffused than in either Egypt or Mesopotamia.

The exomis

The Egyptian and Mesopotamian civilizations had developed in the Bronze Age. Stone had at that time been the principal material used for working tools, while bronze had been used for the more precious fighting weapons.

In the Iron Age, the outcome of wars was determined not by comparatively few well-equipped warriors and chariot-fighters, but by armies consisting of foot soldiers and cavalry.

Primitive democracy became more advanced and widespread in Greece because of the development of a relatively prosperous society with flourishing foreign trade and a worldwide monopoly in oil, wine and pottery. Thus we find the happy combination of a peasant civilization in a country that also maintained trade and cultural links with foreign countries through its merchant shipping. This, combined with Greece's geographical condition as a country divided by mountain ranges into isolated territories, made impossible the founding of larger states or an empire under despotic rule.

The Greek city-state — the polis — had a form of government in which all citizens took part. Their sense of responsibility and their self-reliance were the fruits of individual participation.

Greek street-vendor

Proletarian physiognomy

Status of Women. All that remained of the former matriarchal society was the worship of goddesses, and

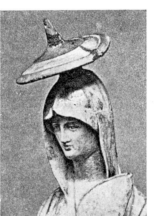

some feel that ordinary women counted for little more than slaves. Goddesses were greatly venerated and played an important part in the Greek religion. The temple on the hill that dominates Athens, the Acropolis, was dedicated to the goddess Athene.

In Classical times, a thoroughly patriarchal relationship existed between the sexes. Women were not permitted to appear in court with their grievances and were not

Grecian woman with a sun-hat of plaited straw

even accepted as witnesses. They were not allowed to take part in political or cultural life. The woman's place was in the home, from which the man himself was often absent. Her entire existence was bound up in her domestic tasks. Thus Homer refers even to a queen who wove and a princess who supervised the washing of clothes. While the wife was neglected, the professional courtesan, the hetaera, was in great demand.

Love between men was generally accepted not as an unfortunate aberration but as something quite normal. Our conception of homosexuality did not exist, and such a relationship was taken for granted. The fact that love was not restricted to love for the opposite sex is also reflected in their dress which did not lay down dissimilar styles for male and female.

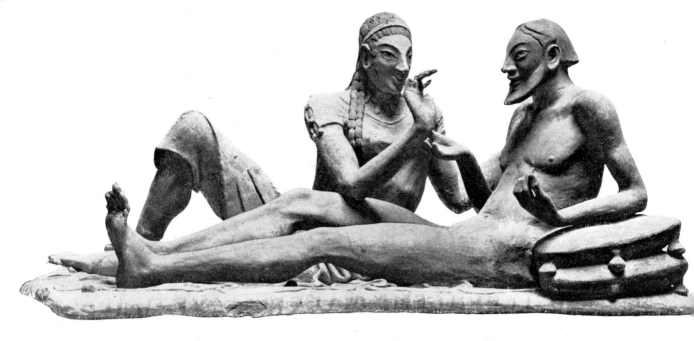

THE ROMAN TOGA

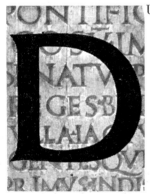

DURING the first period of the Romans' military expansion their territories were bordered by the Etruscans on the north and Greek settlers on the south.

The Etruscans have given their name to the region now known as Tuscany, but the race has been completely merged into the present-day Italian nation. Our impression of Etruscan culture comes mainly from discoveries made in burial places, from graves and from pictures on the walls of tombs. Unfortunately, the inscriptions have not as yet been deciphered, since the script is related to neither Latin nor Greek. The general theory is that people from Asia Minor migrated by sea and settled in this region. Certain original features of Roman art, which in general displays Greek influence, seem to have derived from the Etruscan culture.

The Etruscans were a heavily built people, with short necks and thick arms and legs. Their artefacts give an impression of a peculiar robustness, and of a nature that was violent, sensuous and unrestrained. Their pots were formed with positive looking 'ears', 'noses' and 'beaks'. Their paintings convey a feeling of sensuality which conforms with the Roman con-

Top Etruscan couple. He is naked, while his wife wears trousers and a tunic with short cut-away sleeves. From the 6th century B.C.

Below, Etruscan wall-painting showing a waiter, flute player and harpist. About 480 B.C.

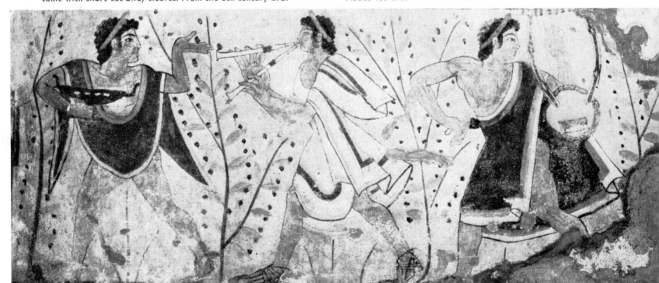

Opposite   A Roman wall-painting of a woman in Grecian dress

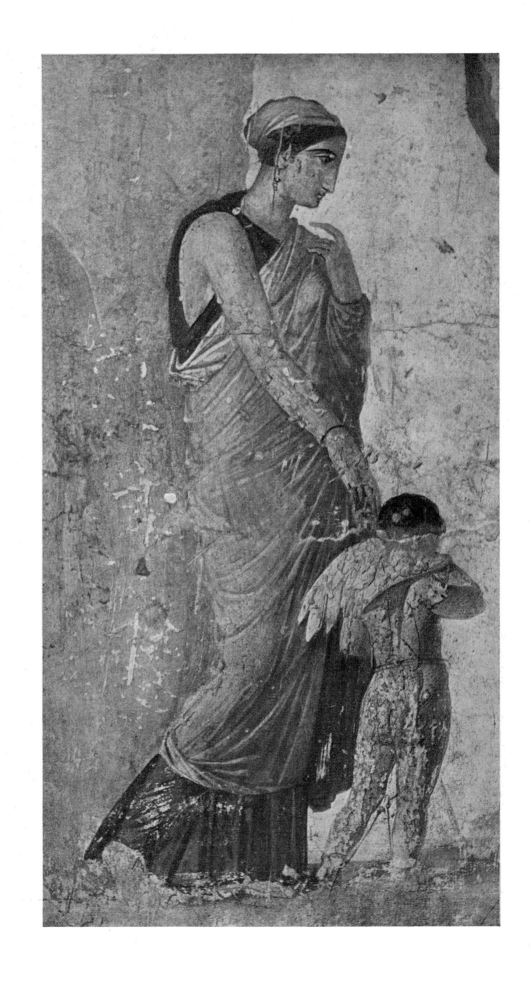

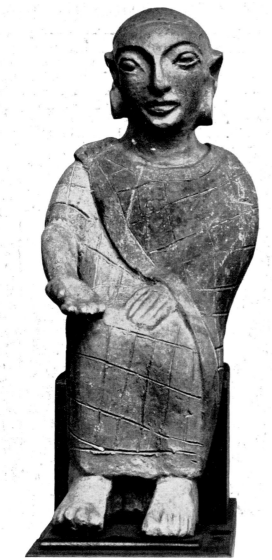

Etruscan woman wearing ear-rings, tunic and cloak from the 6th century B.C.

equally grotesque and overpowering. On the man's urn, rests his helmet and on the woman's is her corn scoop. Man and wife are depicted in a reclining position at table, apparently deep in private conversation, with the woman always of equal prominence.

Women wore heavy necklaces, big chunks of amber, large breast-plates and clasps decorated with filigree of a high standard of workmanship. Their dresses were long, with loose pleats and were sometimes made from the same transparent material as the Egyptians had used, with a shawl or mantle added. Men were clad in loin-cloths or short shifts and their cloaks were draped like those of the Mesopotamians. Both men and women wore pointed caps resembling beehives. Sandals were worn, as well as pointed oriental-type shoes that enclosed the whole foot.

Above, Etruscan shoe from 520 B.C. Below, Gothic shoe from A.D. 1400

The Toga. The Roman Empire was created through military conquest, and the various provinces were linked together by the Mediterranean Sea. Peace and order prevailed within its boundaries for many hundreds of years, and a flourishing trade was carried on with India and China, the two other great empires of the time.

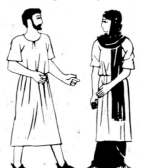

Roman peasants in tunics

The ruling class consisted of citizens of Rome; the remaining majority of the population was made up of slaves. The latter had no rights of citizenship and little is known of their style of dress; it is probable that they wore short smocks and narrow loin-cloths. Freed slaves adopted a felt cap, and the phrase 'appealing to the felt caps' meant inciting insurrection.

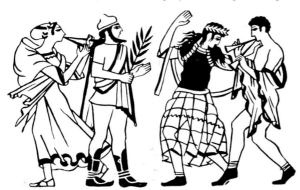

Etruscan dancing couples. About 500 B.C.

tention that the race itself was self-indulgent and ate too much. Music and dance played an important part in the life of the well-to-do and there was greater equality between the sexes than there had been in Greece. Two urns of equal size are always found standing side by side in the graves, their shapes being

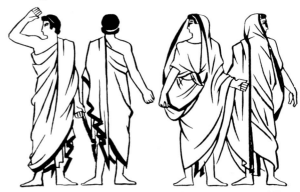

The toga as draped in 400 B.C. and at about the time of Christ

When one speaks of 'Roman dress' one commonly has in mind the toga, which was worn by citizens of Rome for nearly one thousand years. The toga developed from the Greek himation or cloak, in very

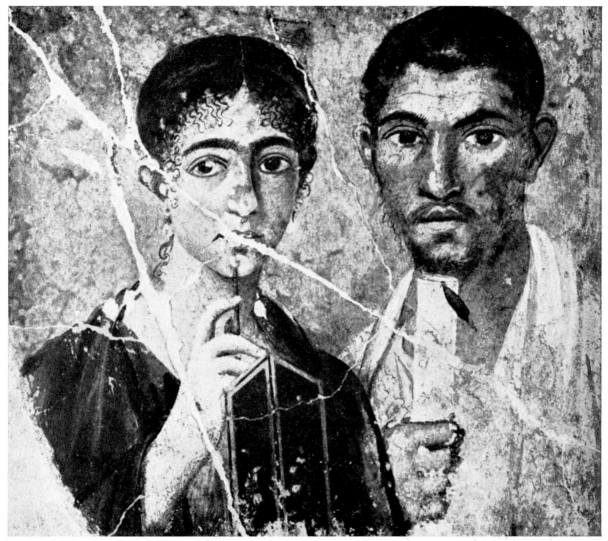

Roman couple from early Christian times. He holds a roll of parchment and she a writing-tablet. Her tunic is red and his toga white

much the same way as Roman architecture imitated the Greek. Unlike the Greek himation however, which consisted of a rectangular piece of material, the Roman toga was cut to a particular shape. The original colour was that of natural wool. A purple border was added to the emperor's toga and also to those of civil servants and of children. The high ranking administrator wore a purple toga embroidered with gold; for mourning the toga was black.

Unlike the Greek himation, the toga was not woven at home. It was a luxury garment worn by

Different cuts for the toga

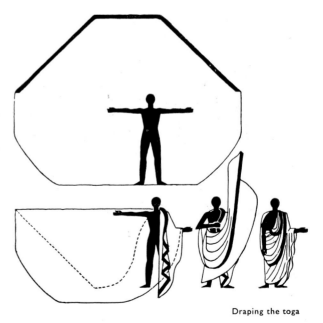

Draping the toga

men of the ruling classes who were waited on by slaves and protected by armed warriors stationed all along the borders.

As lighter materials replaced the original coarse wool, the toga increased in volume and was elaborately cut according to changing fashion, thus becoming much more difficult to drape. To carry the toga was an art, and selected slaves were trained as valets. Instructions survive as to how the orator should arrange the folds of his toga and vary them to suit his speech.

The toga was a work of art, purposely designed to provide expression and effect through the play of light and shade on its folds.

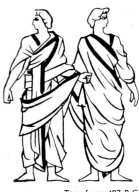

The Tunic. The usual dress at home for both sexes was the tunic. This was similar to the Greek chiton, reaching to the knee for men and down to the ground for women. It sometimes had short sleeves. The colour was grey for ordinary people and white for the upper classes. For festive occasions noblemen wore full-length tunics, with broad purple stripes, called the clavi. In later times, the Roman tunic was decorated with braid around neck and cuffs. In addition to the usual laurel wreath, the victorious general wore a special tunica palmata embroidered with golden palms on a white background, and with it purple

Toga from 428 B.C.

Toga from 487 B.C.

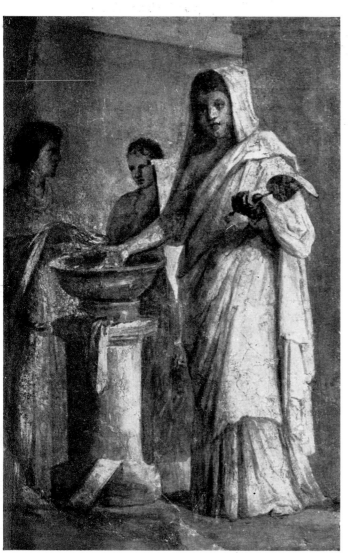

Washing clothes at home. From a wedding scene in a Roman wall-painting

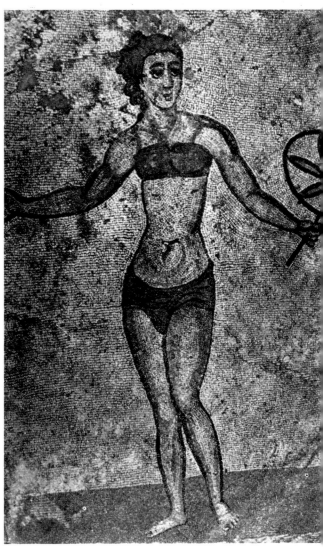

Sea-bathing. A bikini in a Sicilian floor-mosaic of the 4th century B.C.

56

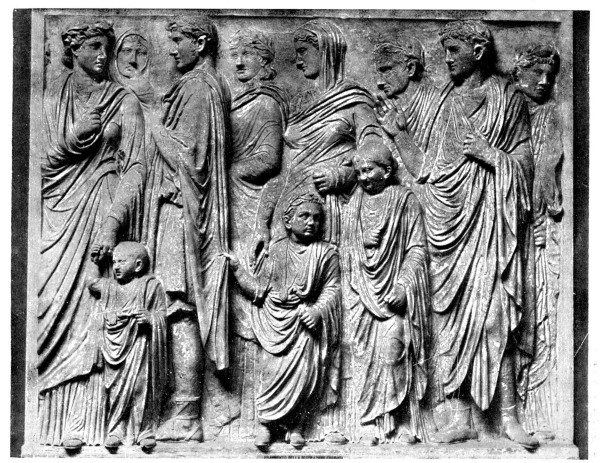
Distinguished Romans with their children, wearing laurel wreaths and togas. Relief on the Ara Pacis erected by Augustus just before the birth of Christ

boots. Nero adopted a flowered unbelted tunic and Commodus wore a white silk tunic embroidered with gold.

In still later times, tunics came to be made of Chinese silk so fine that, in the words of an ancient Roman author, 'our women expose themselves to the world as much as to their lover in the bedchamber'. This fabric was worth its weight in gold and was called 'woven air'.

Women wore an outer garment in the form of a long shawl cut on the same lines as the tunic, and an additional toga (pallium) and head-scarf when out of doors. For travel, both men and women used the old Etruscan cloak (paenula) made of wool or leather, sometimes with a hood. Saint Paul left his paenula behind in Troas and asks in one of his epistles for it to be sent on. Men on horseback wore a blanket wrap (sagum) buckled on the right shoulder; the field commander's sagum was red.

The Romans sometimes wore the Greek type of sandal and sometimes the Etruscan boot or shoe. Footwear was of great importance to them because they not only travelled by boat like the Greeks, but they also marched; slaves did not carry their sandals as among the Egyptians.

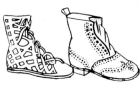
Roman boot, and a modern boot. The decorations on today's boot derive from the pattern of openings in the vamp of the earlier one

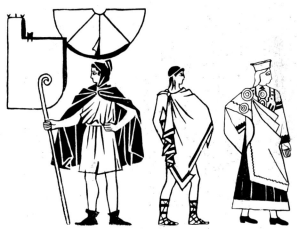
Shepherd's paenula in two different styles, the sagum and modern Lithuanian regional costume with 'sag-sha'

Beauty Culture. In Rome, manual work was done by slaves. Ordinary people did not indulge in much physical exercise, and sport was left mainly to professional athletes. Dancing was merely a form of entertainment as it had been among the Etruscans, and did not involve participation in a religious ceremony, as it had in Greece.

The Romans could not match the physical beauty of the Greeks which had been attained through deliberately working for bodily perfection, the main purpose of all their physical exercise and sport. The baths in

Ancient Rome appear to have been built essentially for pleasure. It is noteworthy that the most famous women of Egypt, Cleopatra and Nefretiti, as well as Helen and Phryne of Greece, are remembered for their great beauty, whereas the famous women of Ancient Rome are remembered for their virtue. Nevertheless, as time went on and a luxurious standard of living developed in the Roman Empire, so general interest in personal appearance grew. We read, for example, of the aristocratic woman in Rome 'who acquires a new face. To attain it, she hides the old one beneath a thick layer of grease. The poor husband receives greasy kisses and sticks to the paste on her face. But when her lover arrives, she emerges fresh from the bath in an atmosphere of Indian and Arabian oils and perfumes. After the greasy crust has been removed, her cheeks are soft as silk and shine as if bathed in asses' milk.'

Great skill was attained in dyeing and bleaching the black hair of Roman women, in emulation of the blonde Germanic slave girls.

Roman Law. In the time of the Republic and up to the beginning of our era, the father exercised complete authority over wife and children, the wife occupying the same position as a daughter. But under the Roman Empire, women enjoyed a greater equality with men. The old Etruscan philosophy had penetrated society, and the pleasures of good food and music had taken precedence over military prowess. Women started to assume an equal place in society. Both at court and in the home, they joined the men when they reclined at table for meals and at feasts. The number of women began to equal that of men at theatres and at the circus.

Women, supported by law, came to exercise full rights over their private fortunes, and divorce was easily obtained. Inscriptions found on tombstones reveal instances much like those in Hollywood, where six or ten marriages had taken place. Marcus Aurelius declared, 'It would be unfair in the highest degree that a man should demand chastity in his wife without practising chastity himself.' Wall-paintings from wealthy homes in Pompeii depict erotic scenes in which women are adopting that position quoted by Robert Graves as a sign of a matriarchal society.

Roman
engagement ring

After Etruscan times, the wearing of gold bracelets, finely engraved necklaces and cameos and delicately cut stones, was confined to women. Our present-day engagement ring, as indeed our whole marriage ritual, originated among the Ancient Romans.

Pax Romana. Looked at from the old Roman patriarchal standpoint, equality between the sexes was a development of dubious value. The reactionary Cato objected bitterly and observed, 'All nations rule their women. We rule all nations, but our women rule us.'

Roman culture developed from that of the Greeks and was not particularly distinct from it, except in the technical, economic and political spheres. The coarse Etruscan attitudes towards human relationships survived among the Romans. They were unable to accept the Greek attitude toward homosexuality, and this practice was never looked upon with favour

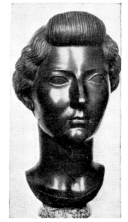

Woman during the
Roman Empire

in Rome. On the other hand, the Romans organized a most practical and businesslike system of prostitution.

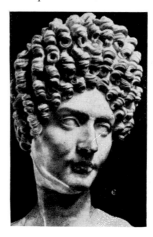

It was during these centuries of Roman supremacy, that a peace prevailed, both longer in duration and wider in territorial sway than any known before or since in the history of Europe.

Hair style
during the Roman Empire

Women's dress
in the home

THE ARAB HAIK

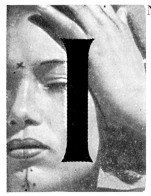

IN THE REGIONS south and south-east of the Mediterranean, the draped form of dress has been retained up to the present day. The white flowing haik worn against the dusky skin of the Hollywood sheikh represents the current ideas of an Arab.

The billowing folds of loose material transform the galloping horseman into a fantastic, fluttering bird. Merely sitting in the saddle, the Arab is an impressive tower of glistening white. The original horizontally draped garments of Mesopotamia gradually assumed a vertical emphasis. A robe such as this, so rich in loose folds, provides perfect protection against the scorching desert sun.

Abstract Sculpture in Cloth. The haik consists of a large rectangular piece of material which covers the entire body in a most graceful and artistic manner. The most impressive haiks are worn in Somalia. Un-

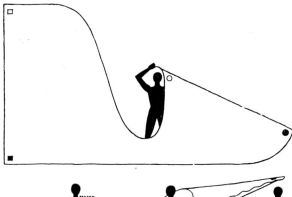

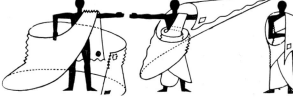

Draping the Somali haik. The cloth is rectangular but the perspective makes it seem indented

like the Arabs, the Somalis do not wear the additional pieces of clothing derived from the Turks, and thus the volume of their haik does not have to be reduced. It is usually made of white woollen material, but is sometimes brown or grey with woven stripes of colour at each end. It can be made of either silk, cotton or wool in natural colour with diagonal stripes. Men

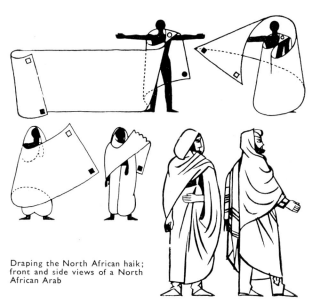

Draping the North African haik; front and side views of a North African Arab

wear only white or natural haiks, but they may have a red or blue border.

The head covering of the Arab consists of a kind of skull cap made of woollen material or of felt. Over this, is folded a triangular piece of cloth, long enough to cover neck and shoulders, and kept together by a cord of camel's hair. Alternatively, a long piece of cloth can be twisted into the shape of a turban thus providing excellent protection against the sun. This headgear

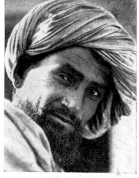

Arab turban

gives the impression of being an abstract sculpture; and its shape is reminiscent of Arabic characters or Moorish ornaments.

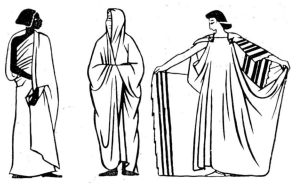

Man from Somalia, Syrian woman, and North African woman's haik

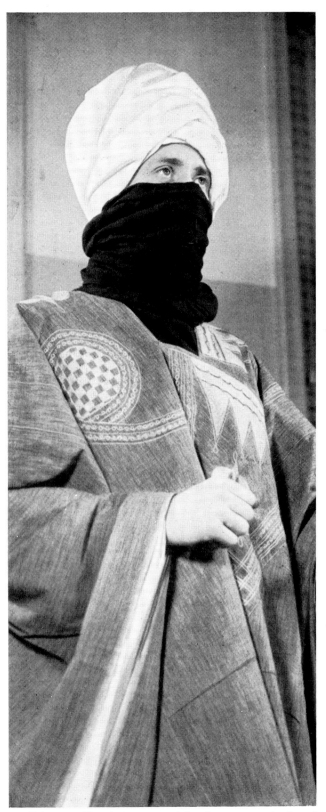

Tuareg man. They do not remove their veils even to eat, but instead use spoons with long curved handles that can go under the veils

To achieve some degree of status and acceptance, the womenfolk of nomadic warrior tribes had to be weak and submissive, outwardly at least. Only by flattering her man and appealing to his superior strength could she obtain recognition. Out of doors she had to be completely covered; even her face was hidden. No other man but her husband and family members could look upon it. So strict was this convention that, if observed by strangers while at work, she would fling her skirt over her head, quite oblivious that this exposed her naked body.

Veiled Men. There is, strange to relate, one Muslim tribe in the Western Sahara, the Tuaregs, where the men and not the women are veiled. The men wear a piece of dark blue cotton round the head, which permits no more than the eyes to be seen. The women of the Tuaregs receive better treatment than other Arab women and have equal standing with the men. When a

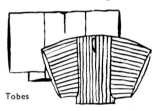

Tobes

man marries a woman of higher social status than his own, the children inherit the rank of the mother. These women are said to be as formidable as the Amazons. They hunt with the men and handle horses and camels skilfully. Their dress, the tobe, is made of narrow strips of cotton woven on small looms. These strips are sewn together to make large squares, leaving an opening for the head, and the sides joined together at the bottom. Alternatively, the square piece of cloth can be worn as a tunic with wide, loose sleeves.

The Dream Women. With the coming of the Prophet Mohammed, the Arabs were drawn into the Muslim faith, which clearly defines the status of women in law and religion. In pre-Islamic times, women were regarded very much as beasts of burden; they were shut up in harems and had no rights in law. The husband could abandon his wife whenever he pleased. If this happened without any fault on the part of the woman, he had to pay for her maintenance for three months and ten days. Among the lower classes, women were not treated quite so rigorously, but their position was really little better in spite of this. The women wove the cloth for the clothes they wore, the rugs they sat upon and the tents that covered their heads. They frequently carried heavy burdens on journeys

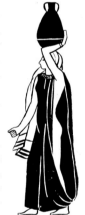

Woman wearing a tobe joined together only at the top and bottom

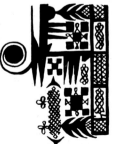

Embroidery on a Sudanese tobe

Women do not drape the haik around the body but wear it hanging from the shoulders, secured by two buckles.

while the men rode, and when camp was set up it was the women who erected the tents and fetched water from the well. Even nowadays Islamic precepts relating to women are frequently disregarded in this region.

Side by side with this practical contempt for women, we find an idealistic worship of the female sex. The somewhat bloodless poems and songs of European troubadours in the Middle Ages were later influenced and enriched by the more lyrical and sensuous poems from Arabia. The sight of a woman's naked body — or merely a part of it — could induce the greatest of ecstasies; a contemporary of the Prophet, writes as follows,

'Beautiful are her thighs, her body small and white. Her bosom is like a mirror and when she turns, her breasts stand out. Her glance is like the glance of the gazelle. Her hair is black as night and falls heavily round her shoulders like date clusters on the palm tree. Her hips are resplendent above her thighs and her legs are slender as the reeds on the lakeshore.'

Arabian Capes. The Arabian burnus is made from wool or cotton. Although it is similar to Roman garments, it did not develop, as some people think, from the toga. The burnus is not a wrapped garment, but falls from the shoulders like a cape. It is open in front and has a portion that forms a covering for the head, much like the Roman paenula.

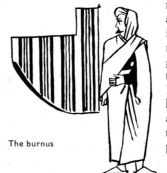
The burnus

A burnus, cut on generous lines and worn by a person accustomed to wearing a wrap, can look almost as impressive as a haik. Brightly coloured material, such as flame red, burgundy or lavender blue, is used on festive occasions, and the burnus is sometimes edged with gold.

The everyday dress of both town or country-dweller is the tunic. It is shaped like a sack and has holes cut in it for the arms and head. Sometimes the tunic is split down the front, and at others a belt is worn with it. Well-to-do people have their tunics embroider-

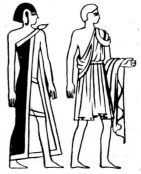
Egyptian drawing of a Libyan cape and Greek exomis

ed and decorated with tassels and gold lace on the breast and shoulders. Poorer people wear plain tunics of coarse material, usually in natural colour; but even the poor wear large geometrically shaped silver ornaments on their simple tunics.

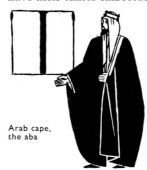
Arab cape, the aba

Muslim Dress. After the rise of Islam, the clothing previously described came under Turkish and Persian influence and dress of a very different type emerged, with trousers, jackets and waistcoats or vests. These garments were cut and sewn to fit the wearer. The effect of this meeting between these two worlds could be rather picturesque. For example, an Arab sheikh in gala dress might look something like this: red burnus with green fringes round the neck; over this, a white burnus with hood; then a haik made of thin muslin and over that a loose white tunic with grey borders. To top it all, he might wear a waistcoat with black edging and blue sleeves and then two more waistcoats in lavender blue embroidered with gold thread. The whole outfit might finally be encircled by a patterned woven belt and worn with turban and red boots.

Arab sheikh with his son

THE INDIAN SARI

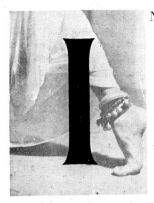

I N A LARGE AREA of the world the beautiful wrapped garment is still worn. The particular countries include India, Sumatra, Java, Bali, East Africa and Madagascar. In more developed countries, however, it has been supplemented by additional articles of clothing. The first invasion of India from the west in about 3000 B.C., brought with it a culture clearly related closely to ancient Mesopotamia, and drove the indigenous population into the hills. The wrapped clothing of Indians and Mesopotamians may therefore have a common origin.

In Mesopotamia, the garment was wrapped tightly, like European swaddling clothes of a later date, whereas in India it was wrapped loosely and easily, rather like the folds of a shawl.

The ancient Indian dress consisted of one or more pieces of cotton taken straight from the loom and not modified in any way. Buddhist figures have been found, however, whose draperies are arranged in much the same way as among the Greeks, and Buddhist monks in India still wear the himation. Indian sculpture of two

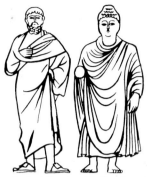

Ancient Greek and Indian draped garments

thousand years back shows men clad in a long piece of cloth draped from the back round the lower part of the body and then drawn between the legs so that graceful folds hung in front. This is the dhoti, a garment that persists unchanged in present-day India. Unlike our trousers, the folds between the legs are loose and airy, providing welcome ventilation in a hot climate. Among all existing classes of society it is not uncommon for the chest and arms to be bare. If, however, men want to cover the chest and arms, they may wear a loose shirt reaching to the hips, or a sleeveless jacket with a semicircular neck opening that does up in front. Coats in the Persian and Muslim styles are also still worn.

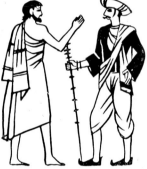

South Indian in a mundu, a draped garment based on the sari, and a Bengali in a dhoti, jacket and shawl

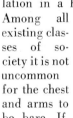

Indian Buddhist monk in a wrapped cowl

The original dress for women is the sari, which consists of a single length of material between five and eight yards long and about one yard

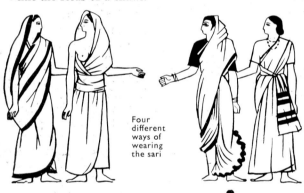

Four different ways of wearing the sari

Stages in draping the third style shown above

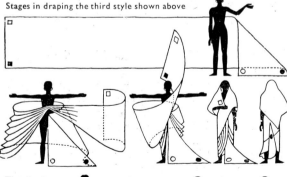

The dhoti

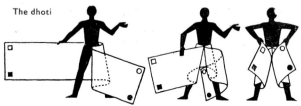

The wrapping of the first style of the four shown on the left

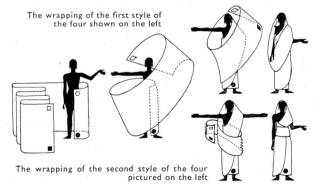

The wrapping of the second style of the four pictured on the left

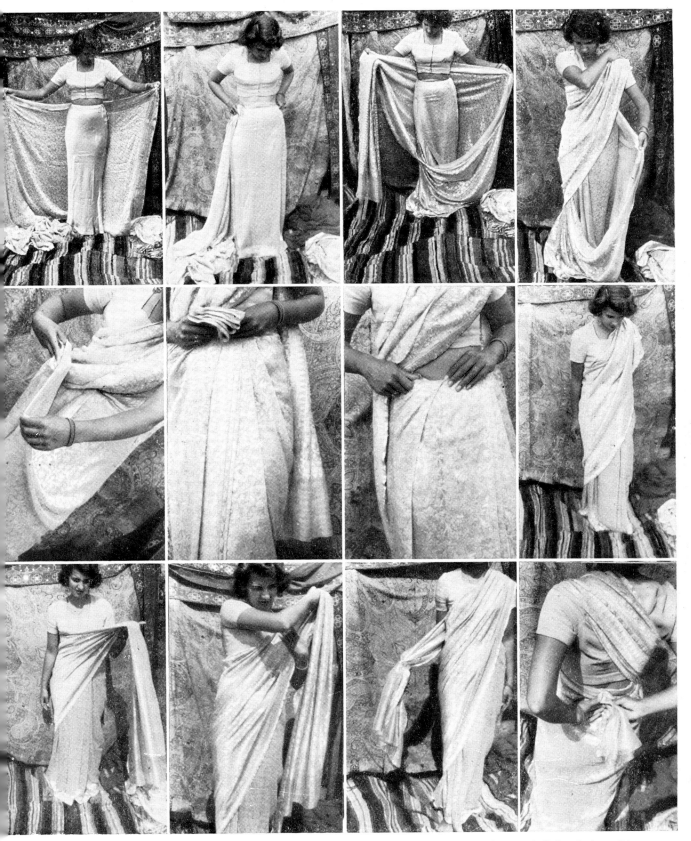

Top row, Beginning over the left hip, the wearer tucks her sari once round her body into the top of a long petticoat; a suitable length of material is kept in reserve to make folds, and the other end of the sari is placed over the left shoulder and hangs loose down the back. Centre row, The upper edge of the part of the sari left loose is gathered in neat folds of a hand's width and tucked into the petticoat, so that the latter is covered by loose folds reaching to the ground. Bottom row, This sari is wrapped in a different way: the end portion does not, as above, hang loosely down the back, but is wound around the waist like a 'belt' and tucked into the upper edge of the petticoat at the back

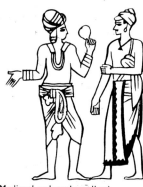
Medieval and modern dhoti

wide. Both the sari and the dhoti are supplemented by shawls, head coverings and turbans. Before the coming of Islam to India garments were simply wrapped or knotted round the body, and were not secured by either buttons, hooks or ribbons. Embroidery was placed only where it could be seen and where it should not interfere with comfort. This restricted the use of embroidery to ends and borders only. The dhoti, for example, carried embroidery at the top and bottom because those parts hang free. The sari, on the other hand, was embroidered at one end only because the other end was enclosed and could not be seen. If the enclosed end were embroidered, it would most likely have caused discomfort since it was next to the body.

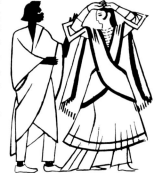
Nubian and Indian shawl

The material used was generally a light airy cotton. Cotton was India's principal textile, just as linen was the principal textile of Egypt and wool of Mesopotamia. To avoid irritating the skin, the cloth was

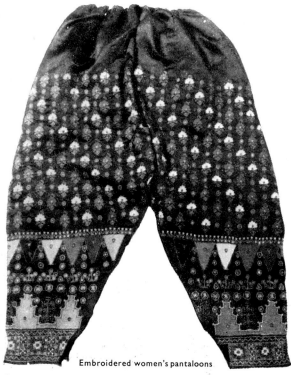
Embroidered women's pantaloons

usually plain and unpatterned but was dyed in rich, luscious colours. Indigo is only one of two hundred and two different colours named in an Indian dictionary.

Muslim and European Dress. During the first centuries following A.D. 1000, when India was under
Muslim rule, civil servants were required to wear tailored garments. Although such clothing was initially held in contempt, it came to be regarded later with admiration and respect. This new style of dress did not allow the same freedom of movement as the old loose garments. Its main purpose was to cover the body completely; even the hands could be concealed within the long

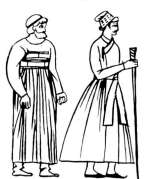
Ancient Ukrainian costume and 17th-century Indian dress

sleeves. The garments we see in sculptures dating from the Middle Ages consist of the sari, worn over a long petticoat, with the short bodice which covered the breasts, and the dhoti which was worn with a shirt. Indians today may often wear clothes in which European and ancient Indian styles have come together. A kind of duel between dhoti and trousers exists nowadays in India, where reactionaries still wear the loincloth, satirically referred to by radicals as 'the nappy'. The distinction between wearing a dhoti

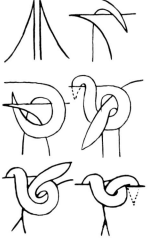
The knot which holds the loin-cloth together

and wearing trousers can occasionally be greater than the distinction between Hindu and Muslim.

Turbans and Jewels. The turban is worn in India by both Muslim and Hindus alike, irrespective of

Hindu turban

caste or sect. But each caste and sect (and even certain families) express their individuality in the way they fold or drape it. The most usual colour is white, but many other colours are worn. A survey has shown that, next to white, red is the most popular, followed by yellow, green, blue and purple. Many turbans are made out of patterned material. Black is seldom worn.

The turban of the wealthy Muslim is decorated with jewellery. On the whole, a lot of jewellery is worn by

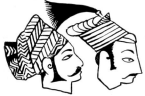
Muslim turbans of 1780 and 1690

both men and women, depending, of course, on their means. Jewellery may be made from platinum, gold or silver, and set with pearls and precious stones, glass, wood, wax or even straw. The women wear more jewellery than the men, sometimes so much that the outline of the body is obscured. The same trend is apparent in the temples, where a great wealth of ornamentation hides the basic lines of the building.

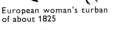
European woman's turban of about 1825

Since Indians so often go barefoot, their feet can be as expressive as their hands, and their walk is as light as a dancer's. Indians are the only people to adorn their toes with rings. The artisan actually uses his toes for his work in the same way that other people use their fingers.

Dance and Sign Language.
The temple-dancers give a unique opportunity of observing the manner in which ancient garments were employed. Only in this way can we even begin to understand the significance of the garment's draping, for it provides a musical and ornamental accompaniment which is in perfect harmony with certain meaningful dance movements. Dancing, as a language, is more restricted than the spoken word, but far more subtle in expression. In the course of his normal education, the Indian of ancient times was trained in the movements and postures which formed an important part

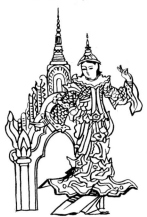
Dancing girl and pagoda, 18th-century Burma

of religious ceremony. The position adopted in Christian worship — kneeling with folded hands — is perhaps comparable. Anyone who has visited Italy will know that gestures can be more expressive than words. It is this sign language which is part of the religious dance of India.

The dancers' hands move in a particular set way, their position assuming a certain significance, in much the same way as when a priest makes the sign of the cross in a Christian church. Control of the fingers, the hands, and indeed of all bodily movement, has been achieved through centuries of careful training, reaching a degree of perfection quite impossible for us to attain. A code or standard of gesture and bodily movement originated inside the temples and quietly spread to the outside world, irrespective of caste or creed.

Position of the temple-dancer's hands that signifies the blooming of the lotus flower. The palms are stained red with henna

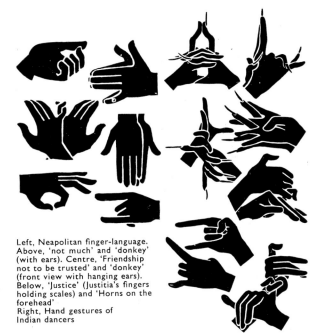
Left, Neapolitan finger-language. Above, 'not much' and 'donkey' (with ears). Centre, 'Friendship not to be trusted' and 'donkey' (front view with hanging ears). Below, 'Justice' (Justitia's fingers holding scales) and 'Horns on the forehead'
Right, Hand gestures of Indian dancers

Rounded Women. The woman's body was influenced by dancing and certain muscles were developed. At the same time, a degree of deliberate body culture was present: Indian women wound strips of material round themselves in order to cultivate the slender and sinuous waist which weaved so seductively in the dance.

In contrast to the Greek ideal of female beauty, the Indian ideal was of a more developed body with full breasts set close together, large rounded hips and a navel set low. While the Greeks admired narrow hips and slender thighs in a woman the Indians preferred amply proportioned women with curving hips and thighs.

It may here be mentioned that some present-day physiologists consider the glamorous long-legged female so much admired now as indicative of sexual frigidity. The production of sex hormones hampers, it seems, the development of long bone formations. Certainly, eunuchs have long limbs.

The Indian woman was regarded as primarily an object for erotic delight and some degree of experience was by no means frowned upon. The figures on the walls of temples provide a detailed study in the techniques of love-making. The devotees study these poses and postures with religious concentration, whereas to the European viewer they probably appear to be pornographic illustrations of fantastic orgies. Certainly the British in India misunderstood the erotic

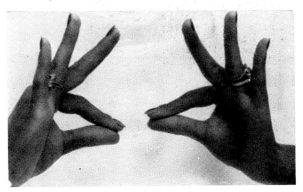

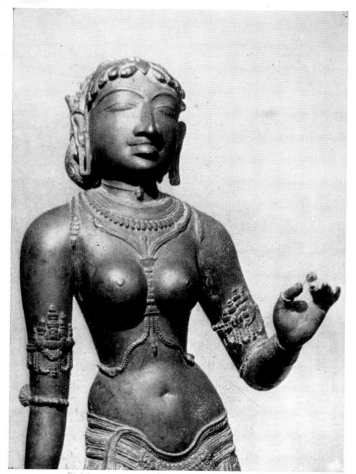

The Indian woman with her slim waist and breasts set close together, wearing elaborate jewellery

Women, of course, had not always occupied such a lowly place. Before the patriarchal society of Brahma came into being, their position was very different. Kali, who gave birth to Brahma and who was mother of all gods 'as the clouds give birth to lightning', is the Mother Goddess from whom all life issues and to whom it all returns.

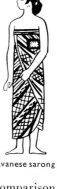

Javanese sarong

The uncovered breasts which long prevailed in India, can still be seen on the Malabar Coast and in Bali. The custom is, in fact, a remnant from that earlier time when women enjoyed a more dominant position. These visible charms demonstrated the superiority of the female sex in comparison to the male, who, particularly in respect to the bosom, was so sparsely endowed. The old epic poets tell us that women took part in making sacrifices and in war.

After that period, women became slaves and their position since then has paralleled the history of their country. When India was under foreign rule, women were subjugated; when India became free they were liberated.

As in other parts of the world, the style of dress in an agricultural society was developed by the skill and the art of the weaver. The simple design combined with the infinite variety of ways of draping the garment exemplify eternal contradiction in female nature.

A European version of the sar

Subsequent history records the defeat of the draped garment by the tailored garment with its complicated cut and reduced opportunity for variety and self-expression.

element in the dance so much that they tried to prohibit all temple dances.

However highly the woman was prized in an erotic context, as a fellow human being she had little status; legally, indeed, she counted for nothing.

The custom of arranging girls' marriages while they were still in the cradle is characteristic of the position of the female in that society.

The Law of Manu legislated that,

'Woman shall recognize no other god than her husband. Even if he is disgusting and wicked and full of failings and vice she will venerate him like a god and serve him with humility. If he beats or cripples her she must kiss his hand and beg his forgiveness because she has aroused his anger. Should the husband die before her, there is no consolation upon earth for her other than to let herself be cremated with him.'

Kneeling woman in a wall-painting dating from the 6th century

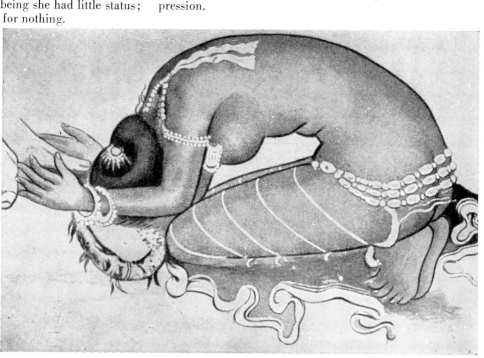

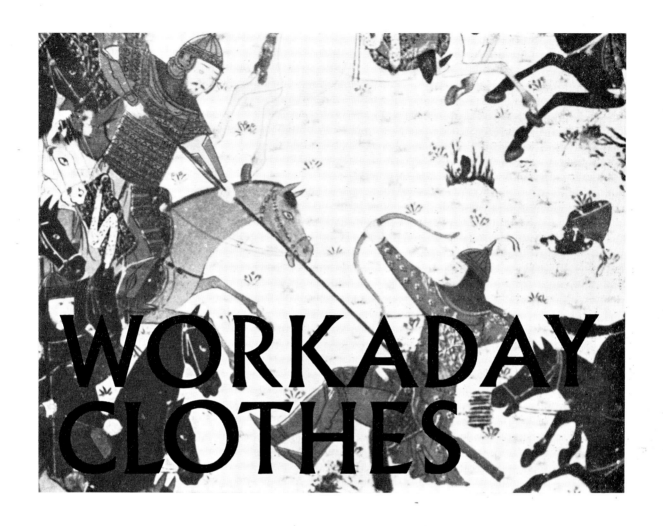

WORKADAY CLOTHES

THE ARMOUR OF ANTIQUITY

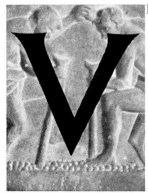

VERY LITTLE is known about the working clothes of ancient times. (Until now we have considered dress mainly as decoration.) There is however the exception of one category which has long been the object of extensive interest and deep-seated admiration — the dress of the warrior. While the leather apron of the blacksmith becomes besmirched with merely soot and dust, the helmet and shield of the warrior are baptized in blood. Most modern ethnologists agree that it is incorrect to regard war as the oldest occupation and the natural way of life among primitive tribes. On the contrary, a peaceable life should be regarded as the norm among such peoples. Organized war did not appear until during a later and more developed period of civilization. Hunting weapons could, of course, be used in family feuds such as those described in Icelandic sagas, but, generally speaking, disagreements between tribes were settled by diplomatic negotiation. The war-paint of primitive times supports this point. The object of the plume flying on the helmet in later times and the colourful uniform was similarly to impress and intimidate. Nowadays, the object is not to create fear but to exterminate the enemy; so brightly coloured uniforms have given way to the muddy colours of camouflage.

Armour. Armour, the first effective war-clothing, did not appear until a civilized society had come into

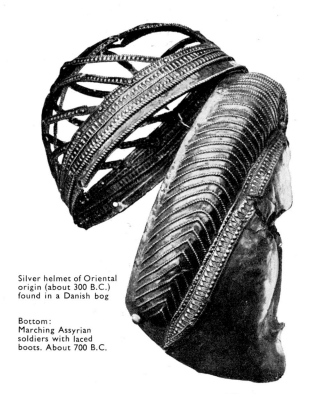

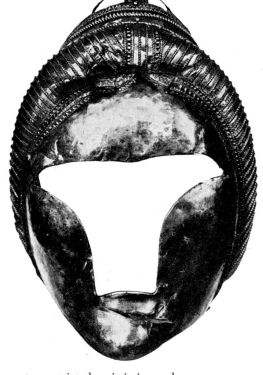

Silver helmet of Oriental origin (about 300 B.C.) found in a Danish bog

Bottom:
Marching Assyrian soldiers with laced boots. About 700 B.C.

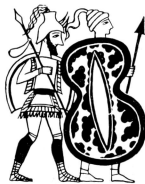

Greek warriors of about 1200 B.C.

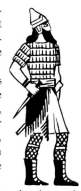

Assyrian warrior of 700 B.C.

existence. The Assyrians, in about 2000 B.C., were using helmets of bronze, copper and, later, iron. Officers were equipped with leather shirts overlaid with bronze scales or plates and with leather iron-studded belts. The rank and file, who had previously fought barefoot, started to wear boots and leggings.

The Assyrian boot was broad and rounded. The front was cut away and a loose leather flap covered the instep and leg. The lacing was loose, so the foot was not constricted as it is in modern-day footwear. Pointed boots were not introduced until the time of the Hittites and the Persians, when they were found to be useful in close fighting.

The Egyptians made breast-plates from leather or padded linen since metal was scarce. The Greek infantry, the hoplites, wore sheets of leather or metal suspended by shoulder straps, protecting their chest and back, with an additional leather section over the abdomen.

The simple woollen cap, dating from the Bronze Age, was worn as a helmet in Denmark. The usual helmet of the Spartans was basically no more than a metal cap, while the Athen-

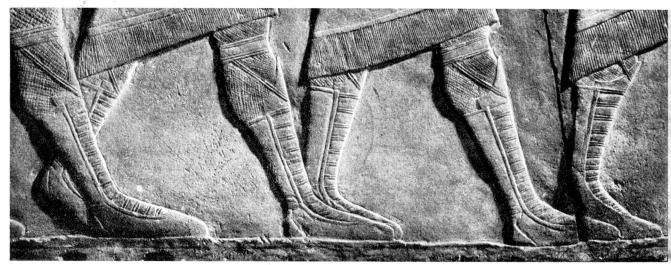

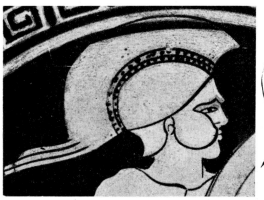

Greek helmet

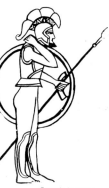

Greek hoplite.

Right: Ancestor figure from the South Sea Islands

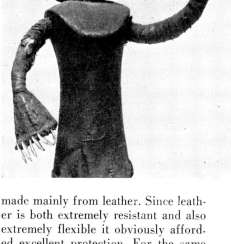

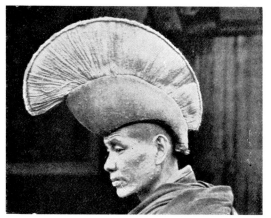

Headgear of a Tibetan priest

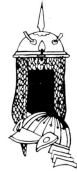

Mongolian and Japanese helmets

made mainly from leather. Since leather is both extremely resistant and also extremely flexible it obviously afforded excellent protection. For the same reason, it is still the principal material for footwear today.

The hoplites wore helmets made of fur, somewhat like bearskins worn by guardsmen nowadays. Fur was also used to cover their arms.

War has its origin in the incursions

ian helmet had the addition of side plates to protect the cheeks and the Corinthian helmet encased the whole head. Both of the latter were reinforced by a central strip of metal, much like the fireman's helmet of today.

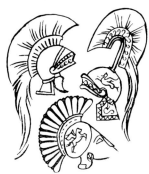

Greek helmets. The type shown at the upper right suggests that an entire animal skin was originally set on top of the helmet.

The leather armour of the Greek hoplites was adopted by the Roman legions at a later date and broad strips of metal added. A well preserved coat of mail has been discovered in a bog in Denmark: it dates from the Late Roman period and is made up of no fewer than two thousand interconnected metal rings. Shields

Danish fireman's helmet

made of metal or wood and covered in leather were used with all types of armour. The ultimate object was to provide protection against the various weapons then in use — swords, spears, lances, daggers, clubs, slings and bows and arrows.

It is interesting that while civilian dress was made principally from woven material, military dress was

Etruscan bronze helmet with protection for cheeks and nose

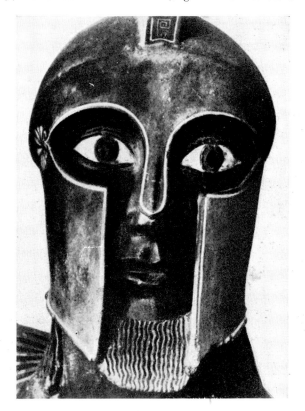

Coat of mail composed of 2,000 rings, dating from A.D. 200–400

Above right:
Spanish soldier in ringed mail, A.D. 1109

Below right:
Norwegian warrior. About A.D. 1250

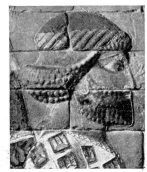
Persian soldier with helmet made of twined material

made by the cattlebreeders of Central Asia who were the first to introduce the idea of armour. The horse was the most important animal for it supplied the speed necessary for sudden attack, a characteristic feature of warfare in ancient time. Most nomadic races formed patriarchal societies, because men were better able to adapt quickly to changing circumstances and unexpected situations. Since mobility was so necessary, the design of armour paralleled the principal divisions of the body. It was constructed somewhat like a doll with movable joints, and thus provided separate protection for the upper chest, the midriff and lower part of the body.

The carriage of soldiers is always more rigid than that of civilians. Precise and controlled movements develop out of an erect military bearing. The movements of these ancient warriors were, however, even more ponderous and restricted, as an inevitable result of the massive armour they wore.

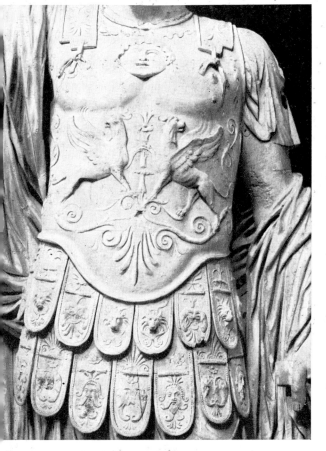
Greek soldier's boot

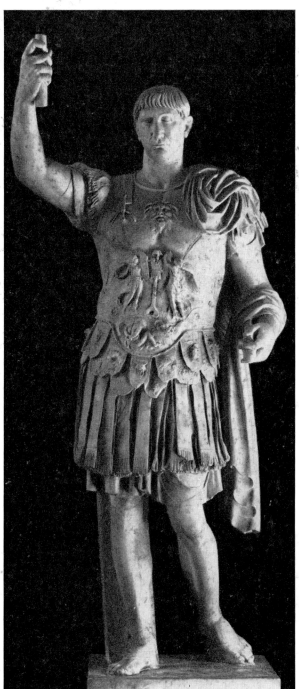
The Emperor Trajan in the uniform of a Roman general

Roman armour

Adulation of the warrior extended to an admiration of his dress and general deportment, which may explain the ultimate victory of close-fitting garments over more comfortable draped ones.

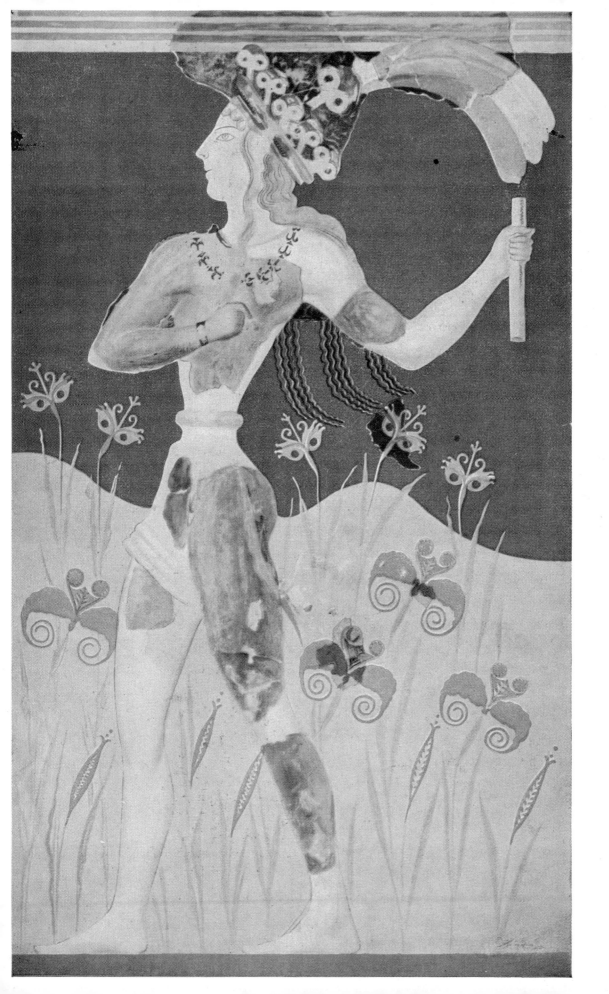

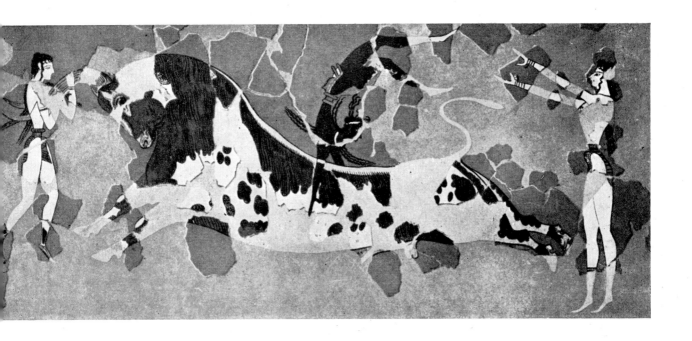

THE GOAT-SKIN SKIRT OF THE AEGEAN

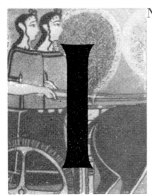

IN the Bronze Age, the islands of the eastern Mediterranean, Crete in particular, were used as clearing houses for the principal raw materials — namely, copper and tin — used in the industry of the time.

Aegean culture, which flourished in these islands and along the coast of the Greek peninsula from 2000 B.C. until the Greek invasion in about 1300 B.C., arose because of local social and economic conditions. Life in Crete was easy and comfortable. Slaves were imported to do the hard work, so their masters were free to develop the decorative arts. On the Greek mainland and in Troy, at the mouth of the Black Sea, circumstances were very different and considerable force had to be shown. The gigantic fortifications with their huge walls and massive war equipment were in harsh contrast to life on the idyllic, sun-drenched island of Crete.

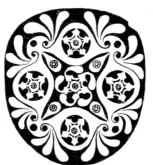

Cretan ornament

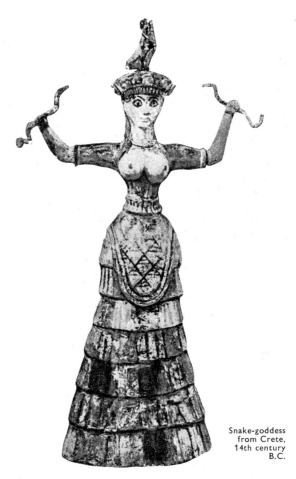

Snake-goddess from Crete, 14th century B.C.

Opposite Cretan youth with crown of lilies. Wall-painting at Knossos   Top Wall-painting from the 16th century B.C. showing a woman about to leap onto the back of a bull where a man is already balancing on his hands

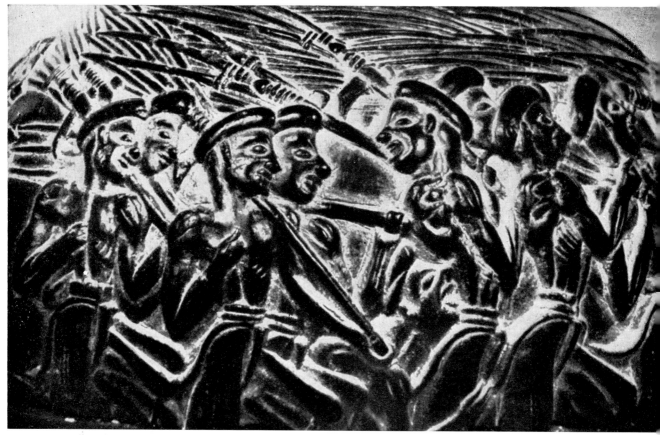

Harvesters with scythes over their shoulders. They wear Basque-like caps, double belts, and 'bathing trunks' with rear aprons

Nature and Culture.

Few cultures have offered more ideal living conditions than those enjoyed by the Aegean peoples. Their houses were provided with drains, lavatories, bathrooms and sun-lounges. Wall-paintings show an industrious, gay people with a great love of nature, flowers and animals. Life was uncomplicated; no vicious wanton gods wreaked havoc on humanity. The outstanding feature of Aegean art is its fresh response to the natural world. It is strange that an awareness of the perfection of nature and the workings of natural phenomena should at times coexist with a rather empty frivolity in other aspects of life. We will come back to this enigma when we deal with the Rococo period in Europe, a time when people tightly constricted by corsets and high-heeled shoes affected great admiration for the natural and unsophisticated. The many porcelain figurines of shepherds and peasant boys and girls dating from this later time illustrate this attitude.

Although an athletic figure was admired by the Aegeans, both men and women wore tightly-laced clothes. The dignity of formal graceful folds was not stressed, since life was casual and no at-

Cretan headgear of about 2000 B.C.

tempts were made to create an impression. The general impression was one of a life of ease. Just as the desert protected the Egyptians from their enemies, so the sea shielded the Aegeans. This freedom from fear permitted them to lead a relaxed life and to wear clothes which were easy and comfortable for work.

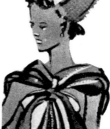

Paris fashion, 1950

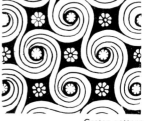

Cretan pattern

Bathing Trunks.

It is clear that trade influenced Aegean dress. The men were naked except for a loincloth which, unlike the white loin-cloth of the Egyptians, was usually patterned. The women wore a longer garment not unlike the wrapped garment of Mesopotamian women. Aegean dress did not consist merely of squares of material draped around the body, but was cut in such a way that it could be tailored to the body. Both sexes wore skirts that hung lower at the

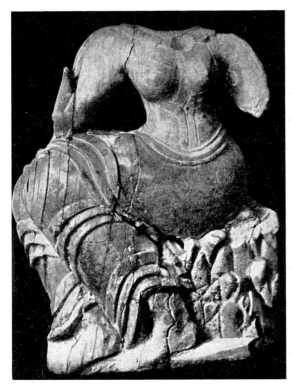
Ivory figurine with a waist that makes it look Indian, but it is actually Cretan

The Open Dress. During the earlier period, all women — except for women athletes — wore a bell-shaped dress cut on a semi-circle which was caught in at the waist by a broad belt. This garment stood high at the back of the neck, forming a distinct collar, and was open at the front down to the waist.

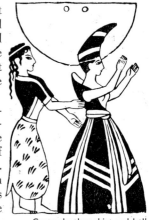
Cretan leather skirt and bell-shaped skirt with the pattern from which it is cut

At a later period, women's dresses acquired patterned flounces or were made from a number of multicoloured squares. These dresses were cut on the same ample lines as the Egyptian dress, since dignified matrons although willing to display their breasts, did not wish to expose their legs. A short-sleeved jacket, open at the front, was worn over the dress.

back and front. Under them, the men wore something like bathing trunks made from a triangular piece of material. Fighting men on the Aegean mainland wore short trousers rather like the shorts worn today.

Both men and women wore laced bodices. Perhaps they had noticed on their travels that their waists were slender in comparison with the square-cut Mesopotamians or the spindly Egyptians and wished to emphasize this characteristic.

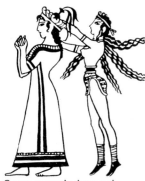
Cretan woman's dress and woman athlete with short skirt

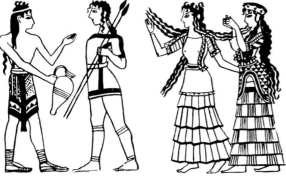
A Cretan as represented in an Egyptian wall-painting, a warrior from the mainland and women's dresses from Crete

The Tailored Dress. Our knowledge of the Aegean tailored dress is limited entirely to paintings discovered during excavations. Leather was apparently the principal material used, usually from goats, the most common domestic animal. The hides had to be cut to a pattern and sewn together to fit the body. There is no doubt that the broad belts were made from leather.

The Naked Bosom. Paintings from the Aegean suggest that women excelled in athletic prowess. There are pictures of women grasping the horns of a bull, vaulting onto its back and executing handsprings. All of this would seem to indicate that women enjoyed greater equality with men than in other areas of the Mediterranean. The custom of baring the bosom and the fact that the deities in ancient pictures were always female, suggest that a type of worship of the Earth Mother existed. Small statuettes also survive symbolizing fertility and these were always in female shapes.

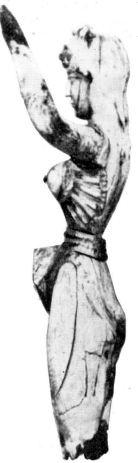
Ivory figurine with apron and corset made of gold-leaf about 1400 B.C.

The Bronze Age in Nordic Countries. The culture of the Nordic countries during the Bronze Age was, in certain ways, connected with the earlier culture of the Aegean.

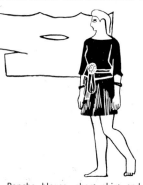

Aegean jewellery with spiral design and Bronze Age buttons from Denmark

The Aegean basic spiral design was developed in beautiful ornaments which were worn by the aristocratic classes who bartered their amber for bronze. The original Aegean safety-pin was developed by Nordic people, becoming the magnificent fibula of that region.

At one time, the Scandinavians followed the custom of burying their dead in hollowed trunks of oak trees. The secretion of tannic acid from the wood acted as a preservative for the woollen garments in which the bodies were clothed, allowing us to see them as they were.

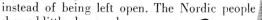

Nordic dress was made in two sections, like that of Aegean women, but the upper part was brought together in the form of a bodice instead of being left open. The Nordic people showed little shyness, however, in displaying their legs. Short split skirts with fringes held together by only a cord have been found in over forty graves.

The Nordic belt-buckle was shaped like a miniature shield and usually decorated with the popular spiral design. The projecting point of the shield formed a hook on which to hang a purse. Only the blouse was stitched; all other garments were draped. Hair styles varied greatly, including short hair worn with a fringe, long hair gathered in a net behind, or wigs.

In death, men and women were equal. Women were buried wearing precious jewellery, with beautiful pottery and glass beside them.

Poncho blouse, short skirt and belt-buckle of the Bronze Age in Denmark

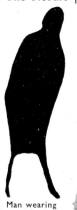

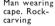

Man wearing cape. Rock-carving

Safety-pin

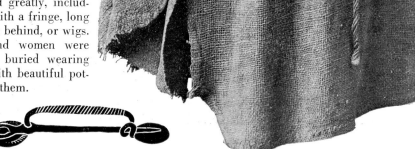

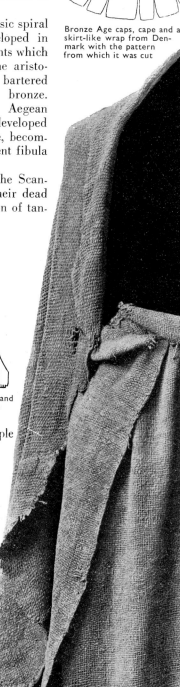

Bronze Age caps, cape and a skirt-like wrap from Denmark with the pattern from which it was cut

PERSIAN LEATHER TROUSERS

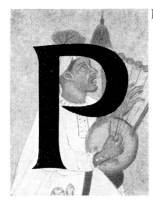

ERSIANS and other related people, such as Hittites, Lydians, Phrygians and Scythians, brought the Indo-European languages to the Near East, Europe and India between 3000 and 1000 B.C. The Persians were great horsemen and fighters; their religion itself emphasized the war between God and the Devil. Their military prowess enabled them, around 500 B.C., to build the first world empire, an empire whose borders touched Egypt in the west and India in the east. It was established by Alexander the Great in 330 B.C. and Persian and Greek cultures merged into one.

The Persians originally came from Central Asia where the climate in winter was so cold that close-fitting clothes were necessary. Nowadays, the temperature in Iran during the wintertime may be as low as –68° F.

The Hide Dress. As would be expected, the material of the earliest cut and sewn clothing was leather. An animal hide in its natural shape can cover the human body, using the skin from two legs to cover the arms and that from the head to form a hood. Evidently the design of these ancient garments followed the original shape of the stripped hide very closely. If the skin was carefully selected for size, very little

needed to be cut off or added to provide quite a well-fashioned jacket.

As previously described, the shirt-type garment evolved from the poncho hide. The Egyptians knew nothing of the tunic until envoys and slaves brought it from Asia Minor (where it is seen in ancient wall-paintings). The tunic did not appear in Greece until after the Persian wars.

The original leather tunic had narrow sleeves which became wider with the appearance of woven material. Loose folds in the cloth made it almost seem as if there were two sets of sleeves.

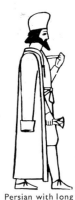

Persian with long sleeved garment, about 500 B.C.

A hole has been made in the ox hide for the wearer's head. The basic pattern for tunic, shirt, pullover and poncho

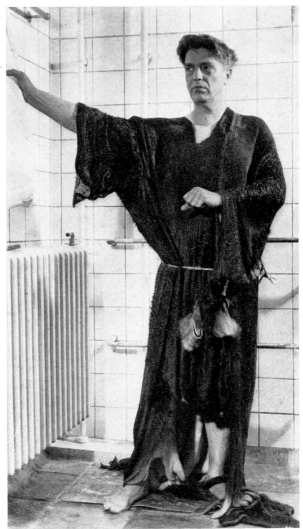

An ox hide used as a garment. The basic pattern for caftan, overcoat and jacket

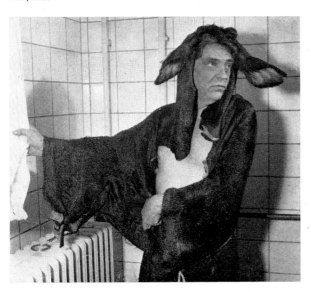

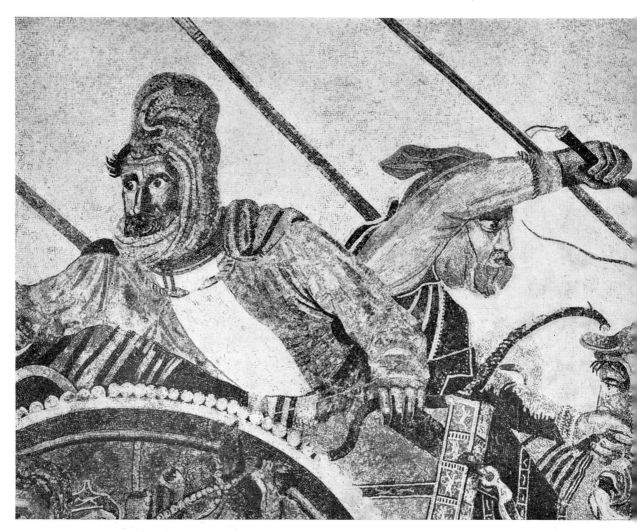

Trousers. A third type of garment was introduced into Persia (and also into China) by people from Central Asia. This garment was the forerunner of our

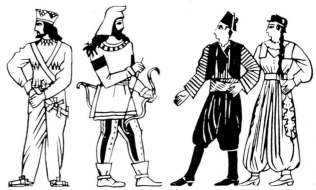

Persian with a crown and Scythian with cap, both wearing long trousers

Couple from modern Bosnia, both wearing voluminous trousers

trousers. Before 500 B.C., trousers were made of leather fitted tightly round the legs. They were attached to a belt at the top and had a flap opening at

Top The Emperor Darius during the Battle of Issus. Both he and his charioteer wear caps which come round the entire head except for the face

The balaclava a modern version of the old Persian cap

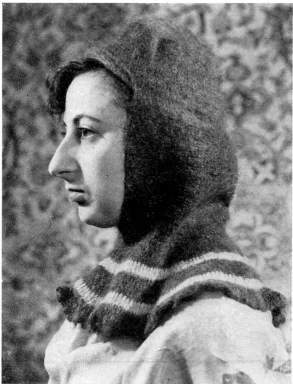

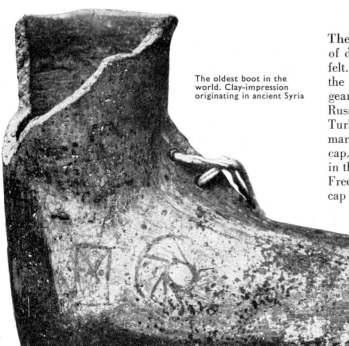

The oldest boot in the world. Clay-impression originating in ancient Syria

The Freedom Cap. Persian men wore a turban out of doors, or a tall brimless hat made of sheepskin or felt. This high-crowned hat was the progenitor of both the head-gear of high dignitaries of the Russian church and the traditional Turkish fez and has also left its mark on the old-fashioned night-cap. Its influence is again evident in the cap worn by the Goddess of Freedom, and in the soft, pointed cap which was worn in Norway

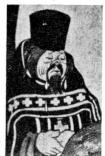

Russian church dignitary

during the German Occupation, a cap that was very similar to those in the earliest Persian reliefs. This so-called 'Phrygian' cap, with its folded-over peak, has always been both a symbol of freedom and a sign of rebellion in certain parts

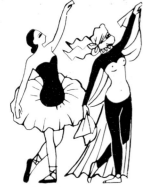

Two kinds of modesty: dancers from Europe and the Near East

the front. As woven material replaced leather, it became possible to make trouser legs wider. Subsequently it was discovered that the two trouser legs could be joined by a drawstring which passed along the top. This made still greater width possible and allowed the wearer to sit cross-legged with comfort. Although trousers have been regarded by Europeans as a male prerogative, they have always been worn by Persian women. In ancient times, Persian dress for men and women was somewhat identical; it was not until comparatively modern times that the 'ballet skirt' was added to the wide pantaloons of harem women.

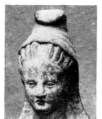 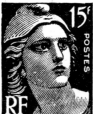 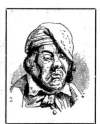

Phrygian cap on Greek Tanagra figurine, on a French postage stamp and as a night-cap

of Greece. The bent-over point reappeared in the toes of Hittite and Persian shoes, and resulted, in fact, from the way in which the shoes were made: the leather was drawn up to a point at the front and then sewn together over the in-step. In Muslim India, a pompom was mounted on the tip, a fashion which is still popular.

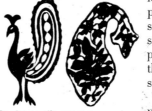

Persian textile patterns

It would appear that the people of Asia Minor introduced not only the pointed toe, but the first heel too. Heels are seen in miniatures from A.D. 1200 in the shape of a low wedge. By A.D. 1500 they were as much as an inch and a half high. Apparently heels were primarily intended to provide horsemen with a secure foothold in the stirrup.

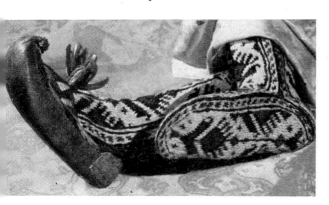

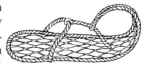

Egyptian pointed sandal from the Hittite period

The sole of the stocking has a pattern which is shown when the wearer sits

Muslim and Mongolian Influence. Persia in the seventh century, was conquered by Muslim Arabs, who introduced Islam as the principal religion. The Mongol-Chinese influence came later as a result of Mongolian invasions in the thirteenth and fourteenth centuries. From these changes developed the form of dress which can be seen in Persian miniatures of the sixteenth and seventeenth centuries and which the clothes worn in Iran today are not unlike. It consisted of a soft, white tunic, which was frequently embroidered and varied in length according to the status of the wearer, and of trousers made in cotton or wool. A cape of camel hair lined with silk or fur was worn out of doors. Women wore a short, open jacket over an embroidered tunic. The material used varied according to the rank of the wearer: coarse and hard for the poor; finely

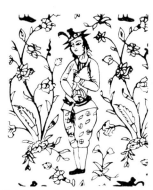

Multicoloured pattern on Persian velvet brocade from the 17th century

woven, soft and colourful for the rich, often with a patterned design. In general, people put colour and decoration as their first criterion, in contrast to Europe where cut was the main consideration.

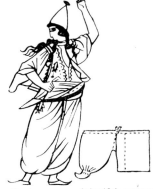

Persian woman of the 18th century

Women of the Harem. The existence of the harem was the direct result of the surplus of women in a warlike society and may thus be regarded as a practical and sensible arrangement. One gets some insight into the king's role from the Book of Esther in the Old Testament. In order to console King Artaxerxes (Ahasuerus of the Bible) for the loss of his favourite wife, whom he had disowned, hundreds of the most beautiful maidens in the land were paraded before him, for his own personal selection. (It was Artaxerxes who coined the well-known maxim, 'Man must be master in his own house'.)

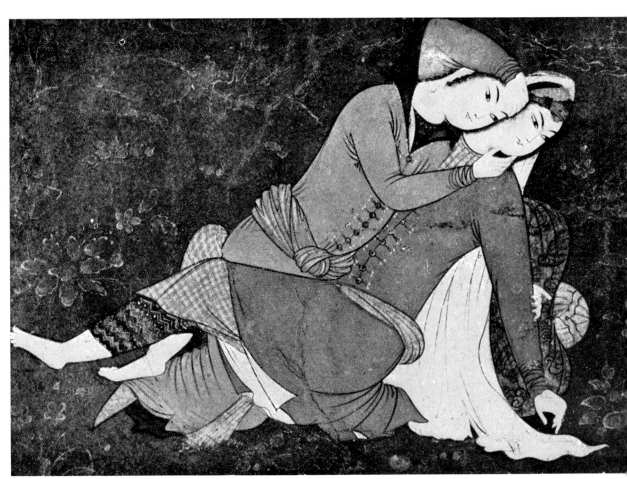

Love scene in a 17th-century miniature Opposite 17th-century Persian miniature of horsemen

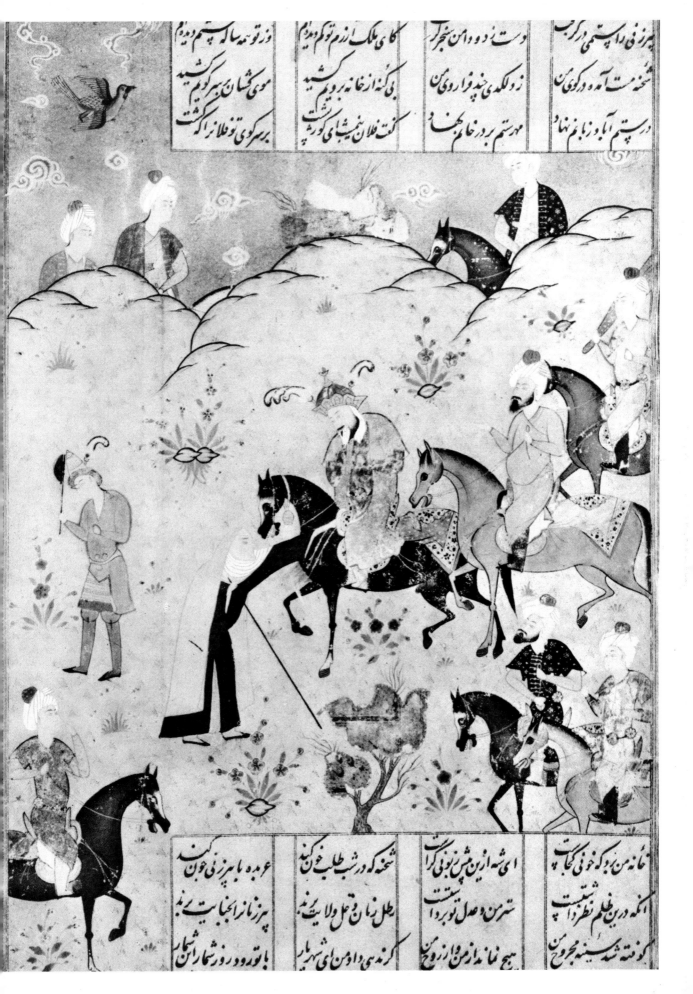

بر زفته را پستی در کرچن | دست نها د و من سنخر چن | کای ملک ازم تو کم دهیم | وز تو مد سالکه اسیم دیدم

شخنه مست آمد و در کوی من | ز دلگه ی چند قرار وی من | بی کنه از خانه بر ودیم کشید | موی کشان بر هر کوم کشید

در پستم آباد و زبانم نها د | مهرستم برد در خام بنها | کفت فلان نمیشای کورشت | بر سر کوی تو فلانرا کرشت

خانه من بر بدکه خونی کجاست | ای شه ازین مش بزوی برگزت | شخنه که در شب طلبی خون کنید | طلل زمان و عل و لایت کنید

انکه درین ظلم نظردا شت | سترمن وصل نو برد و | بر زماز انجبات رند | عربده با بزری زی خون

کوفته ر شد سینه مجروح من | هیج نما د ازمن ازن روح من | کند می واد زمن ای شهریار | با نو رود و روز سشمار این شمار

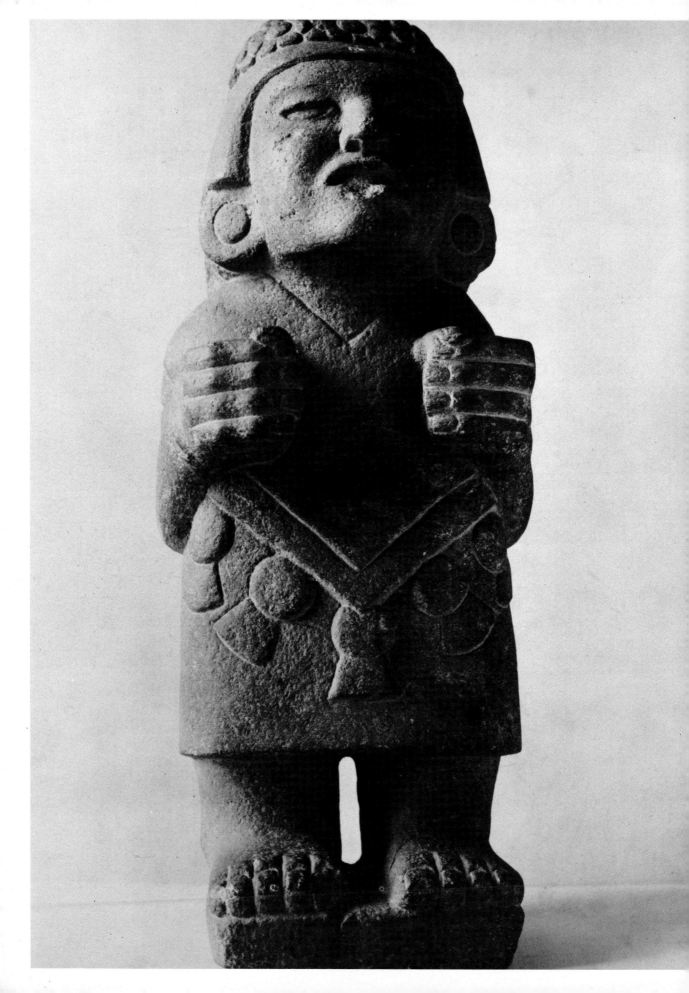

THE INDIAN FEATHER PONCHO

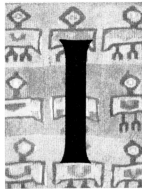

IN ANCIENT MEXICO, the Aztec priests used a human skin as part of their dress; it required no alteration other than a slit with lacing at the back. This skin was stripped from a human body and it fitted as tightly as a pull-over. Neither animal skin nor woven fabric could have provided such an exact fit without being cut and shaped.

The poncho, both in its primitive and its more developed form, was worn throughout North, South and Central America during pre-Columban times.

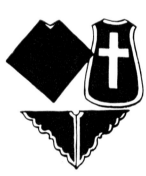
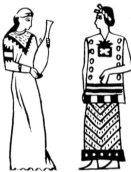

Mexican poncho, Christian chasuble, shoulder covering from Tibet, Persian tunic with poncho-like shoulder covering, ancient Aztec woman's poncho

Advanced Cultures in America. When they discovered America, the Europeans learned that the country was inhabited not only by primitive people, but also by quite highly developed civilizations, such as the Aztecs of Mexico, the Mayas of Yucatán and the Incas of Peru. We are indebted to these early Americans for the discovery of such everyday commodities as maize, potatoes, tomatoes, the cocoa plant and tobacco.

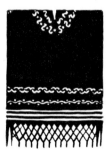

Modern Mexican poncho, the sarape

When the Europeans arrived their chief interest was gold. Cities were burned to the ground, their inhabitants massacred and their works of art destroyed. Only ruins remain of pyramids and palaces still with traces of frescoes and sculpture. Many ancient treasures have been found in Peruvian burial grounds where the dry climate and nitrogenous soil have acted as preservatives.

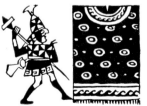

Poncho from an Inca grave

Stone Age Techniques. These were Stone Age cultures in the sense that stone was the principal material used to fashion their tools.

At the same time, the technique of working with softer materials and with metals was understood.

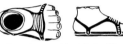

Peruvian sandal with double sole

The people subsisted on the products of their agriculture. Maize was the basic form of nourishment just as rice was in eastern Asia and grain in Europe. The land was cultivated by a scorched earth process. The

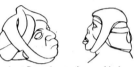

Ancient Peruvian turban and helmet

timber was cut down in a portion of the jungle and what could not be used, destroyed by fire. At the close of the rainy season, big holes were dug in the soil, which was by then fertilized with the timber ash, and maize was sown. After the harvest, the area was abandoned and allowed to revert to its natural state. A new section of forest was then prepared for the following year's harvest by burning more timber.

Ownership of land was communal; no individual rights of ownership existed. The underlying philosophy was that ownership of land, the mother of everything, could not be vested in any one person.

Aztecs, Mayas and Incas. While the Mayas could be regarded as humane, cultured and peace-loving people comparable with the Egyptians, the Aztecs, like the Assyrians, were involved in constant warfare. The Incas of Peru had also created a warlike military state. All strong, healthy males who paid taxes were required to undergo military training from an early age. In time of war, the whole male population was called up.

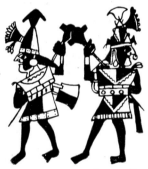

Inca warriors

A sharp distinction existed between the upper or aristocratic class and the lower classes, the former living in palaces hewn from the rock, and the latter in huts built from sun-baked mud and wood. The fruits of the harvest were divided three ways on the basis of one third to 'those who had ancestors', one third to the priests, and the remaining third to the rest of the population.

Notwithstanding the di-

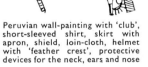

Peruvian wall-painting with 'club', short-sleeved shirt, skirt with apron, shield, loin-cloth, helmet with 'feather crest', protective devices for the neck, ears and nose

Opposite   Aztec stone figurine with poncho

7

83

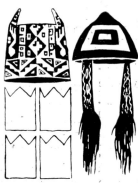

Ancient multicoloured Peruvian cap with basic pattern, and warrior's helmet made from willow around which are wound yellow and brown wool yarn; the tassels are made of wool yarn

vision into classes, the state operated on somewhat socialistic principles. A clear distinction existed in law between robbery for gain and robbery motivated by need. If a robbery or theft was caused by want of food or any other necessity of life, punishment did not fall on the thief but rather on those who had failed to keep him supplied according to his rights as a citizen. Everyone was married and the surplus of women was taken care of by the polygamist upper class. The punishment meted out to an unfaithful wife was death.

Textiles. Silk, wool and linen were unknown among both Aztecs and Mayas. Cotton was the principal material used in weaving, followed by fibre from the American century plant, known as the agave. In Peru, wool from the llama was used for spinning and weaving. Weaving was done on a narrow hand-loom, which restricted the size of the finished material to about one square yard. A number of these narrow strips were sewn together to provide the necessary width for a garment. The natural cloth was dyed in vivid but harmonious colours. Brown and reddish brown were pro-

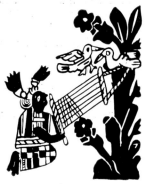

Aztec woman weaver

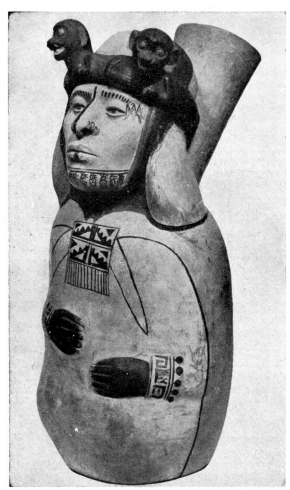

Peruvian water jug showing a fully-dressed man

duced by boiling bark and lichens. Indigo and blue-green were produced by boiling copper in urine. Boiling snails was found to result in a shade of purple. Different colours were placed beside one another to obtain sharp, elementary contrasts, a

Woven pattern, a spider

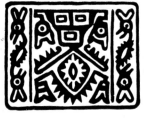

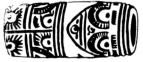

Ancient Mexican stamp dies used to print patterns on textiles

juxtaposition still much favoured by the Indians. Each colour was invested with a particular symbolic significance. Yellow was the symbol for the sun and for ripe corn, blue for aristocracy, red for blood and black for war (their weapons were made from black obsidian).

Geometrical patterns could be woven in the cloth or either painted or printed upon it.

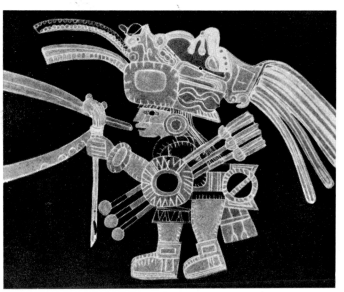

Mexican warrior with head-dress and weapons

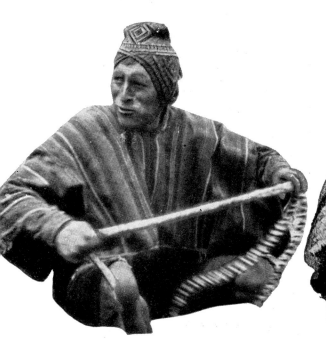

A modern Peruvian in a poncho. Compare his face with that on the water jug on the opposite page

Feather Mosaics.

Garments made up of mosaics of feathers were totally unknown in Europe. Judging by

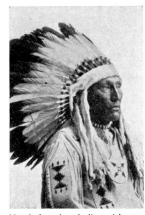

North American Indian with feather head-dress

the few remaining cloaks made in this manner, they were objects quite unsurpassed in splendour. The workers who produced these feather mosaics were held in high esteem and housed in a special quarter of the Aztec capital.

A number of these specialists could work on a single cloak together for several years. The large feathers which formed the foundation were stitched onto the fabric one by one. The smaller feathers were also positioned individually and fixed with an adhesive glue. When the design had been decided upon

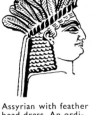

Assyrian with feather head-dress. An ordinary soldier wore one feather, the chief a crown of feathers; a device similar to officers' insignias today

and the proportions worked out, the work would proceed with infinite care; the placing of a single feather so as to produce the desired effect could occupy a whole day. Birds with exceptional plumage, such as the bird of paradise and the humming bird, were kept in captivity on farms in much the same way as the ostrich is today. The killing of such birds was punishable by death.

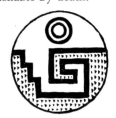

Aztec feather mosaic

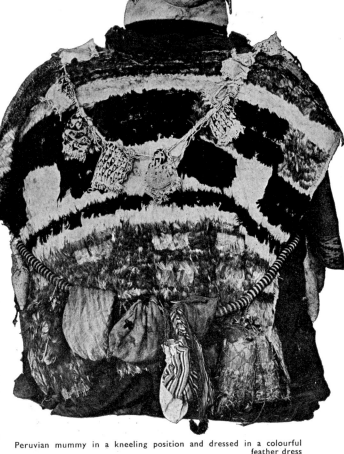

Peruvian mummy in a kneeling position and dressed in a colourful feather dress

Tall Hats and Ear-rings.

Judging by ancient pictures, the headgear was the outstanding feature of ceremonial dress. It consisted of coverings in the shape of animal heads inlaid with metal and precious stones and was crowned with feather decorations of huge proportions. Articles of jewellery in rock crystal and jade have been found, exquisitely worked with stone tools for the adornment of ears, nose and lips. The artistry of the Aztecs has never been exceeded by any other race.

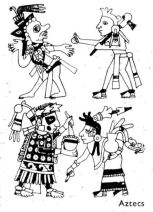

Aztecs

Albrecht Dürer after seeing a collection of this jewellery in Antwerp in 1521, wrote in his diary,

'I have never in my whole life seen anything which has gladdened my heart more than these objects. I have seen these beautifully artistic specimens and I have marvelled at the subtlety and ingenuity of these people of foreign parts. Words cannot express my feelings.'

The Poncho. Maya and Aztec men were dressed in a form of a loin-cloth which hung free front and back, and a poncho, or cape, secured round the neck and falling loosely to knee-level. This poncho was made from the same colourful square used by Mexicans today. Women wore a long sleeveless smock cut on the lines of the poncho, and with it one or more skirts.

The Incas in the coastal regions wore shirts with sleeves, while in the mountain regions sleeveless shirts were to be found. By custom, a member of the upper classes was permitted to wear a set of clothes only once, after which it had to be discarded. A large religious order, the 'Daughters of the Sun', had been assigned the task of making all the clothes worn by the upper classes. The following description of an Inca priest's robing is by a Spanish Conquistador.

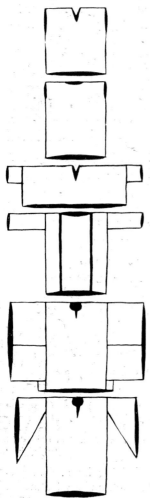

Mexican poncho, Roman tunic, Inca poncho, shirt from Afghanistan, Egyptian woman's tunic, garment from Palestine

'A cloak of red feathers decorated with patterns made from smaller feathers in many colours. A fringe of large feathers mounted on cotton, hanging at the bottom, split and brushing the ground. A tall feather headdress, and a carved wooden sceptre in the hand, to which is attached a bunch of tails from the rattle-snake.'

Strength and Dignity. The men who wore these glistening, colourful garments were of Mongolian extraction. The men were square and heavily built and the women were, by our standards, short and fat. Their yellowish-brown skin was smooth, and stretched so tightly over layers of fat that the outline of muscle and sinew was obscured. Their bodies were springy and resilient and their muscles were well-developed, in contrast to the civilized white races whose muscles

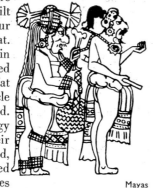

Mayas

Indian girl with poncho. Painting by Diego Rivera

have degenerated through lack of exercise and too much sitting. The Indian used only one single piece of furniture — a plaited mat. This served him as chair, table and bed.

In contrast to the abominable slander of the Spaniards, a type of man emerges not unlike the Mexican peasant of present times. The children had the dreamy eyes which we see today in the work of Diego

Ancient Mexican pattern

Rivera. And there was the same old-fashioned dignity and self-confidence, the same sense of colour, design and rhythm which exists among Mexican Indians today.

Human Sacrifice and Flowers. It is difficult to understand the Aztec philosophy and to reconcile ourselves to their cult of human sacrifice. We should remember, however, that more lives were taken in the short period during which Christianity was introduced by the Spaniards, than in all the centuries of human sacrifice.

To understand the strange and colourful dress of the Aztec Indians, we must take into account the sombre background of an existence dominated by force and cruelty. A vivid contrast emerges when we compare the background and culture of the Aztecs

86

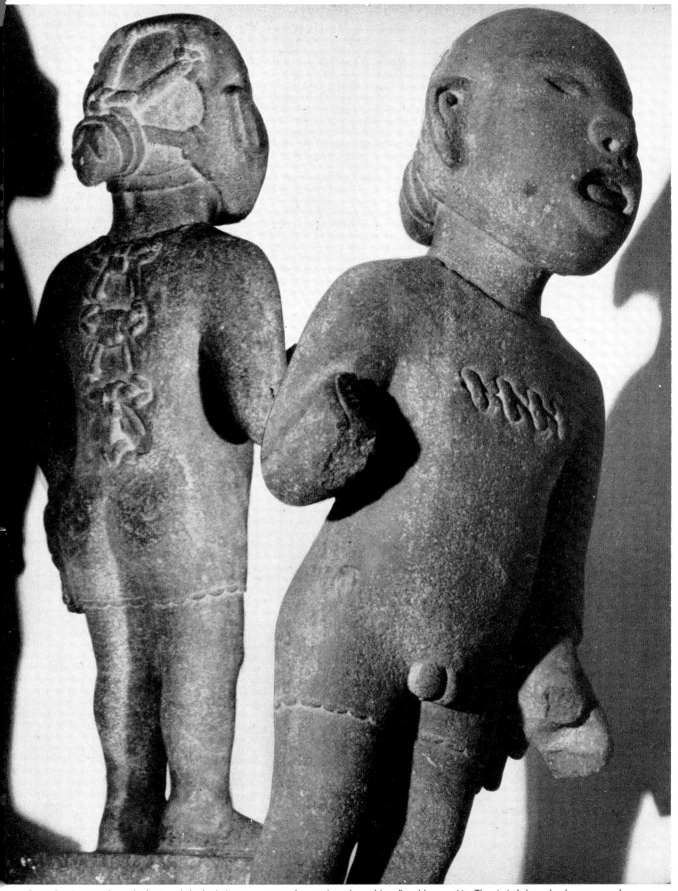

Stone figurine seen from the front and the back. It represents an Aztec priest, dressed in a flayed human skin. The victim's heart has been removed through the opening on the chest which is then sewed together. The legs have been cut off and the facial skin serves as a mask

with their counterparts in China. On the one hand, we can visualize the sun blazing down on the pyramids, priests clad in grotesque garments with masks, feath-

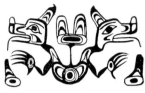

Textile pattern popular among Indians of the North-west of the American sub-continent

ers and fluttering snake-tails enacting rituals involving human sacrifice. On the other hand, we have the cool atmosphere of China. Here, people clad in simple robes of silk worship their ancestors in quiet, restrained ceremonies at the foot of their private altars. Tea is sipped and the room is wreathed in the subtle fragrance of incense.

Flowers played a great part in all Aztec ceremonies. Even the priests would plait flowers into their unkempt and evil-smelling hair, matted with the blood of human sacrifices which had never to be removed.

Spanish Central America. The Central America which emerged as a result of the Spanish Conquest

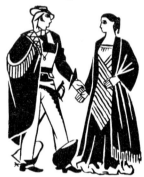

was dominated by a different spirit, a spirit both of good and evil. In place of the old social system, where freedom had, to some extent, prevailed, we find subjection to the tyranny of Spanish land-owners. The people were deprived of their land and treated as beasts of burden. The cult of hu-

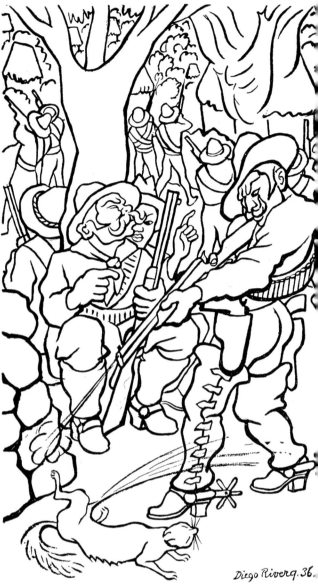

Spanish soldiers taking Indians captive. Drawing by Diego Rivera

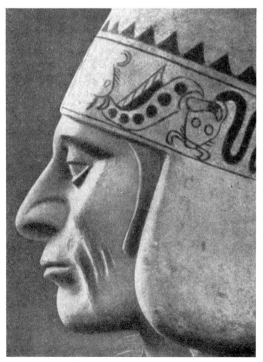

Profile of a Peruvian clay jug

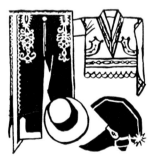

Pieces of Spanish Mexican apparel

man sacrifice did not cease entirely but was practised with a difference. The victims were no longer decked with flowers and regarded as demigods until such time as they were offered up in sacrifice. Instead, massacres were carried out in rebel villages, the people shot and their homes burned down.

The peon sandal with a double thong between the toes was worn about this time by native slaves only. Their masters adopted high-heeled riding boots with spurs.

Modern Mexican sombrero

THE MONGOLIAN SILK KIMONO

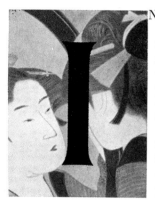

IN EARLY TIMES throughout eastern Asia, a garment designed as a cape that hung from the shoulders was the form of dress most prevalent. This later formed the basis of all subsequent fashions. Indeed, examples of this form of dress have been found all over the world; some of the earliest examples, dating from the Bronze Age have been discovered in graves in Denmark. In countries between the Caspian and the Pacific, no dress or undergarment exists which has to go on over the head. The form of dress worn in Mongolia shows that the culture of these people has been more widely shared by all classes than have the cultures of western countries. Social classes among the Mongolian peoples were divided by strict traditional etiquette, but from an aesthetic viewpoint all were similar, whether high or low, rich or poor.

In the main, the plain style of dress is the same for both sexes and for all social classes. It is worn by old and young, in winter and in summer. The garment — a bit like a surgeon's dress to look at — is easy to work in despite a pleasantly loose cut.

A contemporary Chinese author, who has lived in both Europe and America, asks,

'Is it really necessary for a person to give any reason for objecting to being encased in tight collars, waistcoats, belts, braces and suspenders, when at home he is accustomed to wearing loosely cut garments?'

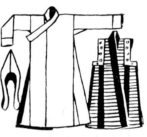

Caftans from Syria, North Africa, Syria, China, Iran and Turkey

far back as 2000 B.C., a civilization based on agriculture and horticulture had developed, which made extensive use of artificial irrigation. These large cultivated regions received shelter and protection from mountains on the north, south and west, and from the sea on the east. The nomad tribes from time to time invaded the area and made their own rulers emperors. Their fashions certainly had an influence on the upper classes, but numerically, however, the nomads were few and they had no effect on social or economic conditions.

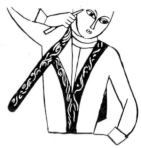

Shawl collar from South China

It was understandably in these densely populated areas, at that time the most densely populated in the world, that a degree of privacy came to be regarded as desirable and, indeed, as the basic right of an individual. It became necessary to draw a line in one's association with the rest of the world. We see indications of this feeling in the Chinese manner of shaking hands — never touching each others hands — when welcoming or saying goodbye to a guest. We see it again in the inscrutable smile of the oriental, the flicker of the wrinkled face and half-closed eyes, in such contrast to the open-faced, toothy grin of the American and European.

Tibetan hood, caftan and waistcoat

Lin Yu Tang has written that Western dress aims to reveal the contour of the human body, while Chinese dress seeks to conceal. Why should we, he says, tell the world if our waist measurement is very large. If we are above normal, surely this should be regarded as our own personal business.

The simple style of dress from ancient China, folding from left to right and fastened only by a belt at the waist, is still to be seen in the Japanese kimono. This came from China in about A.D. 700 and the same style in Korea derives from the time of the Ming dynasty, from A.D. 1350 to 1650.

Men wore an ankle-length caftan over jacket and trousers; women wore a skirt in addition to the usual jacket and trousers.

Both caftan and jacket were fitted with a draped collar, and the opening of each held together by a cord on the right side. During the last few years this style has been introduced in European dress.

China. The main centres of ancient culture were situated in the large river valleys of China where, as

Silk.

Silk is the foundation of all clothing in East Asia; as soft, smooth and expressive as the golden skin of the Mongolians themselves. For thousands of years, natural silk, with its beautiful and subdued butterfly colourings, has been used by these people for everyday dress. Many of the traits which we regard as characteristically 'Chinese' have originated in the relationship between the silk-worm and the breeders of this little creature.

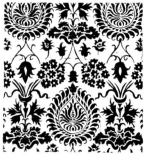
Chinese pattern with lotus flowers

Breeding silk-worms calls for the highest degree of hygiene, which therefore becomes a practical necessity for the Chinese peasant and his family. In films the Chinese pad around in felt slippers. This custom springs from the silk-worm larva's antipathy to noise.

In Japan the people go barefoot or in stockinged feet inside the house. The thick carpets on which they walk by day they sleep on at night.

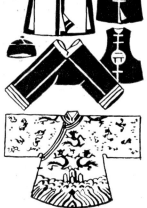
Caftans opening on a slant and in the centre; waistcoats, caps and trousers

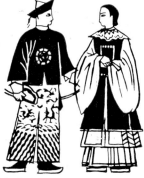
Mandarin couple; he wears felt slippers and she has baggy sleeves to her dress

Discretion in Dress.

Buttons, hooks and pins are practically unused in Japan, whether for practical or decorative purposes, and the kimono is worn unfastened. Buttons and pins are sometimes used in China, but more often laces or ribbons are employed.

The various layers of clothing are worn in such a manner that they open outwards. The outer garments have larger openings at the neck and

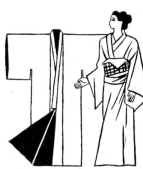
Japanese kimono

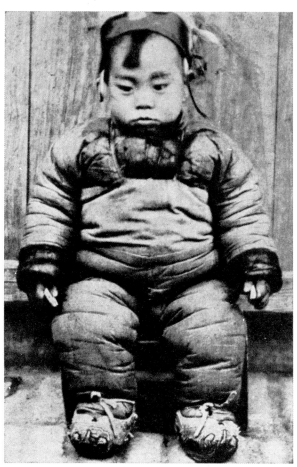
Chinese child in wadded clothing

chest, and shorter sleeves, to provide the greatest possible freedom of movement.

Cottonwool (wadding) is placed inside the material for additional warmth in winter; this is removed in spring when the weather gets warmer. During very cold winters, as many as thirteen or fourteen kimonos are worn, one on top of the other. In this way, the Chinese in Northern Siberia can be as warm and comfortable as natives in their furs.

Sleeves are frequently made long enough to cover the hands. Having one's hands covered is regarded as friendly and well-mannered in China, in contrast to our part of the world where it is considered unmannerly to keep one's hands in one's pock-

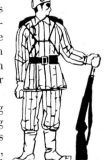
Modern Chinese soldier in wadded uniform

ets. The wide sleeve can serve the same purpose as a handbag.

In Japan, small articles are suspended from the belt by a thong terminating in a small carved knob known as the netsuke, often a work of art in itself.

Golden Lilies.

An unusual chapter in the history of Chinese fashion lies in the bold attempt to change the course of nature by altering the shape of women's feet

Opposite Tang dynasty figure of a dancer, A.D. 600–900

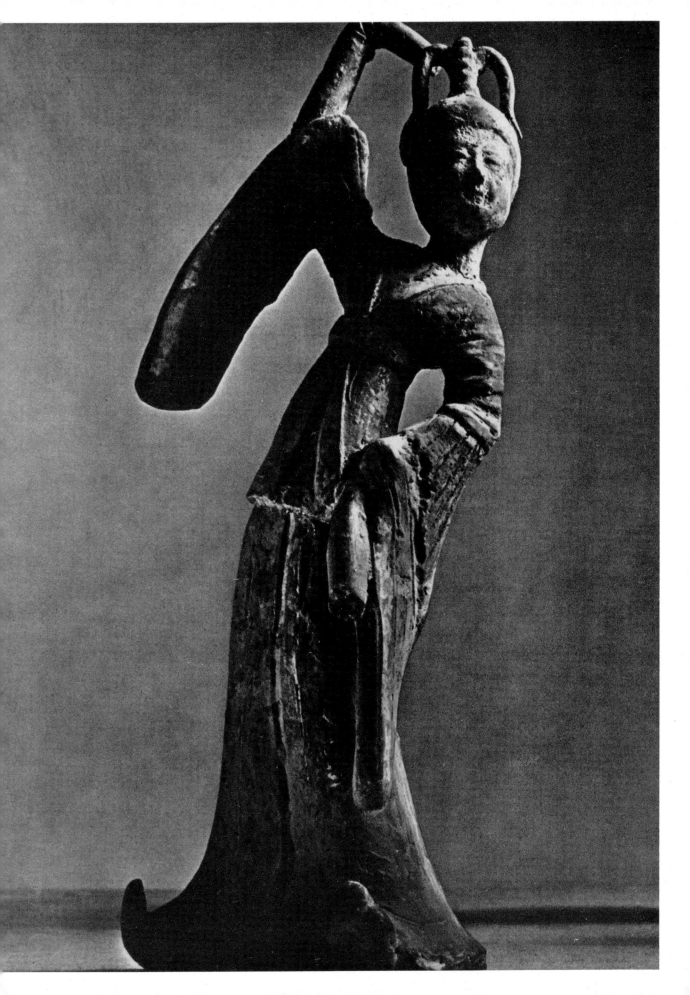

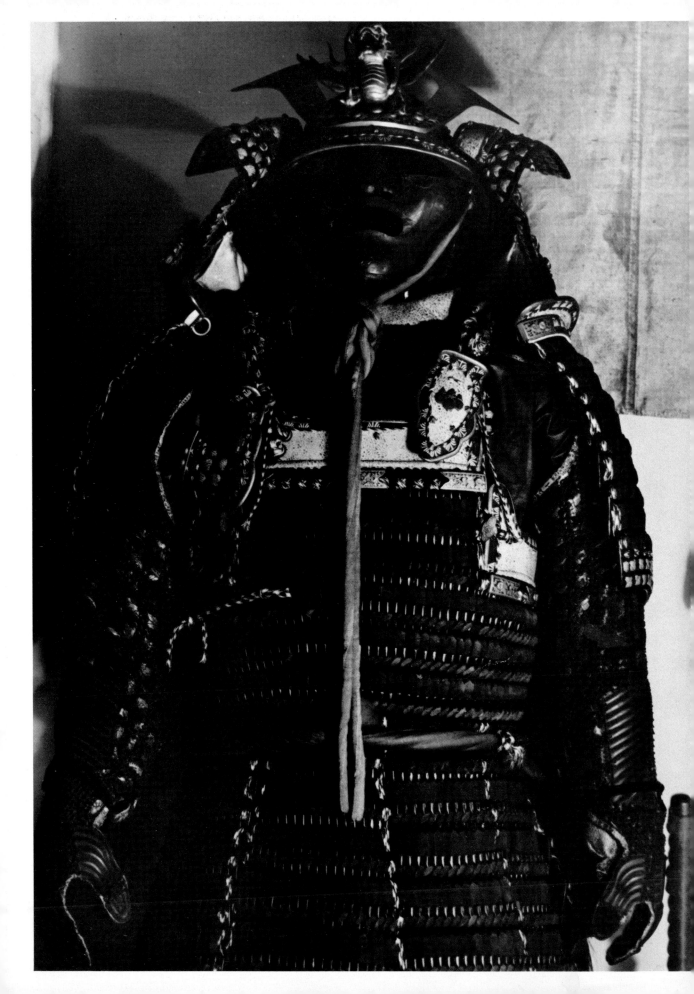

(known as 'golden lilies'). The purpose was to provide visual evidence of inability to work and consequently of the ability of the husband to provide all necessary money. The size of her foot determined the commercial value of a woman. This is manifest in the custom of exhibiting the shoes of the bride-to-be during the marriage negotiations in order to establish the price. Deformation also provided a guarantee of matrimonial fidelity, in that the wife's perambulations were restricted to a minimum. It is interesting that only women's feet were subject to malformation. The custom of 'golden lilies' disappeared with the Revolution and the overthrow of the Mandarin system. The social implications of this practice are even more marked when we realize that, in the main, the Far Eastern foot has retained its natural shape and suppleness. Artisans use their feet as an extra pair of hands; each toe can move independently of the others. During the last war,

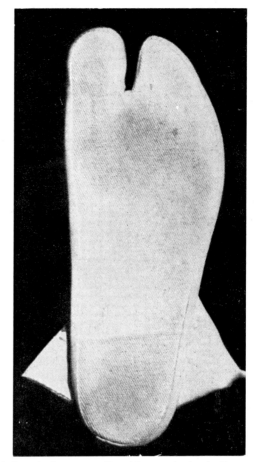
Everyday Japanese stocking with separation for the big toe

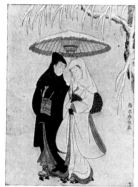
Japanese women in a snowstorm

the Japanese used their feet in climbing and scaled obstacles which defeated the Europeans. The blue and white socks used in Japan are made with a separate compartment for the big toe which prevents the toes from being squeezed together. The flat sandal is kept on by only two thongs, one between the big toe and next toe, and the other passing over the front of the feet. Such a sandal can be shaken off with a single movement when entering the house, where the carpet serves as both sitting place

and bed. Clogs made of thick blocks of wood take the place of low sandals when the weather is wet.

Japanese clogs

Red Happiness — White Sorrow. In the same way that, in the East, material is more important than cut, colour is more important than material itself. The meanest dress can be made more attractive by a few brightly coloured borders.

The magnificent decorations and colours originating in ancient times are no mere casual adornment but carry symbolic meanings, ranging from red for marriage to white for mourning. The blue of night, the scarlet of the sun, the pallor of the moon, are more than just colours. They carry with them a legendary and symbolic significance, that refers to history, religion and politics.

The privilege of wearing golden robes was reserved for members of the Imperial family. The Imperial kimono, as used on ceremonial occasions, was invested with a philosophical significance whereby the circle repre-

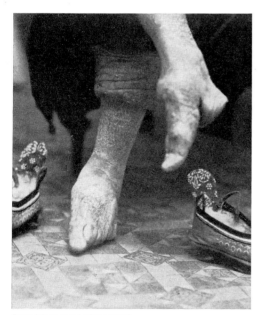
Bound feet, the 'golden lilies'

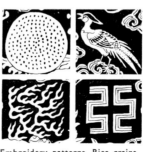
Embroidery patterns. Rice grains, golden pheasant, fire, two bows

Opposite Armour of a Japanese samurai

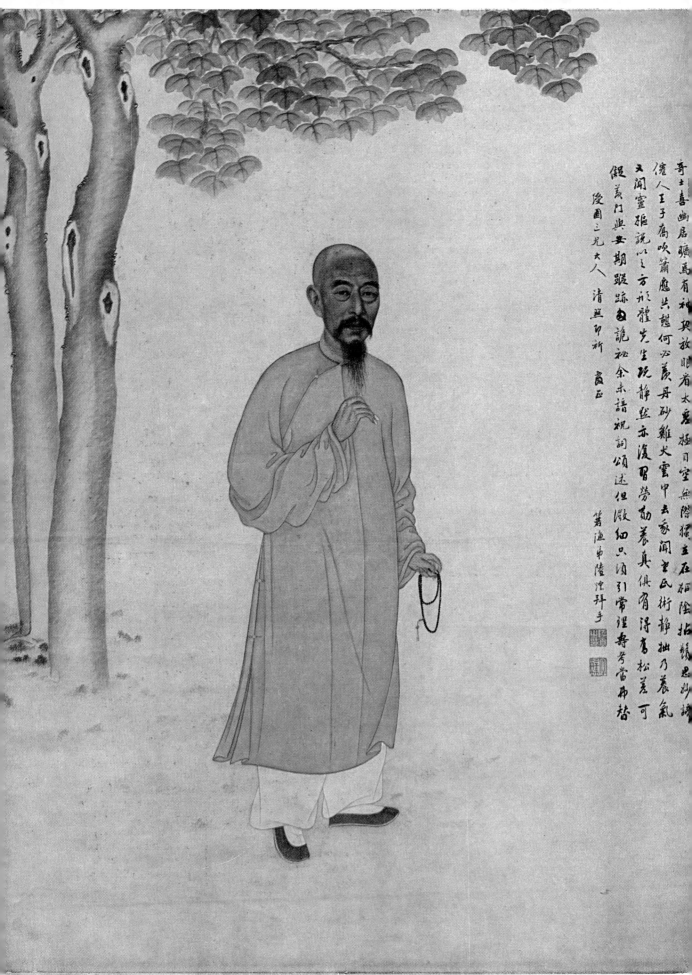

sented the completness and perfection of the Universe and the square betokened the limitations of worldly existence. Symbols existed for sun, moon and stars, as well as for fire, dragons, pheasants, temple vases, axes, water-cress, rice. The sun symbolized active strength while the moon was an emblem of passivity.

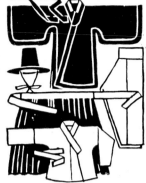

Embroidered garments are considered effeminate in European countries; not so in ancient China. The servant of the state had a picture embroidered on his gown. The student was indicated by a salmon swimming through a pool

Korean outfit. Caftan, shawl collar, cap, skirt, trousers and short caftan

towards a waterfall. After the first examination was passed, the salmon was replaced by a dragon. A second class civil servant had a golden pheasant on his gown, one of the fourth class had a wild goose. An embroidered lion denoted second class rank in the army, a tiger denoted fourth class. Proficiency badges in the scouting movement today follow much the same pattern.

The Japanese kimono bore the largest pictures, such as enormous dragons and large landscape embroideries. The latter made great use of symbols, such as the magnolia tree for spring, the lotus flower for summer, the chrysanthemum for autumn and the blossom of the prunus tree for winter. Paintings by eminent artists were also reproduced in their original size in finely executed embroideries.

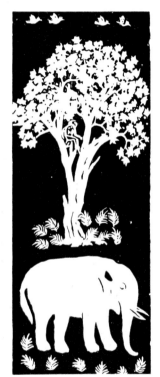

Chinese textile pattern

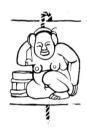

Knob of Japanese belt, netsuke, made of ivory

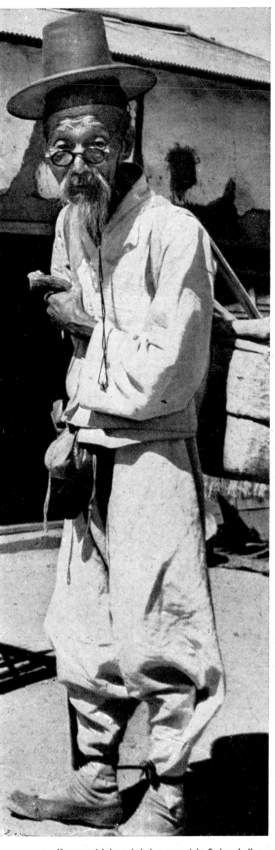

Opposite   Chinese caftan. Painting on silk

Korean with horsehair hat over tight-fitting skull-cap

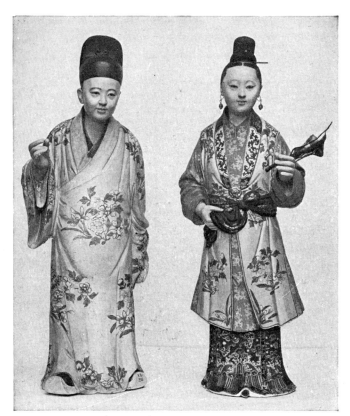

Chinese couple. Porcelain figures from the 18th century

'The unselfish wife permits her husband to take a concubine without feeling insulted. A man of principle will never sleep with another woman without permission from his wife and no true lady would ever deny him such permission.'

On the other hand should a husband catch his wife in the act of adultery, he had the right to kill her. Adultery by the husband was not regarded as an offence by law. If a wife remained childless she was liable to be divorced, as she also was if she was disobedient to her mother-in-law or even if she talked too much.

Technique of Love-Making. In Japan, it was customary to send girls to brothels at the age of fourteen. Here they were educated in the trade and when they had saved enough money they would return to their villages to get married and become respected wives and mothers.

Poetry and erotic art formed part of life in the brothels, and prostitution was regarded as a perfectly respectable calling. Love and marriage were not connected in the accepted sense, but the

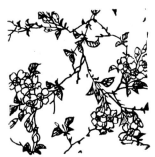

Japanese printed textile pattern

marriage relationship had been developed with an admirable regard for its ethical aspect, its elegance and its dignified grace.

Family Life It has been said that a woman in ancient Chinese society was governed by three commandments: obedience, obedience and obedience. When a child, she had to obey her parents, when a wife, her husband, and when an old woman, her son. Even in well-to-do families, sons and daughters were brought up together, but the sons always took precedence over the daughters in every respect. Father and son sat together at table

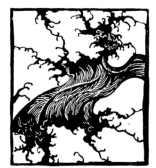

Japanese printed textile pattern

waited upon by wife and daughter. Brother addressed sister by name but was addressed by her as 'Mister Brother'. Monogamy was normal, even in the wealthy classes, but the husband was at liberty to take one or more concubines should he so desire.

We gain an impression of the marriage relationship from a contemporary author, Ku Hu Ming,

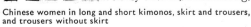

Chinese women in long and short kimonos, skirt and trousers, and trousers without skirt

Japanese woodcut with descriptions of a court lady's many charms

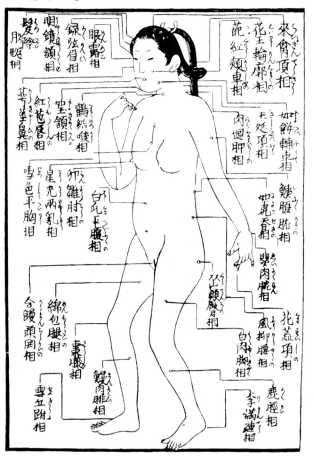

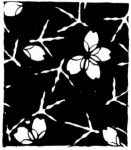
Printed textile pattern by Hokusai

The Japanese girl was presented with *The Bridal Book* by her fiancé before their marriage. This provided her with full details of what she would be required to do, supplemented by vivid pictures in colour, and formed a manual of procedure and etiquette not lacking in humour.

The general attitude toward nudity is somewhat contrary to European feeling. Up to the present day, men and women have bathed together; on the other hand, pictures of naked people are regarded as indecent. When the first Jesuits introduced pictures of the Virgin Mary and the Saints, even these were considered pornographic because the arms and feet were exposed.

The Flat, Snow-white Bosom. Sexual characteristics are less marked in the Mongolian body than in the European. The sparse growth of hair we find on the men would be considered effeminate by European standards, and the slender hips and flat posteriors of the women would be considered boyish. Women's breasts, while rounded, are not very developed and are not regarded with much interest. It is characteristic of the patriarchal attitude of China and Japan that poems will speak of womanly beauty in great detail but hardly mention the breast at all. A well-developed bust might perhaps be excused, but broad hips and a protruding bottom would be regarded as positively indecent. Consequently, the Japanese woman wraps her middle tightly with a broad silk scarf which is tied in a large bow.

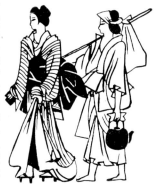
Japanese women's attire

The Mongolian head has always occupied a larger proportion of the body than the European head, and the only way to balance it is by straight hanging dresses. This applies particularly to the Japanese with their artistic and ample style of hair arrangement. The pigtails of the Mandarin in the China of the Manchus were regarded as a sign of rank, as were the long finger nails protected by silver casings. This custom is the

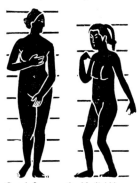
Greek figure – the Medici Venus – whose head is $1/_8$ of its height, and a Japanese woman whose head is $1/_6$ of her height

male counterpart of the 'golden lilies' feet of the women, and provided visual evidence that the wearer had no need to engage in manual work.

Walking and Sitting. Walking with out-turned feet was regarded as well-bred in Europe until a few generations ago. In the East, this custom is reversed and the feet turn slightly inwards. The latter is really more natural and produces the gliding movement of a body in motion which enhances the elegant effect of the kimono.

In Japan, people sit on the floor with one knee bent upwards and the other touching the floor, with the weight resting on the sole of one foot. This sitting posture is taught from childhood and results in the beautifully developed shoulders so much admired in Japanese women. The absence of any support for the back produces strong muscles in the shoulders and neck. The ankles grow sturdy through this position, particularly in the case of the women, who have more leisure for sitting than the men. This becomes such an essential characteristic in the conception of physical beauty that one is inclined to regard the Eastern sitting position as a refined form of bodily exercise purposely designed to obtain such a result. It is certainly

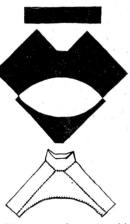
Chinese woman's trousers with the basic pattern

undeniable that a large head would not go well with spindly legs and ankles; there is no doubt that the slender ankle, regarded as normal and desirable in Europe, has developed through the habit of wearing high heels and the consequent alteration of the leg muscles.

The low sitting position is normal in many Indian and African Negro tribes. The peasants of Jutland adopt a squatting position, resting the back on the heels of their clogs. The Chinese also like a low sitting position, most frequently using a small stool.

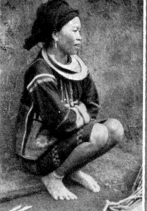
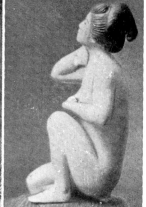
Chinese and Japanese sitting positions

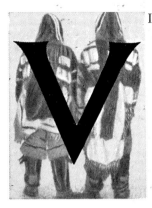

VISUALLY recognizable characteristics link the inhabitants of the north — the Eskimos of North America and Greenland and the Arctic tribes of Soviet Russia — with the Mongolians; they have the same narrow hips and broad faces. The Eskimo has an enormous capacity for chewing, and it is natural to relate this characteristic to the preparation of their hides, in which mastication plays an essential part.

Living, as they do, in a frigid temperature for most of the year, body heat must be conserved. This is achieved in two ways: by a diet having a high fat content and by covering the body with hides. These hides are cut to shape and stitched together. Here, in a rudimentary form, begins the art of tailoring, where the important thing is not the material but the cutter's knife or shears and the dressmaker's needle. Some knowledge of the way these primitive

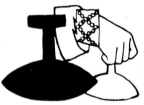

The Greenlander's knife resembles the saddler's knife of today

people tackle their skins is necessary before we can understand the processes they use. It may be the Berber in the Sahara Desert who repairs his sandals every evening without the help of either thread or tacks. Or it may be the Lapp in northern Finland and Scandinavia who turns and pummels a piece of hide for days on end to make himself a pair of shoes. Before he begins work on them at all he speculates and experiments to work out which method would be best, and when one shoe has been made he starts all over again to discover the basis for the second shoe. The art displayed by Eskimo women in working hides puts all other forms of handicraft to shame.

The Life of the Hunter. The Eskimos, before being influenced by Western civilization, lived in small tribes. They moved about from region to region depending on the prospects of good hunting and fishing. The dog has always been their only domestic

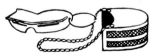

Eskimo snow glasses made of bone

animal and is used for pulling the sledge, their sole means of land transport. The kayak was used on the

water and also another larger type of boat. During the winters of continual darkness they lived in earth and sod huts or in domed huts made of snow. Heat and light were provided by means of oil-burning lamps. In the summer they moved into tents made of hide. Hunting and fishing, their means of livelihood, were pursued on a cooperative basis and governed by traditional rules. Food obtained was shared among all members of the tribe in the settlement. They worked well together and life was peaceful. Family feuds were not unknown, but even so the general atmosphere was amicable. In Greenland and Alaska, these violent feuds were settled by verbal exchanges, each side singing malicious and insulting songs addressed at the other.

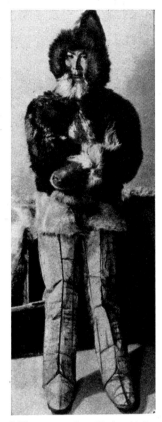

Eskimo woman from Thule with fur parka and short pants of blue fox fur and long sealskin boots

Obedience was (and still is) required of the woman, and a temporary exchange of wives between husbands could be transacted without formality. Marriages were arranged by the parents of either side and girls were given in marriage at a very early age.

Decorations and Patterns. Eskimo men fashion their own hunting weapons which they frequently decorate with pictures of the chase. They carve wooden or bone handles with crude but lifelike human and animal figures. The women cut and stitch their clothes to which they attach small colourful geometrical designs. Coloured square patches of hide are sewn on. Holes are made in the hide and laced with leather thongs, and fine embroidery is executed in reindeer hair.

The love of elaborate

Design embroidered on a kamik, or boot, from northern Greenland

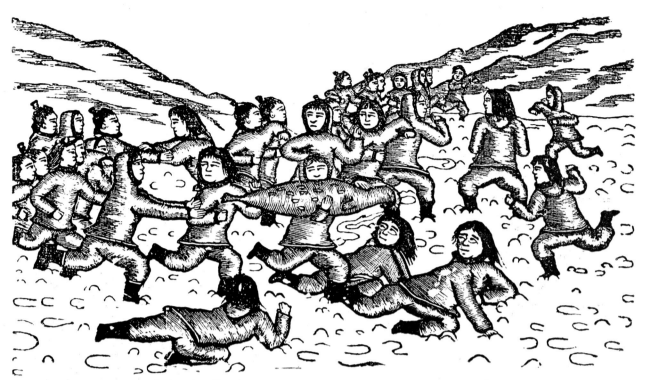

Greenlanders at play. Woodcut by Aron from Kangek

decoration is characteristic of the Eskimo. A normally utilitarian garment can be embellished with the most elaborate and colourful decoration. Coloured beads were always being used to great effect. They sew them close together in traditional patterns making wide borders that cover the shoulders and chest. Thus we find the Egyptian fashion of the collar repeated among the Eskimos.

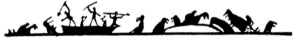

Eskimo bone-carving from Alaska

Preparation of Hides. Sealskin can be used to make clothes but it tends to lack pliancy and does not provide much warmth. The hide of the blue fox is better in these respects, but reindeer skin is the most satisfactory. The intestines of seal and bear provide an excellent waterproof material, rather like plastic in appearance, but even tougher. Skin taken from birds is much softer and is suitable for undergarments. The skin of the hare provides a fairly satisfactory material for stockings, but otter skin is even better.

The general preparation of hides and skins is the responsibility of the women, even though the men

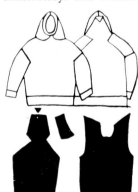

Eskimo sealskin blouse from front and back, with pattern below

may occasionally lend a hand. It is the women also who cut and stitch the materials with a skill almost beyond description. The pieces are sewn together edge to edge with a horizontal stitch. A particular kind of stitch is used for the finer material taken from the intestine, and to produce waterproof seams the needle is actually passed through half the thickness of the skin.

When at work, the women sit on the ground with their legs outstretched and the material spread over their laps. A similar sitting position is adopted by the men on the sledge or in the kayak.

Clothing. Even to this day, dress for Eskimo men and women is very similar. It consists of a shirt, hooded blouse, trousers, stockings and boots. The blouse is similar in shape to the shirt but has the covering to pull over the head.

The woman wears a flap hanging down front and back which looks like shirt-tails. This is also worn by the man in certain tribes. The male blouse is shorter, perhaps because the kayak's opening is so narrow. Gussets are inserted at the armholes to provide freedom

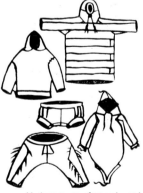

Various types of anoraks and trousers worn by Eskimos

of movement, and the hood is securely tucked inside the neck of the blouse. The borders of the hood and

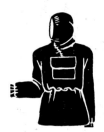

Modern European parka (anorak). Both the name and the pattern, but not the pocket, originate in Greenland

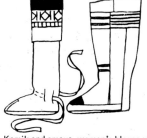

Kamik and amaut, woman's blouse with bag for carrying a baby

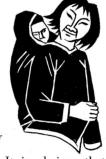

sleeves are trimmed with wolf or dog fur to give protection against the wind and extra strength.

The trousers worn by both men and women cover the legs only as far down as the knee, again for freedom of movement. The close fit emphasizes the slender hips and flat posteriors of these people.

Indoors, both sexes used to wear only a pair of pants and were otherwise naked; skirts are not known.

other to enable him to see out. It is obvious that Eskimo dress is a kind of armour, even though it is designed for protection against no human foe.

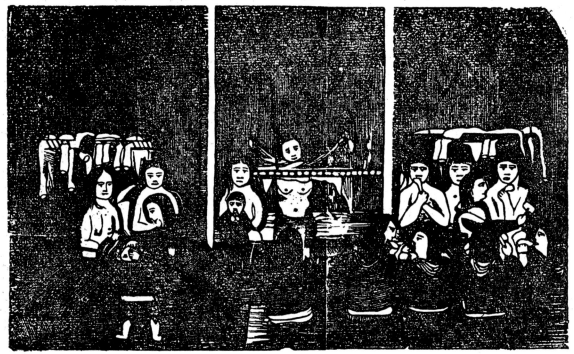

Greenlandic hut and the inhabitants. Woodcut by Aron from Kangek

Kamiks, or boots, are cut in such a manner that they can be worn on either foot. A double sole is fitted and between the two soles a layer of dried grass can be inserted.

Combinations. Children frequently wear trousers and stockings made in one piece. Alternatively, they may wear a one-piece garment with an opening at the back or with a wide opening at the top to get into.

The hunter's all-in-one outfit in Greenland comprises hood, shirt with sleeves, trousers, boots and gloves, all together. This combination garment has two openings only, one through which the wearer gets in and out and an-

In contrast to the tough, dry leather which protects the warrior of southern climes, the Eskimo is enclosed in soft pliable skin, which seems to retain some of its old animal warmth. It is a fitting frame for their friendly natures.

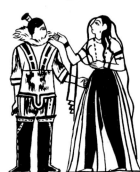

Eskimo and Indian women in trousers

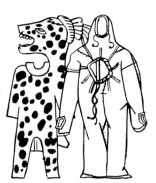

One-piece suits: Aztec priest's attire made from jaguar skin and Greenlandic hunter's outfit

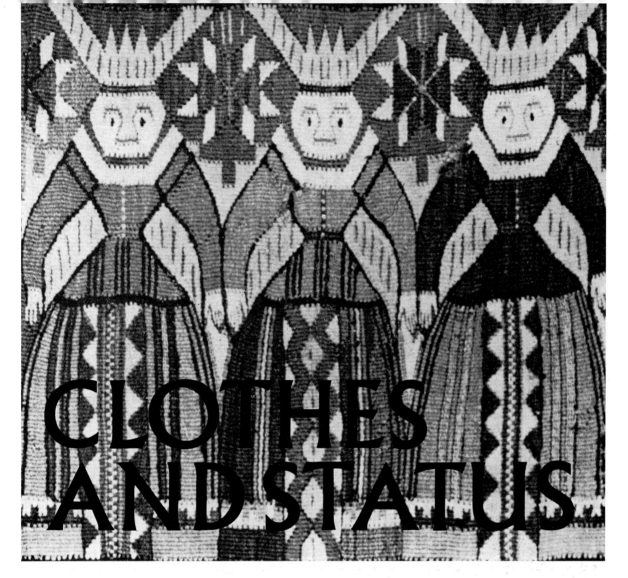

HISTORICAL COSTUMES

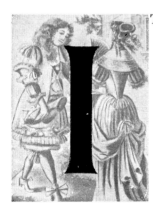T IS ONLY in comparative-
ly recent times that new
materials have been in-
troduced, nor has the
climate of Europe changed
greatly over the centuries.
During the period be-
tween the Great Migra-
tions and the French Rev-
olution the practical re-
quirements of clothing
underwent little change.
Change was taking place,
however, in and between
the different levels of society, bringing with it a corresponding change in ideas and calling for new forms
of expression in art as well as in dress. As the tempo
of social life quickened, so the spirit of fashion followed suit.

Up till now, our description of development may be

likened to a series of static magic lantern slides. But
from now on, it should be visualized as a cinematogra-
phic film in which pieces of clothing move about in
changing dimensions and perspectives, sometimes con-
flicting with one another, at other times joining together in harmony. During the last thousand years or
so, the style of European fashion has become gradually
more and more international in character.

National costume is a comparatively modern phenomenon, dating from the nineteenth century. History
relates that the first fashion doll was sent to the queen
of Richard II of England in the year 1391 to show her
the latest designs from France. In Rococo times, dolls
were dispatched all over Europe every month. In 1716,
a certain Louise Rosset was granted a monopoly in
staging exhibitions of fashion dolls in Copenhagen.
When fashion magazines started, towards the end of
the eighteenth century, style became syncronized over
the whole of Europe.

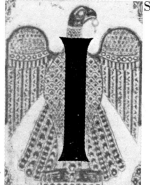

ISTANBUL, then called Byzantium and later still Constantinople — was made Nova Roma or second capital of the Roman Empire by Constantine the Great in the year A.D. 330. One hundred and fifty years later, when the western part of the Roman Empire was overrun by Germanic invaders, Byzantium became the centre of the civilized world and remained so for a thousand years. Greek tradition was developed under strong Asiatic influence, with Christianity as the State religion. Christ was regarded as the favourite god of Constantine, who was baptized on his deathbed and was buried with symbolic graves of the twelve apostles surrounding his tomb.

In Byzantium, Christianity was used as a political weapon in the quest for imperial power. The Russian Nestor Chronicle describes the impression the religious ceremony in the Church of Santa Sophia made on envoys of the Tsar, who were then engaged on a foreign tour; on returning, they gave such enthusiastic reports that Russia joined the Eastern Church. Byzantine

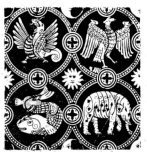

Brocade in white and gold from the 8th or 9th century A.D.

furnishings and ceremonial robes are still found in Russian churches, and Byzantine influence could be seen in Western European courts and religious institutions till about 1000.

Ceremonial Dignity. The style of clothing at the Byzantine court and in the churches reflected the ceremonial occasions on which it was worn. Many-coloured, dignified robes with full, sweeping lines, embroidered with gleaming pearls and precious stones were displayed on the dignitaries. The purpose was born to impress and to symbolize an unconquerable, unchanging system.

For the most ceremonious occasions, such as coronations, weddings and funerals, the oldest and most traditional forms of clothing were worn. Evidence may be seen of the partly Asiatic origins of Byzantine dress, whose general effect was somewhat reminiscent of gay Babylonian festival robes.

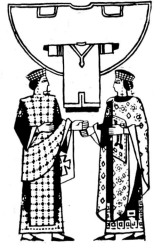

Men and women's attire from the 11th century with patterns above. The woman's tablion is worn on the front of her cape, its two halves being shown in the pattern

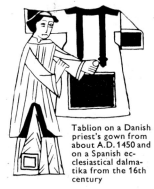

Tablion on a Danish priest's gown from about A.D. 1450 and on a Spanish ecclesiastical dalmatika from the 16th century

The general cut was very simple, the most important part being the T-shaped tunic. This reached to the knee for the lower classes, and down to the ankles for the well-to-do and upper classes. It was made of white silk with colourful embroidery and was encircled by a belt embossed with precious stones.

Egyptian crown of silver with inlaid precious stones. About A.D. 600. The 11th-century Hungarian crown of St. Stephan. Crown of the Russian Tsars from the 13th century but based on an older model

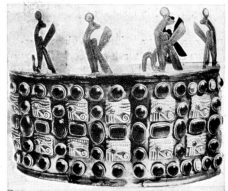
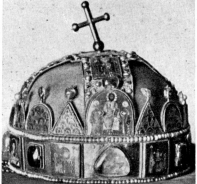
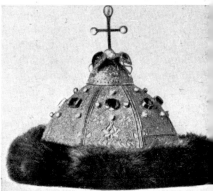

Opposite Empress Theodora with her retinue. Mosaic from the 6th century in Ravenna. The men are wearing large tablions

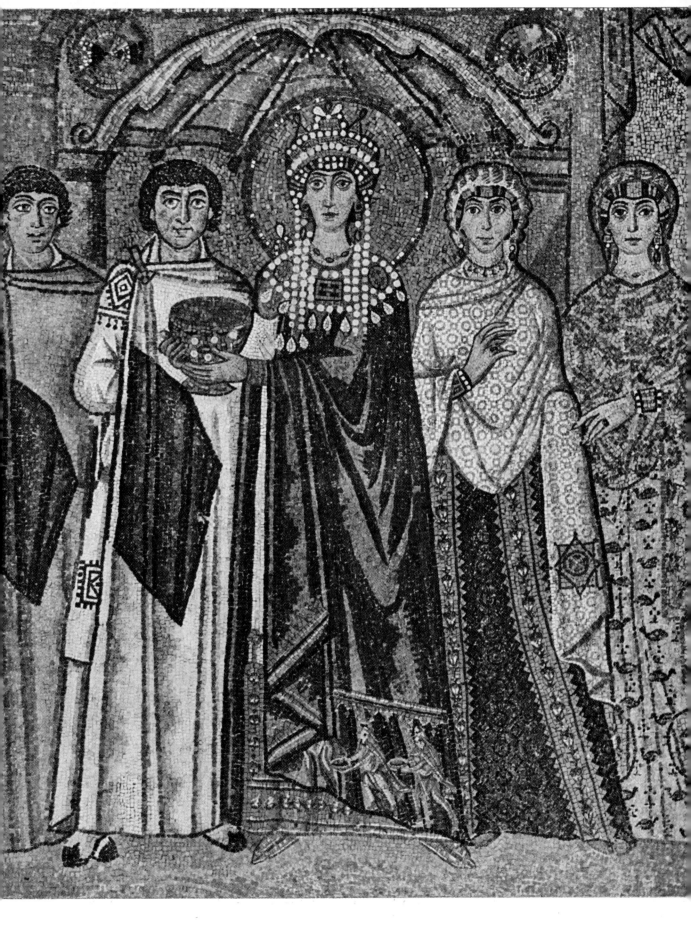

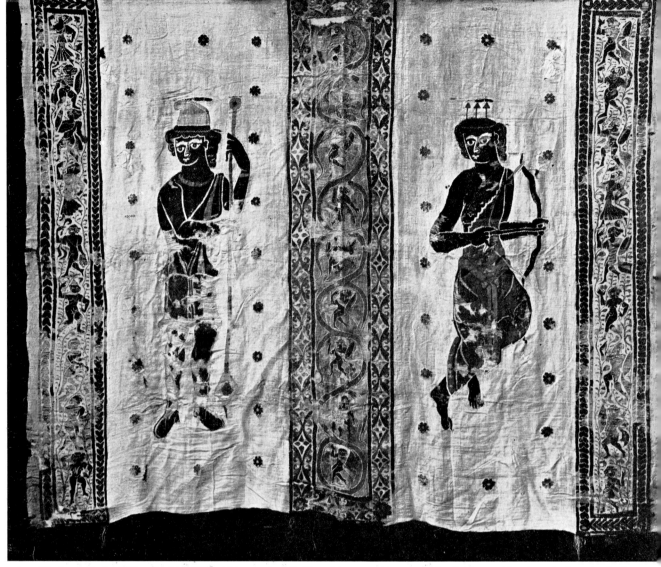

Woven textiles from Alexandria of the 5th and 6th centuries A.D. Alexandria exported large quantities of such material to the entire Byzantine Empire

The wide-sleeved dalmatika could be worn over the tunic or instead of it. The cape was worn over the

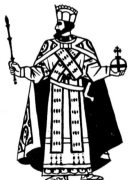

Byzantine emperor of the 11th century with diagram showing the draping of the pallium

right shoulder and had a tablion, or small square picture panel embroidered with pearls, sewn on the front. This served to indicate the rank of the wearer, in much the same way as the motifs on the gowns of ancient China did. Noblemen and priests also wore the pallium, a narrow embroidered band, on top of the cape and a round jewelled hat on their short, cropped hair.

During the early part of this period, women wore the embroidered Roman stola and tall collars set with jewels. The stola, and later the dalmatika, were encircled by a leather or metal belt worn high on the waist. The coat was put on over the head, and long hair was enclosed and almost hidden by silken ribbons and elaborate jewelled diadems.

The Sinful Body. Breeding silk-worms and weaving silk for clothing has been known since about A.D. 500. Stiff brocades could not produce the sculpturesque folds of linen but they conveyed a colourful dramatic impression. At this time, many artists turned away from sculpture and concentrated on mosaics.

With the tendency towards magnificence and splendour went a general sense of modesty, a desire to conceal the body. Christianity in the Byzantine Empire went far towards developing a bureau-

Emperor of about A.D. 1100, in full regalia

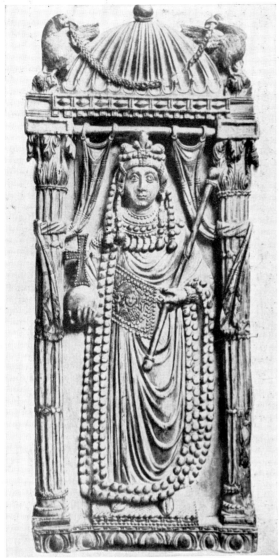

Byzantine empress of the 5th century with diadem of ostrich feathers, strings of pearls and ornaments, and jewelled tablion. Ivory carving

cratic state, but at the same time it nourished a fear of the naked body that amounted almost to panic.

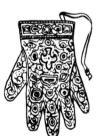

Embroidered glove, about A.D. 1100

Theological reasoning followed the teachings of St. Paul, even though the circumstances in which they had been formulated were so different. In Tarsus, St. Paul's native town, women covered their faces and their hands. When Chrysostomos visited Tarsus, in about A.D. 100, he recorded that 'women kept their faces covered but left the souls wide open'. St. Paul felt that much of the conflict in the world resulted from the different ways in which women dressed themselves in comparison to the way in which his mother and sisters in Tarsus were clothed.

Trousers, modelled on those in Northern Europe and Asia, were an accepted form of dress from early

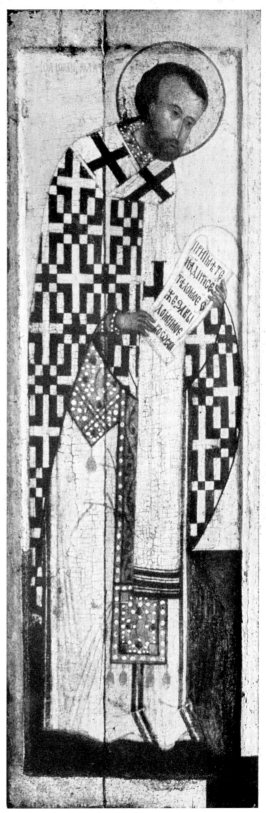

Russian icon representing a 13th-century bishop who was canonized after his death, dressed in tunic, cape with cross, and long, narrow pallium with crosses woven into the material

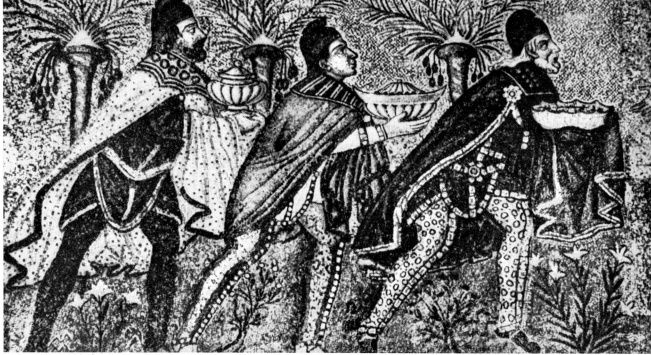

The Three Kings. Sixth-century mosaic in Ravenna. The kings are wearing red caps, violet and green capes with red dots, tunics and tight-fitting stockings

times in Byzantine society, although prohibited over and over again in Rome.

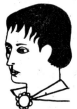

Byzantine hair style

The body vanished completely beneath the lavish folds of soft cloth. Holy men and women appear in elongated forms suggesting that straight lines and slimness were a characteristic of piety. Sublime holiness and long limbs were synonymous.

The course of all human action was laid down in the paragraphs of the corpus juris, and outward appearance was controlled by strict conventions in which the wearer, as an individual, played no part. The mere fact of wearing emperors' robes made a man emperor. An individual clad in a primate's cape became primate. No established form of ecclesiastical dress existed during the first three hundred years of Christianity, but from that time until A.D. 1000, the usual Byzantine court dress was adapted for church dignitaries and indeed is still used in much the same form today.

Dressed in Jewellery. The Emperor Charlemagne dressed, except on special occasions, like his subjects in shirt, smock and trousers, with a short fur coat and cape during the winter. The laces of his shoes were criss-crossed above his ankles. When he visited Rome in A.D. 800, he was compelled by the Pope to wear a long tunic, but this was discarded as soon as he returned home.

About this time, Byzantine dress was spreading into Western Europe, where it gained marked success. A description by a monk of a royal hunting party reminds us of Byzantine mosaics — stereotyped, stylized people, and much glitter and gold.

'At last Charles arrived, his noble head encircled by a golden ring. The blonde Rotrud rode in front of the women wearing a bright jewelled diadem in her hair. A beautiful buckle secured her mantle. The thoughtful Bertha followed behind wearing a golden band around her forehead. Her blonde shining hair was plaited with golden braids and her exquisite neck was covered by a costly marten skin. Her dress was emblazoned with topazes set in gold and other precious stones. Then came the beautiful Gizela wearing a veil woven with purple threads covering her slender neck. Her hands were snowy white, her forehead bright as gold, and her eyes shone brighter than the rays of the sun.'

The Dress of the Viking Age and the Period of Great Migrations. While the Byzantine Empire was growing in Eastern Europe, migrations were taking place over Northern and Western Europe, and the Viking invasions were in progress. These sunbronzed barbarians with their fair skin and blue eyes, who robbed and plundered their way southwards, had their own ideas of suitable attire, very different from the standards of the cultured priests and statesmen of the Byzantine Empire. We have a description of the everyday dress of these Teutons given by a Roman historian at the beginning of the Christian Era. They wore — he says — only a cloak held together by a buckle on one shoulder. Several

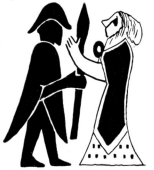

Swedish warrior of the 8th century and Norwegian woman of the 9th century

Danish cape from the Iron Age

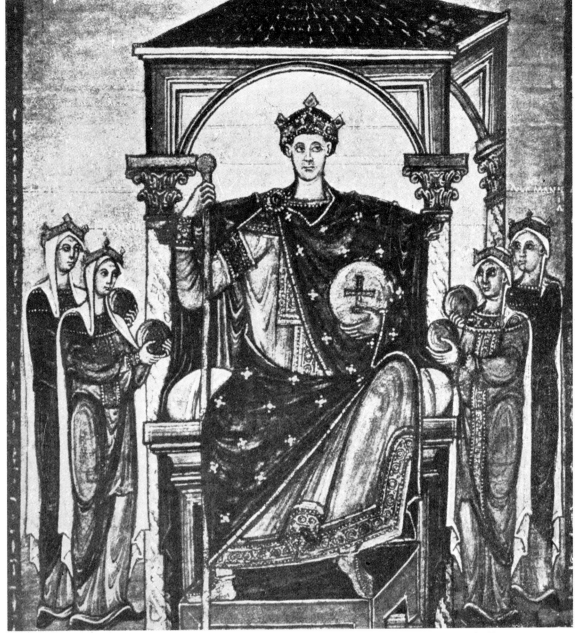

Emperor Otto enthroned in about A.D. 975, dressed in a tunic with wide embroidered borders under a purple mantle. The women are wearing tunics and virgin's crowns

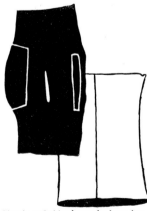

Mantle and skirt from the Iron Age in Denmark

examples have been found of rectangular or semicircular cloaks which produced a curved hemline that reached to the ground at the front and back but only to knee-level at the sides. Both Teutons and Celts wore trousers under the cloak. Early trousers reached to the knee and had wide tops and narrow legs. These became longer as time passed, and stockings were attached. The next addition was a kind of shirt worn tucked inside the trousers or hanging loose outside. The earliest examples were made from a square of material folded over and stitched down one side. This garment was worn from the shoulders and had no sleeves until A.D. 400, when long sleeves were added.

Female dress comprised a cape or shawl fastened in front with a buckle and one or more skirts held up by shoulder straps. Shoes made of leather and folded over the foot were worn. They were sewn

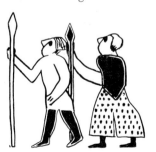

Norwegian styles in the 9th century

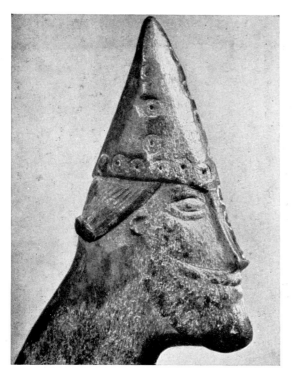

Swedish Viking with pointed helmet and nose-guard, carved from an elk's antlers

together at the heel and laced over the instep. Around A.D. 800, the Norwegians designed boots with sewn-on soles, the same for both feet. Ornaments were fashionable throughout the Viking Age. They were frequently in the form of buckles decorated with animal motifs. Heroes in battle were presented with heavy golden armlets.

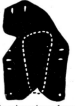

Leather shoes from the Iron Age in Denmark

Teutons and Celts. A Roman historian recorded that Teuton women were held in high regard; there was felt to be something sacred and even prophetic about them. 'Therefore neither disdain their advice,' he writes, 'nor omit consideration of their demands.'

The Celts elected female judges, and it was the woman who chose her husband and made the proposal of marriage. No man could enter into a contract without his wife's approval and Celtic gods were usually female. The Celtic paradise was known simply as 'the land of women', and here it is important to note that the adoration of the Virgin Mary originated among the Celts.

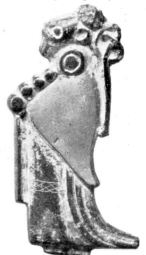

Viking housewife with train, ear-rings and hair ribbon

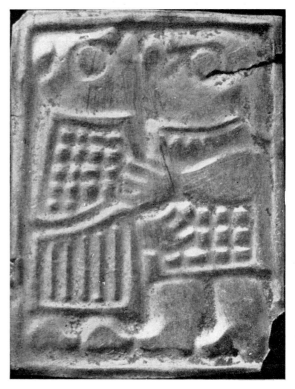

Trousers, dating from the 3rd or 4th century A.D., that covered the foot like present-day tights. They were found in a bog in Slesvig

Wedding amulet of gold showing a man and a woman kissing. She seems to have on a split dress and he a knee-length shirt

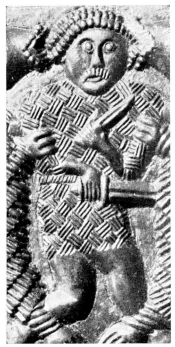
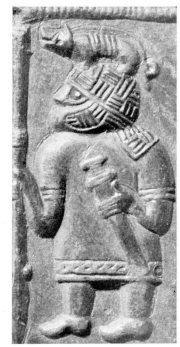
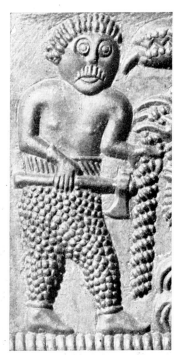

Bronze reliefs from the island of Øland, showing Swedes of the 7th century. Left, roughly woven tunic shirt. Centre, A helmet with chin and neck-guards topped by a wild boar. Right, Hairy animal skin trousers. All three man have moustaches but clean-shaven chins

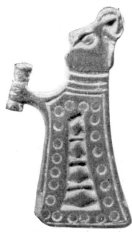

Housewife in a full-length robe

In Chartres, where Fulbert built the first church to Our Lady, the matriarchal conception of religion had existed for centuries before the birth of Christ. On the other hand, the Celts had no equivalent of Aphrodite and the naked woman had no place in their art comparable to that of the naked man. Since it was the woman who chose her partner, the arts emphasized those manly charms which influenced her choice.

Barbarians and Byzantines.

It was common practice for Teuton soldiers to be roped together before battle lest they should break rank. A Roman historian has described how the women dealt with men who fled the field: one woman would kill her husband, for example, another her father or brother. If a battle was lost, they would strangle

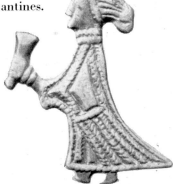

Woman of the Viking era offering a toast of welcome

their children with their bare hands or cast them beneath the chariot wheels or horses' hoofs, before taking their own lives.

This philosophy had no similarities with the precise, deliberate, old-fashioned dignity of the Byzantines. Here there was no nonsense. What had to be done was done quickly and efficiently and this was reflected in Teuton dress. There was, however, some interrelation between the Vikings of the North and the Byzantines of the South. The latter were referred to in Nordic languages as 'Myklagaard'; it was from the Nordic countries that the Byzantine emperors obtained their bodyguard.

The Nordic bard in the saga, the Hávamál, made caustic reference to the Byzantine theory that fine feathers make fine birds, as he set up two scarecrows and sang,

'I gave up my clothes to two wooden figures in a field and when so dressed they appeared like heroes.'

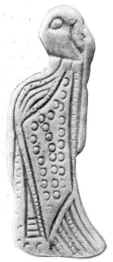

Viking woman's attire in Sweden

Under the mellowing influence of Christianity, the Nordic peoples came to appreciate soft materials and comfortable garments. A dislike of long sweeping garments had been in evidence for some time in Western Europe. As late as the tenth century, we hear of a bishop travelling in the Near East and strongly dis-

109

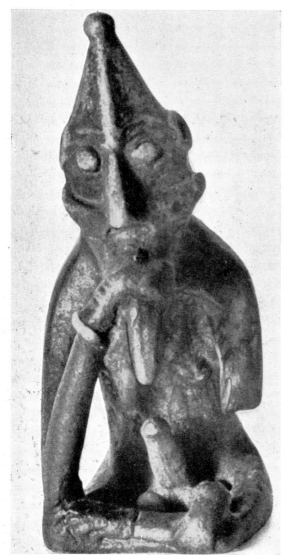

The only known pagan idol from ancient Scandinavia. It represents
Frey, the god of fertility, and dates from the Bronze Age in Sweden

Two Philosophies. Byzantine fashion was adopted
by the Barbarians for reasons quite unrelated to the
original function of the clothes. Roman logic and the
purity of Greek humanism were completely obliterated
by passionate mysticism, in the same way that Church
ritual became an abstract performance to be observed
by people who did not understand the language in
which it was spoken, whether it were Latin or Greek.
If we compare the beautiful Nordic coins, the brac-
teates, with the equivalent Roman coins stamped with
the head of the emperor, we can see at once the fundamental difference in the outlook of these two peoples.
The Roman coin was a practical article in everyday
use, bearing an impression which everyone could
understand, in itself a useful form of propaganda for
the Empire. It was something to look at, something to
value, something to handle from time to time. In contrast, the Nordic bracteate conveyed a feeling of mys-
tic charm and mysterious significance. The pattern
took the fanciful shape of the head of a horseman
mounted on a horse with horns and surrounded by
sacred symbols.

The Byzantine mantle or cloak was not merely a
beautiful and costly piece of clothing. As seen through
northern eyes it became a heavenly garment, woven
by the angels and fallen from the heavens.

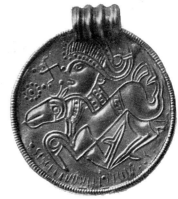

Bracteate. A chased gold pendant from Bornholm

approving of the wide sleeves and long trains worn
by courtiers. A Father of the Church sighs,

'Cursed be the long clothes which tempt to sensual thoughts.'

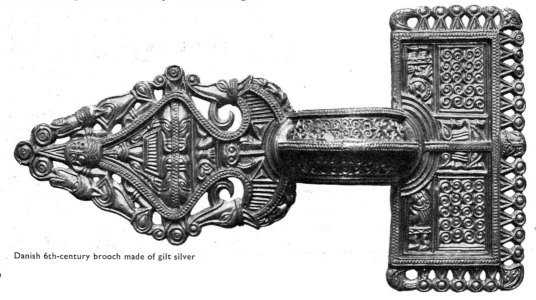

Danish 6th-century brooch made of gilt silver

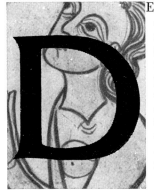

DEVELOPMENTS that came after the Crusades included a change in the role of money, which now came to assume increasing importance. Previously landowners had lived comfortably. But with more widespread possessions, the cost of travel increased, and consequently the need for money. Not everyone approved of this trend; an anonymous poet wrote in about 1050, 'Money now rules and also sits in judgement'.

Knight, Cleric, Burgher. The social order of this time was represented by the feudal system. The knights

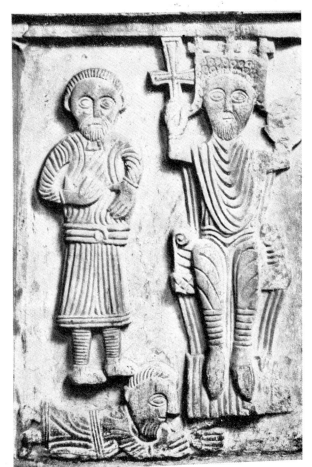

Croatian king of the 11th century. His cape is arranged on his shoulders in such a way that his back is completely covered. The standing and the lying men both wear belts fastened with a button in front. Stone-carving

were the privileged class in this society and obtained their property and possessions from their higher feudal lord, emperor or king. Trade was developing and cities were expanding. In order to secure stable markets and prices, and to counteract the influence of the knights, frequently 'robber knights', guilds came to be formed by the merchants. With them emerged an important and influential social class made up of ordinary citizens or burghers.

Noblewoman of the 11th century with pattern for her tunic and sleeves

Normans of the 11th century in the Bayeux Tapestry. King and bishop wear long tunics, and persons of rank wear mantles. All wear their hair short and are clean-shaven

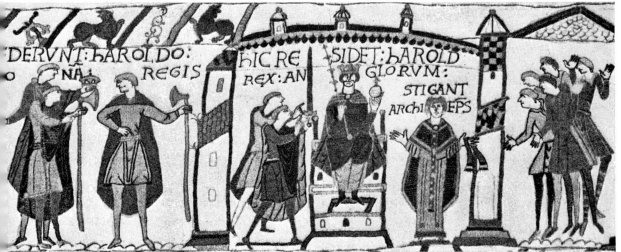

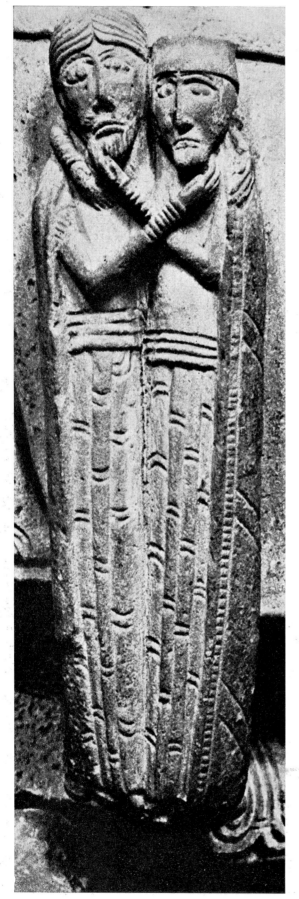

In the twelfth century, a woman from a mercantile background would have been punished if she had dressed like a noblewoman, but two hundred years later women could not only dress like noblewomen but even excelled them in array. At the same time, another kind of collective enterprise, represented by the monasteries, made great advances. It should be understood, however, that the greater part of the population consisted of artisans, peasants and serfs.

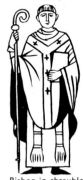

Bishop in chasuble, A.D. 1120

At this time, the more affluent section of society occupied themselves with tournaments, hunting bears and wolves, dancing courtly dances in their castles, bending over the chessboard. Interiors were lit by torches, tallow candles or shavings from fir trees. Clerics went about their placid duties officiating at the religious pageants in which all citizens took part and surrounded at home by their books and musical instruments.

The Dawn of the Middle Ages. When we study the Middle Ages, we can perceive a general awakening in the air. The Icelandic saga of Eigil Skallagrimson gives this same impression, as do the letters written in Paris during the same period between Héloïse and Abelard: letters that are so pregnant with feeling and so expressive of love — the latter almost adolescent in tone, and yet so true-to-life. Abelard was subsequently castrated on the orders of the girl's guardian, whose trust he had betrayed.

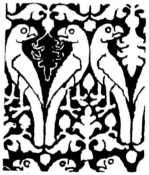

Silk pattern, ca. A.D. 1160

We are confronted at this time by a magnificent resurgence of art, architecture and theology, in contrast to the simultaneous rebirth of a Christ-like disdain of wealth and power. St. Francis, in the midst of the victorious progress of art and philosophy, exposed the inner hollowness of worldly pomp and directed people's mind to love of the poor and lowly and to the undefiled elements in nature: Brother Sun, Sister Moon, Brother Wind, Sister Spring, Brother Fire, Mother Earth.

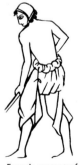

French peasant of the 13th century naked from the waist up

Adam's Clothes.

St. Bernard wrote,

'People who admire themselves because of their clothes are like the sinner who boasts of being branded, in that the guilt of Adam first made clothing necessary.'

Man and woman of the 11th century on a baptismal font in Scania

Opposite, Detail from the Bayeux Tapestry

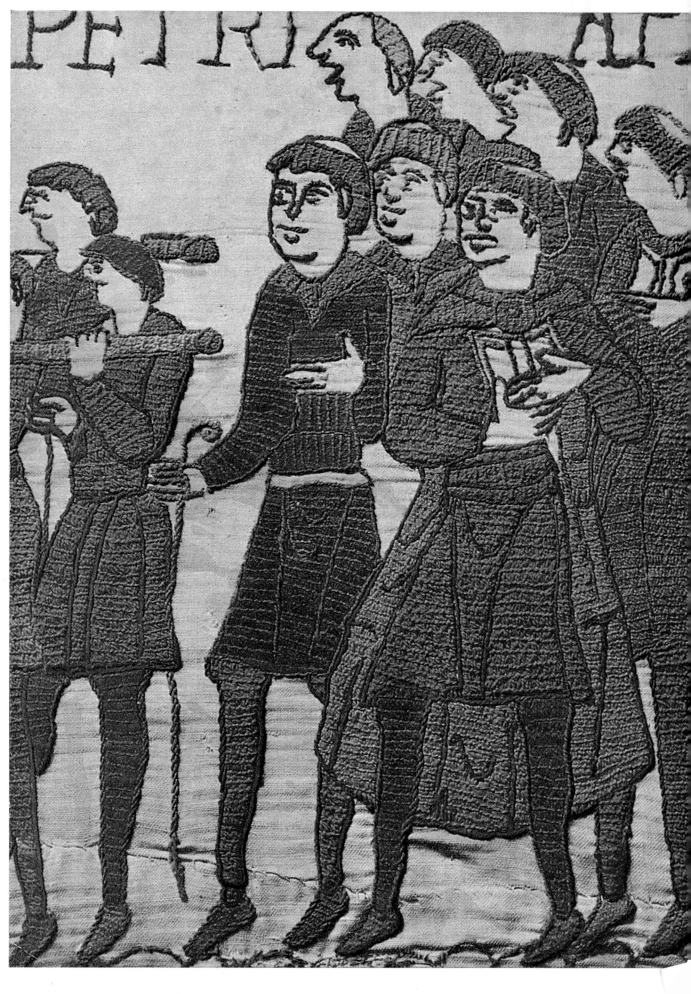

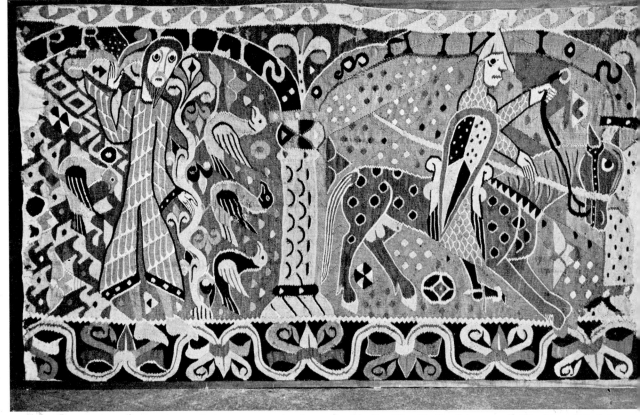

Norwegian tapestry of the 12th century with pictures representing the months of April and May. The bearded man on the left with a split tunic is listening to the birds' song while the young clean-shaven knight in chain-mail and helmet, carrying a shield and lance, is riding out to seek adventure

In accordance with this point of view, nakedness came to be regarded as the body's heavenly state, the true image of God. Adam and Eve were depicted naked as a central decoration in all churches. Lady Godiva, who founded several churches in England, rode naked through the city of Coventry in 1043 as a protest against taxes imposed by her husband on the poor. This act was greatly acclaimed and an annual pageant still takes place through the streets of Coventry to commemorate it.

Sinful man was not considered worthy during life to expose his naked body, but the puritanical horror of nudity did not yet exist. On one occasion, St. Francis removed his clothing during a sermon in full view of the congregation, to demonstrate the unimportance of such mundane things.

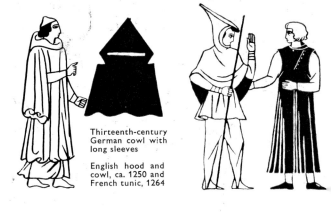

Thirteenth-century German cowl with long sleeves

English hood and cowl, ca. 1250 and French tunic, 1264

Mantle, Shirt, Trousers and Socks. Clothes were made in the home. The women of the house spun, wove, cut and sewed the garments for the whole household.

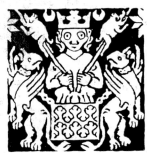

Thirteenth-century brocade pattern

For thousands of years, the mantle had been the principal item of clothing for everyone. It was only at the very top level of society that a shirt was worn underneath. After A.D. 1000, the mantle became exclusively an item of upper-class dress, and the

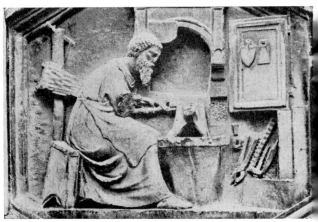

Italian smith with leather apron, 14th century. Florentine stone relief

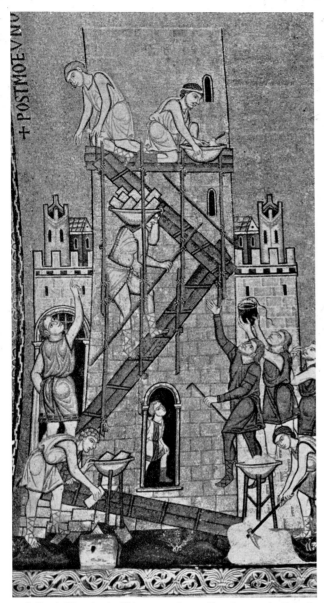

Italian builders in the 13th century from a Venetian mosaic. Only the architect, holding a T-square, wears long hose and sleeves. The laces of his sandals are tied high up on his legs

only reached to the knee; longer clothing was reserved for church dignitaries and priests. Towards the middle of the twelfth century, long clothes as a result of Byzantine influence, came to be worn more and more by all classes in Western Europe. By the end of that century the fashion was universally accepted both there and in the Nordic countries. Narrow belts were worn round the waist, secured by a buckle or tied in a knot, with the ends hanging loose. After 1200, the shirt came into common use. A contemporary maxim advises,

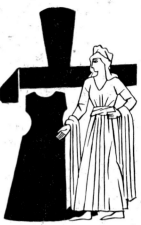

Twelfth-century French lady's gown with the pattern for the gown and sleeves

'Always cut your shirt considerably shorter than your mantle as no well born man can appear in flax or hemp.'

The legs were covered by long trousers to which socks were attached. Wide linen trousers dating from

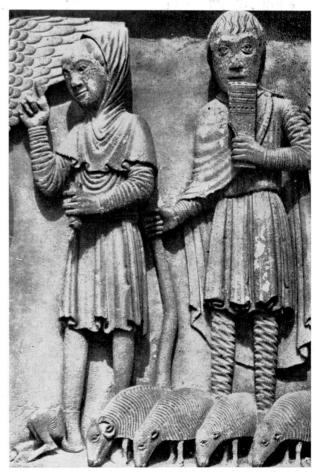

French shepherds from the 12th century. One wears a hooded cape and the other hose that hang in folds. Stone-relief at Chartres Cathedral

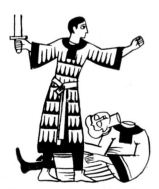

German executioner wearing fur-trimmed tunic, composed of many pieces of fur, with a long belt. The sleeves are funnel-shaped

courtier was required to remove his mantle when he went before the king. This mantle could be either oblong or circular in cut, and was fastened on the chest or shoulder by a buckle or strap. Ornamentation consisted of decorated borders around the neck, sleeves and hem; this could be woven, embroidered or attached in the form of appliqué. In 1050, the mantle and shirt still

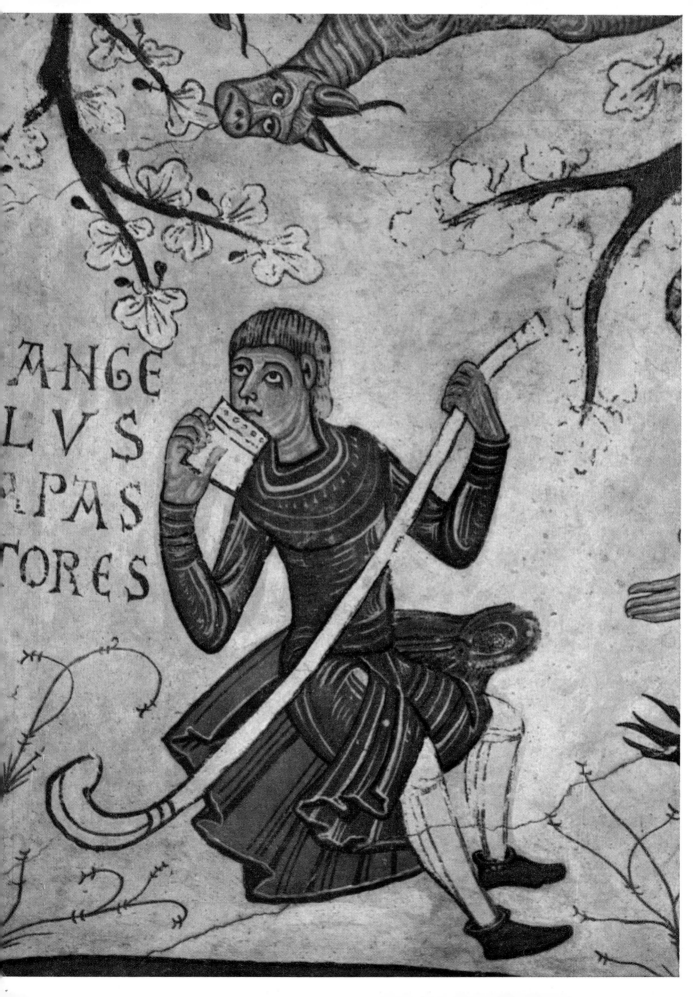

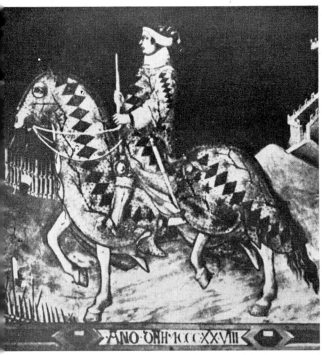

Italian military commander, 1328. Both the mantle of the horseman and the trappings of the horse are made from cloth with woven patterns. Painting by Simone Martini

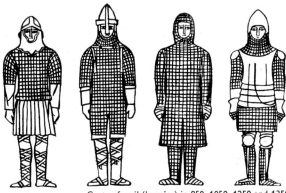

Coats of mail (byrnies) in 850, 1050, 1250 and 1350

or coat of mail, a ringed metal shirt, was worn with a hood attached to cover the entire head. The pointed Viking helmet and broad-brimmed metal hat were also used. During the thirteenth century, it became customary to wear a shirt over the byrnie, perhaps to help keep the metal dry.

Hair styles were also influenced by war; a luxuriant head of hair or beard could provide an all too easy

Sudanese warriors have used the medieval horseman's outfit to the present day. The wadded material protects the wearer from arrows and spears

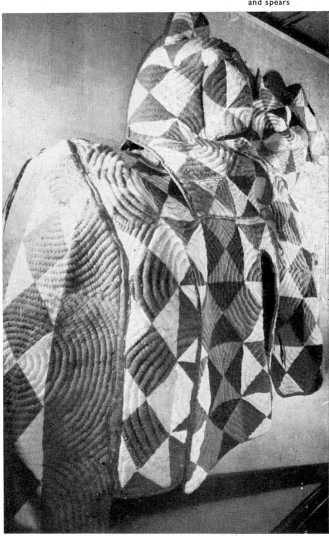

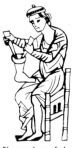

Shoemaker of the 13th century

the Viking Age (and still worn by sailors and fishermen in Denmark and Holland) were excavated at Oseberg in Norway. They also feature in the Swedish Skog Tapestry which dates from the early twelfth century. In cases where socks were not attached to trousers, they were strapped and laced criss-cross up the leg.

As the shirt became longer, so the trousers became shorter and gradually changed into being underwear. At the same time, socks and stockings began to be shaped to the leg and made large enough for the trouser bottoms to be tucked in. Shoes of the eleventh century came up over the ankle, and were later secured by a buckle. Boots were laced on the inside of the leg.

Headgear usually took the form of a small skullcap, but after 1150, a hood was used for travel. This was usually attached to a short cape and became the normal headwear of the period. Fifty years later the low-crowned hat with a broad brim, made its appearance.

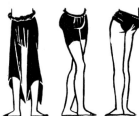

Breeches in 1200, 1425 and 1475

Byrnie and Helmet. No less than seven crusades took place between the years 1100 and 1250. Thus, military dress assumed great importance. The byrnie

Opposite, Shepherd, fresco in the Church of St. Isidor, León, Spain, 1150–1200

117

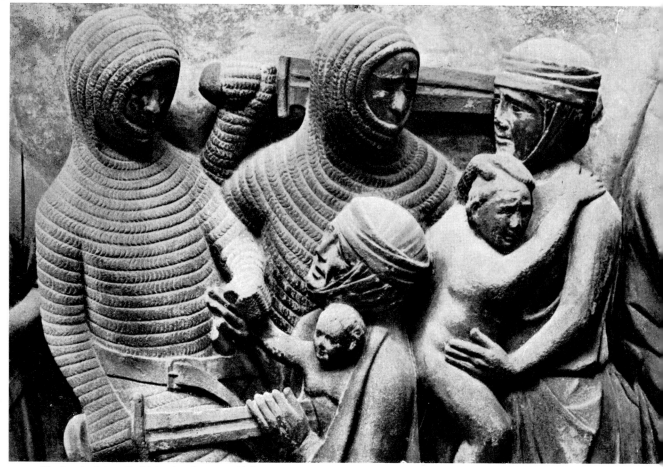

Warriors in chain-mail with hoods and women with bands encircling their forehead and chin. The Massacre of the Innocents, stone sculpture at the Cathedral of Notre Dame, Paris

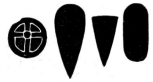

Shields from the period 1050–1250

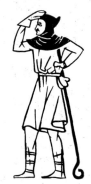

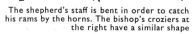

The shepherd's staff is bent in order to catch his rams by the horns. The bishop's croziers at the right have a similar shape

grip for the opponent in hand to hand fighting. The Norman warrior was always clean-shaven and had cropped hair. During the comparatively peaceful time following this period, long hair and beards again became fashionable, but the Crusades put a stop to such extravagances. After about 1200, bobbed hair with a straight-cut fringe and occasionally a lock of hair combed forward below the ear became popular.

Silk Shift and Head Covering. Women, as well as men, wore an overshirt and undershirt. The undergarment was nothing more than a shift secured by a buckle. This was everyday wear at home and at work. The outer garment, or overshirt, was a good deal shorter and shaped more like a blouse.

Around 1150, enormously wide sleeves which reached the ground came into fashion, but fifty years later they returned to normal proportions and were laced at the sides. Capes were worn by men and women alike. The hair style for women at this time consisted of a centre parting and long plaits interwoven with silk ribbons that fell over the bosom. Young girls could either wear their hair loose, kept somewhat in place, perhaps, by a comb, or in plaits coiled on top of the head. Men and women wore similar conical or flat topped hats. From the beginning of the thirteenth century, married women covered their heads with a thin veil made of linen or some other fine material. This kind of head covering was arranged so that it fell over the forehead and covered the sides of the face and the back of the neck. A piece of material like a wimple, covering the throat and chest, was also worn.

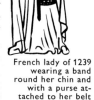

French lady of 1239 wearing a band round her chin and with a purse attached to her belt

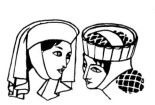

Head and chin scarves of about 1250 and hair-net

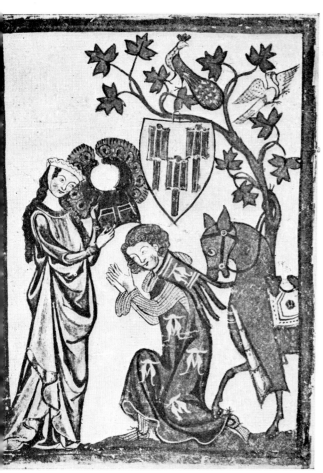

Swiss troubadour miniature from 1330 based on a picture a century older. The man's and woman's attire are identical

Fresh Perceptions and Expressive Bodies. Paint was used on houses in towns; church buildings were

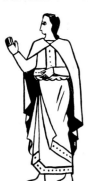

decorated with frescoes and mosaics worked in glass or precious metals inlaid with enamel, and created a symphony of colour. Bright clothes were worn by priests and laymen alike. From 1000 on, it was fashionable to have trouser legs made in contrasting colours, one green and one red, for example. Another fashion divided all clothing vertically into two different colours, one for the left side and one for the right; this fashion persisted all through the Middle Ages. Wealthy people wore outfits in many different colours.

Mantle and tunic, 1241

Here is a description of a royal wedding in England in the thirteenth century,

'The guests were dressed now in green, now blue and grey and purple. They changed colours in accordance with their mood or the fancy of the lady to whom they had pledged their love.'

The people of the Middle Ages were endowed with healthy bodies and a fresh outlook on life. This is

German noblewoman about 1250. The mantle with large collar is held together by bands fastened to the brooch on the shoulder. Stone sculpture in Naumburg Cathedral

clearly seen in the frescoes of the time which capture the expressiveness of gesture and movement, and also demonstrate how carriage and stance can tell us more about a person than facial expression alone.

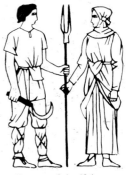

Peasants of the 13th century

The paraphernalia we find indispensable for sitting down and resting, our sofas and armchairs, (designed, it would seem, to put our muscles out of action) had not yet been devised. One sat on the floor, on the doorstep, chest, or bed, whichever was most convenient. One was always close to one's fellow human beings. In church, one knelt on the floor, the stone bench along the wall being reserved for the sick. Ancient paintings of the enthroned Madonna provide an apposite example of good posture in which a person sat upright instead of leaning back.

At this time, the beginning of the thirteenth century, a new etiquette of behaviour gained ground which disapproved of any exaggeration of bodily movement or gesture. We learn that,

'The maiden must lower her eyes and not look wildly about her. She must slowly allow her eyes to wander over the objects which are nearest to her, neither too quickly nor too slowly and without moving her head.

'She must conceal her hands beneath her cape. She must walk with short steps while lifting her dress so that it shall not trail in the dirt. And when she sits she may not cross one leg over the other.'

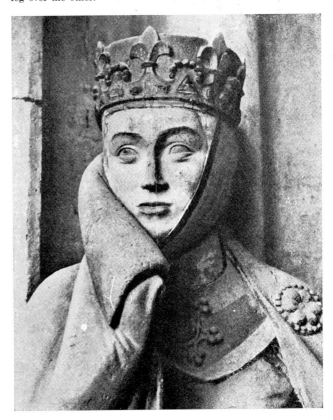

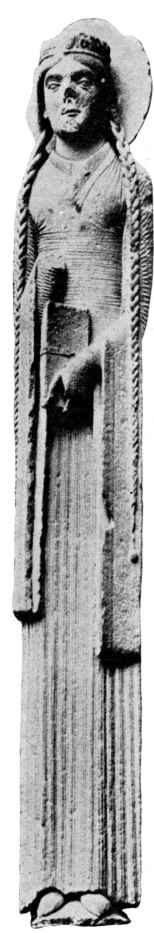

The Poetry of the Troubadours.

The songs of the troubadours expressed a new concept of love, almost transforming women into objects of religious adoration. This marks the birth of romantic love.

It had been ruled in 1174 in a French 'Court of Love', that love between husband and wife was impossible. These authorities reasoned that lovers would of their own free will give themselves to each other, whereas between husband and wife this became a duty. Chastity belts are a harsh reminder of this rough distinction. When the poetry of later times linked springtime with love, it was largely because fine weather made it possible to roam abroad, and thus provided better opportunities for clandestine lovemaking than their overcrowded houses allowed in the winter. The Church held that sexual passion, in its power over the reason, was a result of original sin. But the love poetry had no power to change prevailing social conditions or establish love in its rightful, natural place in human society. Religion thus gradually lost contact with human reality.

A harsh reality was disguised by a romantic fiction, in which men became heroes and women assumed the role of goddesses. Over his chain mail the knight wore a shirt embroidered in the favourite colours of his beloved.

The Church and Women.

Women were regarded by the priests as unclean creatures. They were provided with a separate entrance to the church, situated to the north whence all evil derives. Sin entered the world through a woman's action. Woman was the eternal cause of sinful lust, and for this reason the source of all wickedness. The most pious men were tempted by demons in female form. Some priests with a senile and perverse fear of women went so far as to agree with Odon of Cluny when he wrote,

'A beauty which consists of slime, bloom lymph and gall. One must consider that behind the nostrils, in the throat and in the stomach nothing exists but the entrails. And if one finds it difficult even with the tip of a finger to touch excrement or slime how then can one desire to be embraced by a sack so full of filth . . . .'

Notwithstanding such views, the Church of the Middle Ages veered away from patriarchal attitudes. Worship of the Virgin Mary assumed a central part in services, and nuns in convents became the equal of their counterparts in the monasteries.

The Church as Unifier.

During the Middle Ages, sharp contrasts were developing between the different aspects of society: soft sunshine and heavy rain; primitive force and gentle poetry; virile sensuality and vapid fantasy; coarseness and refinement — all of these were mixed together and inseparably intertwined. The role of the Church was to guide these various tendencies in the right direction. Whatever else it failed to do, it could at least provide the unity of a Christian Europe.

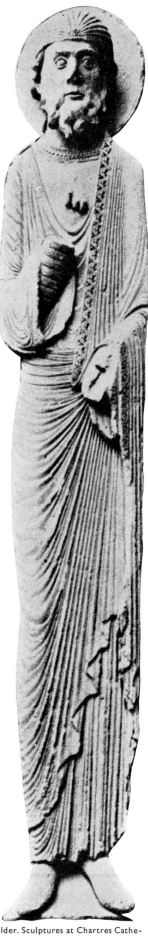

French man and woman about 1150. Her dress has a scarf and loose sleeves, his mantle is draped over the left shoulder. Sculptures at Chartres Cathedral, representing the chaste ideal of the early Middle Ages

GOTHIC ARMOUR AND POINTED SHOES

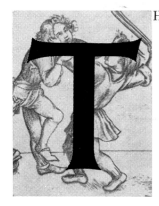

THE FEUDAL system and an agriculturally based economy dominated the early Middle Ages. Later, the centres of life and communication began to move away from monastery and manor house to the big towns and cities.

The citizens of these new centres became the leaders of society and the arbiters of culture. Unlike the feudal overlords, whose power and wealth lay in the ownership of land and the control of labour, the new ruling class was rich in actual money — money which was essential for the feudal lords, and indeed even for kings, in conducting wars and building fortresses. The big merchant interests ranged over vast areas. The Hanseatic League, centred around the large ports of Northern Germany, became complete master of a trading area which extended from London to Novgorod. In a similar way, trade in the Mediterranean area was entirely controlled by the big merchants of North Italy.

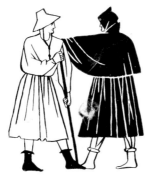

Italian shepherds, 1305

The end of the Middle Ages was, in many ways, eventful and significant. Dante wrote *The Divine Comedy* which expressed the spirit of the Middle Ages in the form of a magnificent dream-vision. He died in 1321, the year in which gunpowder was introduced. The Black Death swept Europe and exterminated nearly half the population. In 1431, Joan of Arc was burnt at the stake. Printing was invented. The year 1483 saw the birth of Martin Luther, and in 1492 Christopher Columbus discovered America.

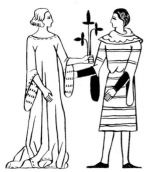

Free-hanging sleeves, England, 1350

Soaring Gothic. The new merchant aristocracy, attempting to vie in importance with the feudal lords and the representatives of the Churchs began to develop a sense of nobility and piety far exceeding

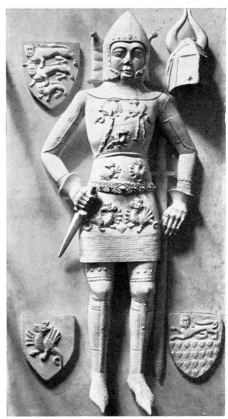

Danish duke in plate mail with pointed shoes and horned helmet. Sculpture on coffin in Roskilde Cathedral, 1363

that of the true nobles and priests. A strict code of honour was established and religious fervour reached what was virtually a state of hysteria. Altogether, there was something unrestrained and excessive about the forceful single-mindedness of the Gothic Age. The upward surge of temporal power and the aspiring fervour of religion were reflected in all forms of art, from church steeples to dress.

A communal spirit still existed within individual sections of society; peasants grouped together for cooperative farming; merchants banded together in

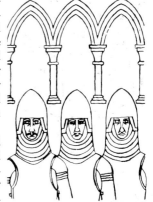

Gothic arches and helmets

guilds; the artisans formed their own fraternities. But there was by no means a unified system. As money began to dominate the economy, the old class ties were broken down and a strong feeling of individuality and self-awareness developed. The era in which the Gothic style was dominant is characterized by a series of conflicts between the principles of collective feudalism and the new ideas of individualistic capitalism.

The Triumphant Progress of the Scissors. Shaped garments made to cut-out patterns appeared during the latter part of the Middle Ages. The primary factor which made this type of clothing possible was the invention of the button. Buttons found in use among the Turks and Mongols by the Crusaders were copied, and they soon displaced the buckle, always up to then the most splendid ornament of dress.

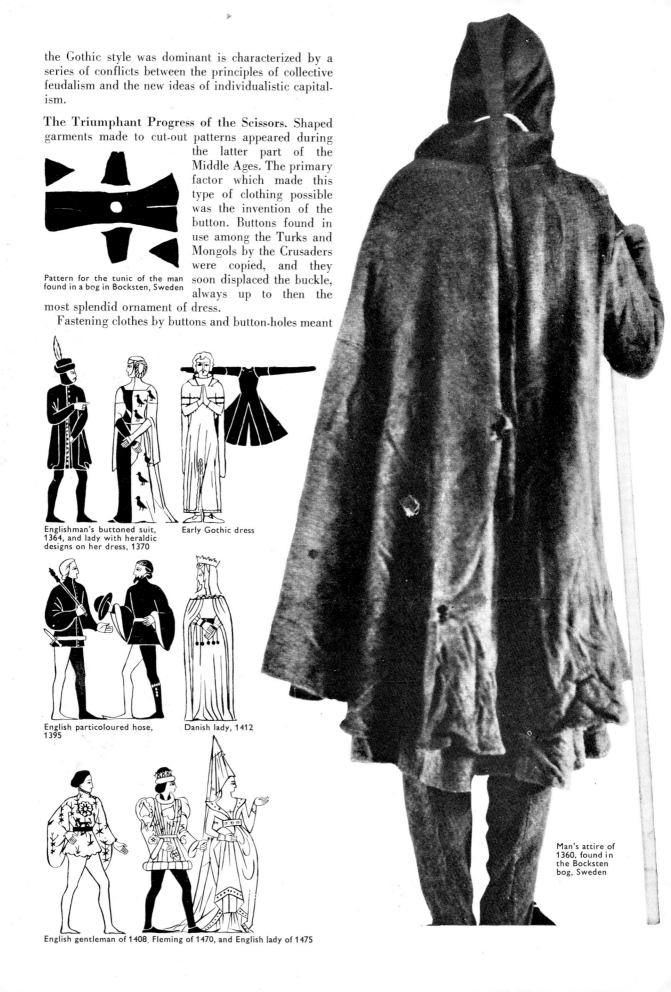

Pattern for the tunic of the man found in a bog in Bocksten, Sweden

Fastening clothes by buttons and button-holes meant

Englishman's buttoned suit, 1364, and lady with heraldic designs on her dress, 1370   Early Gothic dress

English particoloured hose, 1395   Danish lady, 1412

English gentleman of 1408, Fleming of 1470, and English lady of 1475

Man's attire of 1360, found in the Bocksten bog, Sweden

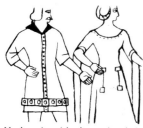

Man's suit with decorative belt worn on the hips and woman's dress with free-hanging sleeves

that the dress had no longer to be sufficiently roomy to pull on over the head. With the development of the close-fitting garment came the art of cutting to shape and the insertion of the wedge-shaped piece of material known as the gusset. The new design permitted the more affluent to swagger about in close-fitting jackets and shaped trousers, while the more lowly continued to wear the old-fashioned long shift. This development also marked the first real difference in the design of male and female dress.

Chaucer's Pilgrims. The English poet, Geoffrey Chaucer was born in about 1340; the exact date is not known. His *Canterbury Tales* provides a vivid picture of a band of pilgrims journeying to Canterbury at the end of the fourteenth century.

There was a *Knight*, a most distinguished man ... Speaking of his appearance, he possessed — Fine horses, but he was not gaily dressed. — He wore a Fustian Tunic Stained and dark — With smudges where his armour had left mark ... He had his son with him, a fine young *Squire* ... He was embroidered like a meadow bright — And full of freshest flowers, red and white. — Singing he was, or fluting all the day; — He was as fresh as is the month of May. — Short was his gown, the sleeves were long and wide ... There also was a *Nun*, a Prioress ... At meat her manners were well taught withal; — No morsel from her lips did she let fall, — Nor dipped her fingers in the sauce too deep; — But she could carry a morsel up and keep — The smallest drop from falling on her breast ... There was a Monk, a leader of the fashions; — Inspecting farms and hunting were his passions ... I saw his sleeves were garnished at the hand — With fine grey fur, the finest in the land, — And where his hood was fastened at

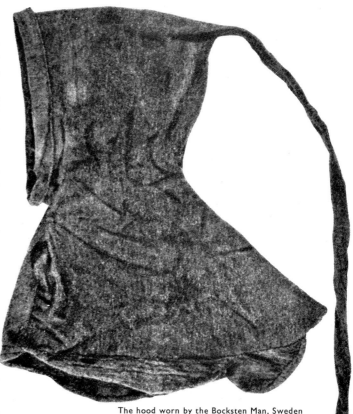

The hood worn by the Bocksten Man, Sweden

his chin — He had a wrought-gold cunningly fashioned pin ... A *Doctor* too emerged as we proceeded ... In blood-red garments, slashed with bluish-grey — And lined with taffeta, he rode his way ... A worthy *woman* from beside *Bath* city — Was with us ... Her kerchiefs were of finely woven ground; — I dared have sworn they weighed a good ten pound, — The ones she wore on Sunday, on her head. — Her hose were of the finest scarlet red — And gartered tight; her shoes were soft and new.

It is interesting to note that the cape or mantle, which had earlier been extremely important, is not mentioned at all in this poem. By this time, it was worn only on ceremonial occasions.

Plate Mail. Armour undoubtedly played an important part in shaping the new fashions. During the thirteenth century, protection in battle was provided mainly by flexible chain-mail, but as time went by and weapons became more deadly, chain-mail gave way to the more solid armour-plate. This, unlike the byrnie, had to fit close to the body and joints provided flexibility. This necessitated redesigning the clothing worn underneath the armour, and the original shirt and tunic were replaced by jerkin and tight-fitting hose.

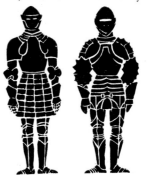

Armour in 1440 and 1460

The Jerkin and the Full-Sleeved Coat. From 1300, clothing became more tight-fitting. Buttons were used. Much emphasis was laid on showing the full length

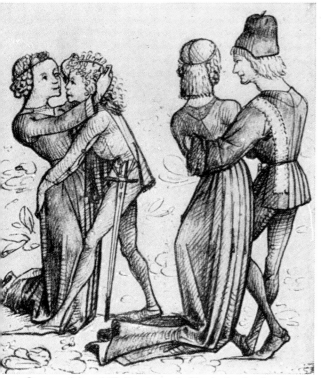

Germans of about 1475. Drawing by the 'Hausbuchmeister'

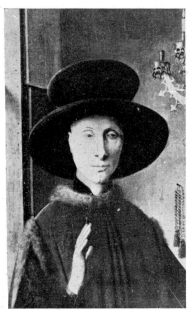

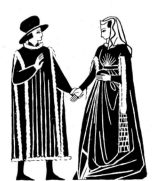

Left, a detail of Van Eyck's Arnolfinis's marriage portrait, 1432. Above, Drawing based on this painting

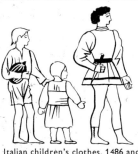

Italian children's clothes, 1486 and 1461

of the leg. The short jersey type of garment first appeared in France in about 1350. Some thirty years later, it found its way to the Nordic countries. The old-fashioned, loose shift was metamorphosed into a shirt, over which was worn a jerkin that closely fitted the upper part of the body. Whereas the shift had comprised a length of material front and back, often made in one piece, the jerkin had stitched seams front and back. And as the jerkin had an opening down the front and did not have to be put on over the head, the top portion could be cut high at the neck. Tails at the back sometimes reached below the knee.

A full-sleeved coat was worn over the jerkin which, until about 1450, was cut high at the neck. Slits were made in the side of the coat for access to the purse or sword which hung from the belt of the jerkin. In time,

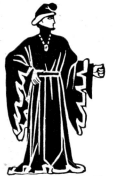

Coat with long wide sleeves

small bags were fixed inside these slits and referred to as 'false purses'; they were, in fact, the first pockets. It is interesting to observe that while pockets have remained an essential part of male dress, women still carry handbags, as in the Middle Ages.

Fashions from Burgundy. In the fifteenth century, England and France were considerably weakened by a succession of wars. The court of Burgundy became the leading centre of fashion in Europe, while control of the Flemish weaving industry was in dispute. Burgundian clothing became excessively close-fitting and shaped to the body. Trousers were so tight that a codpiece, a wedge-

Codpiece

shaped piece of cloth, had to be inserted in the crutch to enable the wearer to move about at all. Waists were laced in, chest and shoulders were built up with padding. This tight-fitting style of dress persists today in the costumes of circus acrobats. Finely sewn pleats appeared at the back and front of coats, and sleeves were fashioned in absurd shapes, bellying out like barrels or tapering like pears. After 1450, sleeves became narrow again but where they joined the shoulder were puffed out with wadding. Necklines were cut away to expose the shirt, in the same way that suit jackets do today. As more of the shirt was visible, it

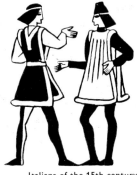

Italians of the 15th century wearing the sleeveless jerkin, the giubberello

came to acquire elaborate embroideries of coloured silk or gold thread and was secured with a cord round the neck. The full sleeves were of various patterns. Slits were made in them through which the arms could emerge, leaving the rest of the sleeve hanging free.

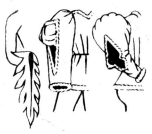

Sleeves with slits and padding

Stockings become Trousers.

Trousers were worn with the short coat of the Viking period, but as the coat became longer trousers became shorter, until they looked like short pants. Consequently, when short coats reappeared, the thighs were left largely uncovered; an historian from Mainz records in 1367,

'Fashion became so ridiculous that young men wore coats so short that they failed to cover their private parts front or back. When they stooped they exposed their bare posteriors. What a scandal!'

An old English law, passed in 1475, suggests that exposure of the private parts was a privilege reserved for the upper classes.

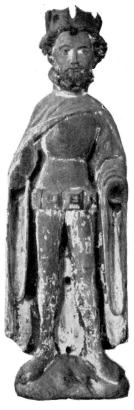

Swedish 14th-century dress featuring the mantle, wide sleeves and decorated belt

Opposite   Young Flemish girl, about 1450.
Painting by Petrus Christus

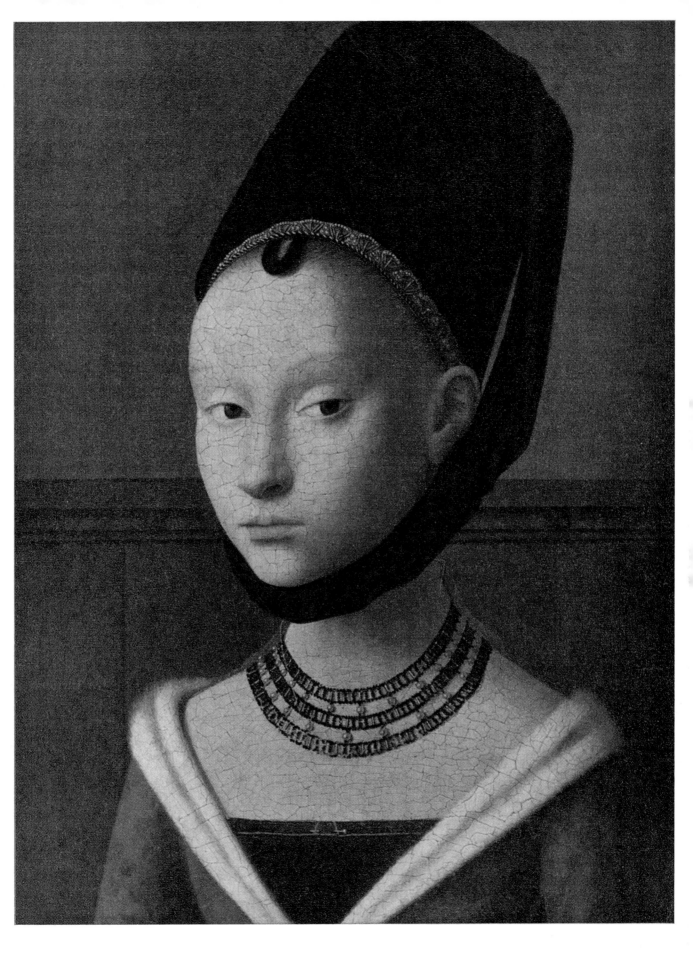

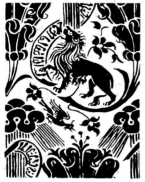

Italian brocade of the 14th century, yellow and red on white

'Nobody below the rank of Lord, Esquire or Gentleman may wear a coat, cape or smock so short that when he stands erect it fails to cover his private parts and buttocks, in which case he pays a fine of 20 shillings.'

This problem was solved by adding a piece of material to the hose and the result was that trousers

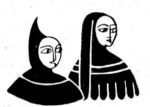

Long hose with leather soles

reappeared much as they were worn during the Iron Age. Long hose was fitted with leather soles and short hose was worn with shoes. The short trunks became underwear.

Heads and Hair Styles. After 1300, it was deemed incorrect for people of rank to appear out of doors without some head covering. When Gothic styles prevailed the usual headgear was the hood. From 1350 on, more and more material was used for the back of the hood so that it hung down over the back and could be used as a scarf during cold weather. The Burgundians varied this fashion: their extended hood was coiled on top of the head like a turban, with a tassel at the end. This tassel was used as a balance weight which could be thrown over the shoulder to keep the head covering in position. In addition to the hood, and gradually usurping its position, was the red pointed cap which remained peasant headwear for several centuries. It survives today in the traditional headgear of the Scandinavian Santa Claus. The cone-shaped cap of the early Middle Ages was now worn only by men, and hats were coming into general use. The latter had high crowns and broad brims encircled by ribbons whose ends hung free; in some cases, ribbons were decorated with ornaments or feathers.

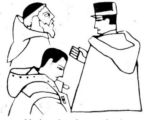

Modern hoods: monk, airman and French gendarme

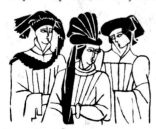

Burgundian headwear

Fashions in hair styles changed frequently and considerably. During the 1300's, hair was worn part-

ed in the middle. Around 1400, it was worn in a roll at the back of the head. In 1410, it was cut pudding-basin fashion and shaved in a straight line above the ears. There were objections to beards in 1329, since they made 'men appear like cats and dogs'. Several town authorities, in 1350, forbade the wearing of beards within town boundaries. Such directives must have been in vain, since it is known that all the kings of Europe were bearded until the end of the fourteenth century; by the beginning of the next century, however, men were universally clean-shaven.

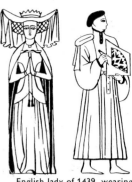

English lady of 1439, wearing 'Hell's windows' and head-dress, and Frenchman of 1440 with hood resting on his right shoulder

Up to 1350, women's faces were framed by bands of fine linen placed over the forehead and under the chin. In northern Europe, women later wore something like a bonnet, made from crimped linen or fine metal mesh, which framed the face and covered the back of the head.

The high, pointed head-dress, brought from the East by the Crusaders, appeared in Europe after 1400. It was built on a frame, or even a number of frames, and assumed fantastic shapes like horns, hearts or ice-cream cones, with fine veiling draped on top.

Young girls and brides, until 1420, wore their hair loose and uncovered, but after that time adopted the head-dress. The hair on the forehead and temples was shaved, and each eyebrow was plucked to make a thin arch.

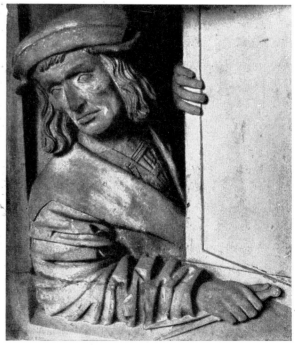

Austrian master-builder, 1512. Carving on the pulpit of St. Stephan's Cathedral

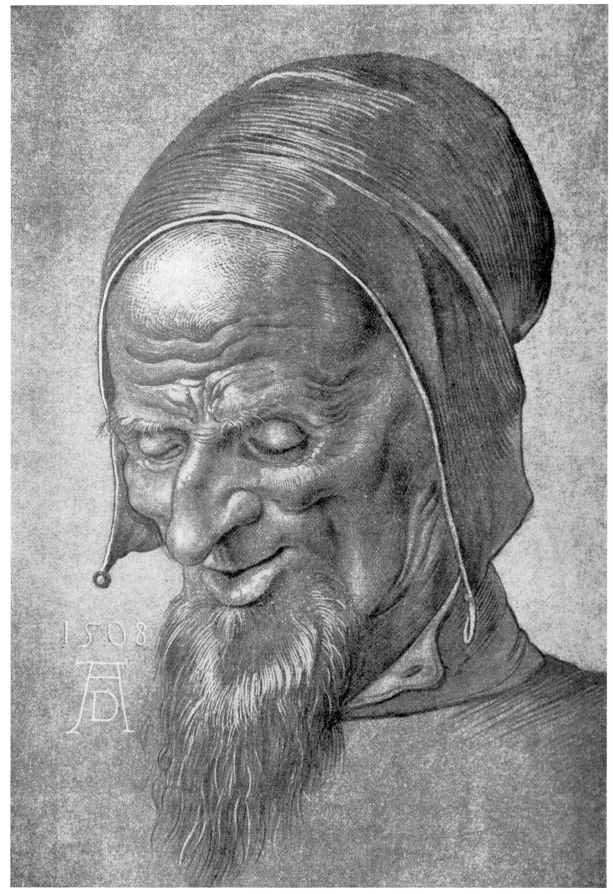

Old man with hood that fastened under the chin. His upper lip is shaven, but he wears a beard of the type once favoured by old sea-dogs. Drawing by Albrecht Dürer

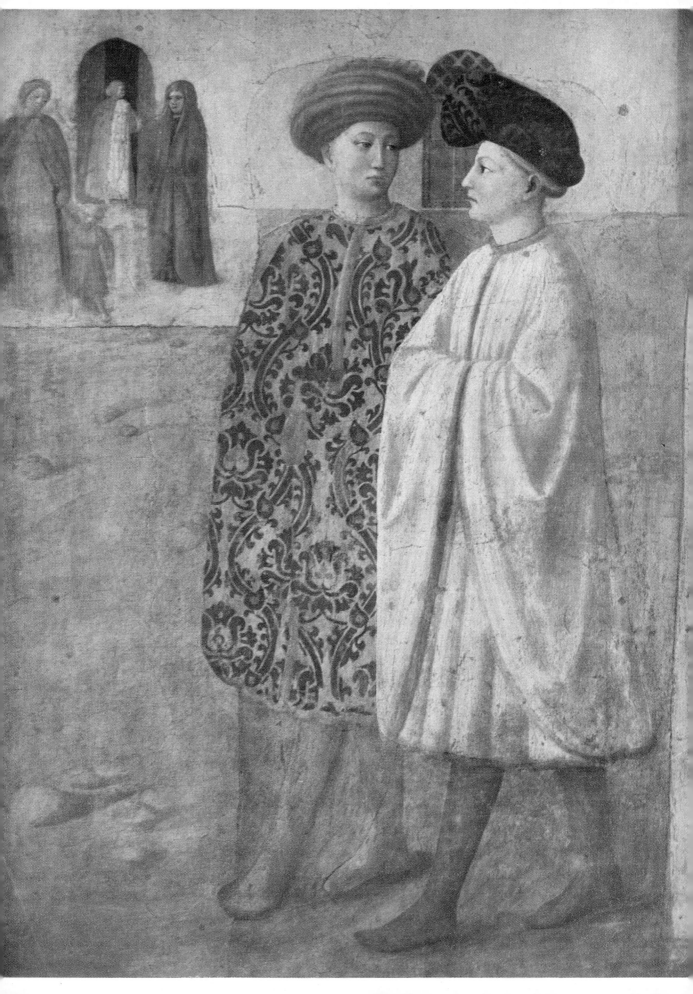

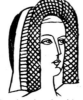

Early versions of women's hats: headband and linen band under the chin, hair-net of metal wire and cap with linen piping

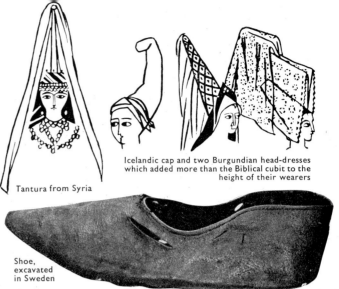

Icelandic cap and two Burgundian head-dresses which added more than the Biblical cubit to the height of their wearers

Tantura from Syria

Hell's Windows.

Around 1330, the loose shift worn by women became less voluminous and more close-fitting. Instead of concealing, it tended to emphasize the contours of the body. Eventually, the upper and lower sections of women's dress were made separately and then sewn together; the upper part was fastened with buttons. The blouse and skirt of that time were the forerunners of traditional female dress. The fashion

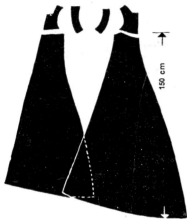

Pattern of Queen Margrethe of Sweden's dress in Uppsala, ca. 1400

developed further during the Renaissance and continues in the present day.

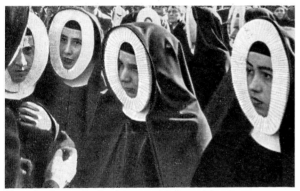

Nuns of today wearing head-dresses with linen piping

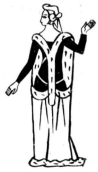

Fur-trimmed and lined overshift; an undershift in a different colour is worn underneath

High-born women wore an undershift with long sleeves and an overshift with full, elbow-length sleeves. After 1330, the shorter sleeves of the overshift disappeared, leaving a wide opening, 'Hell's Windows', through which it was possible to see the close-fitting undergarment. A train was added to the overshift at the beginning of the fifteenth century. In the case of noblewomen, trains could be so long that page-boys were employed to carry them. These long trains were referred to by monks as 'the dance floor of the devil'. Soon afterwards, women's dresses adopted the fur-trimmed sleeves of the men.

Opposite Florentine youths of about 1425. Painting by Masolino

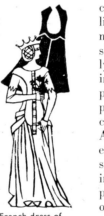

French dress of about 1375 with its basic pattern

Shoe, excavated in Sweden

Devil's Horn.

The type of footwear then worn, whether it was the close-fitting hose or the leather covering sewn round the foot, left little or no room for the toes to move. In about 1360, it was possible to establish social status merely by the shape of a person's foot: in the case of the well-to-do it was pointed; in the case of poorer people, who had gone barefoot since childhood, it was square and flat. As a result of this acquired difference, pointed footwear, designed specifically to emphasize it, came into fashion. Dagger-like toes appeared around 1400 and then went out of fashion. But they appeared once more some sixty years later looking like pointed horns. Since then, except for a short time during the Renaissance, the pointed shoe has remained fashionable throughout Europe. At least one English foot-specialist has recorded his disapproval of the natural foot,

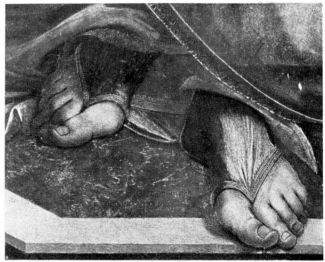

'Perfect feet' painted by Botticelli, ca. 1500

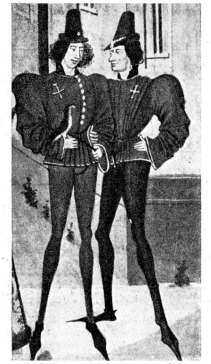

Fifteenth-century Burgundian dandies in tall hats. Flemish miniature

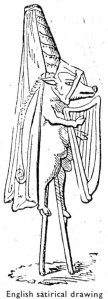

English satirical drawing of the 14th century, deriding the tall head-wear and the high stilt-like wooden sandals

'The truth is that the feet of children who have been accustomed to go barefoot become broad and coarse and far from the ideal foot as envisaged by the great painters and sculptors.'

Man's Armour and Woman's Dress. It is remarkable how difficult it was to get away completely from the long loose dress. One part or another of clothing was continually singled out for development or exaggeration — veils, trains (sometimes nineteen yards long), immense outrageous head-dresses looking like tops of wedding cakes, shoulders puffed out like balloons, shoes so long that the tips had to be bent back and tied to the knees. The Byzantines, for instance, were not even aware of such a concept as a train. Might all these extravagances have been a revolt against the rigid ideas of the time?

Let us compare the basic dress of the woman with the male's casing of steel armour.

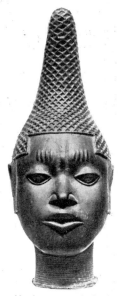

Headwear worn in Benin, West Africa

Garments as close fitting as an eel's skin can give the wearer a strong sense of self-control and inviolability, manoeuvring in them seems easy. Women, however, perhaps more aware of their own personalities than men — elected to express themselves through the medium of fantastic head-dresses, pointed shoes, puffed shoulders and billowing sleeves. Their light voluminous draperies provided a counterpart to the iron-clad male severity. The same elaboration characterizes the jewellery of the time. From 1350 bells were frequently attached to their dresses, suspended from belts and from garters, hung on chains around the shoulders. They could even be so arranged and tuned that they produced a tinkling melody when their wearer moved. Well-born young girls, however, wore a simple golden virgin's crown.

The dress of this time indicated the distinction between the sexes far more clearly than during the earlier Middle Ages. By now, both male and female dress was associated with sex appeal. Women had acquired more influence in the choice of husbands, or at least in the choice of lovers. Previously the initial stages of love and the ritual of love itself had been brief, arbitrary and stylized. Among the Germanic and Celtic races women had never danced. But now dancing and ball games became quite a usual form of entertainment for both sexes.

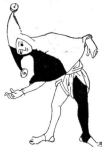

Court Jester with bells on his cap, late 15th century

Male attire excelled female attire in beauty and in colour, but women's dresses now showed the first signs of decolleté. John Huss deplored this fashion when he wrote in 1400,

'Women wear their dresses so open round the neck laying bare almost half the bosom, whether in God's House, in view of priests and clerics, in the market place, or even in the home. And what is hidden of the bosom is artificially enlarged and pressed upwards until it seems that they have two horns on their bosoms.'

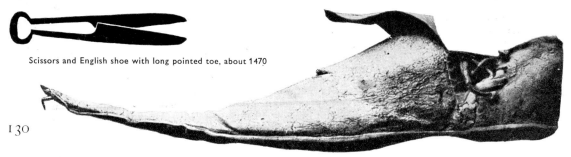

Scissors and English shoe with long pointed toe, about 1470

Twin-horned Flemish head-dress of the 15th century

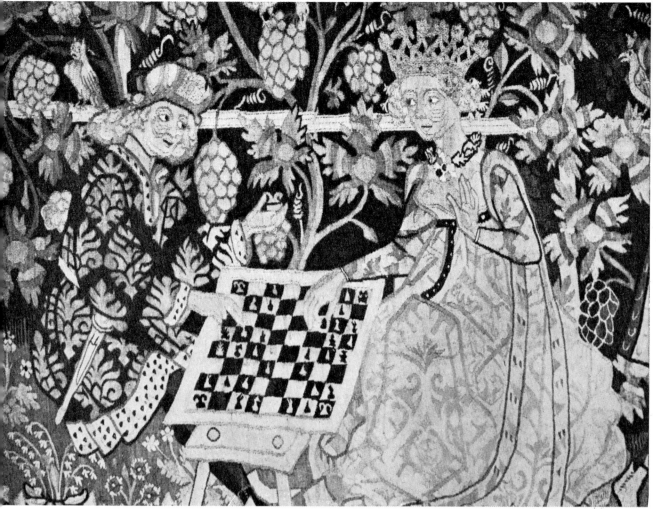

Swiss chess players on a mid 15th-century tapestry. His palmetto-patterned coat has sleeves and is trimmed with fur; she wears a sleeveless over-shift and virgin's crown

Women had now discovered a weapon which could be employed in two ways: they could assert their power by either revealing or concealing their bodies.

customary for men to sit on the right and women on the left.

Differences in Male and Female Dress. Certain basic distinctions between male and female dress are still in existence today. For example, men button their clothes on the right and women on the left. There appears to be no very good reason for this; however, one theory is that a man can keep his right hand, his fighting hand, warm by placing it inside the front of his coat. A woman with a baby on her left arm can feed it more modestly at her breast. In the churches of many countries, it is still

English lady of 1488 and Danish gentleman of 1496

Deportment. Deportment also served to mark the difference between the sexes. Men of the Gothic period stood with shoulders back, chest out and stomach in. Their female counterparts stood with shoulders sloping backwards and stomach thrust forward. Men threw their heads back whereas women drooped theirs forward. This S-shaped stance may be seen in pictures of women throughout the later Middle Ages. The protruding stomach, of course, indicated pregnancy, which was considered a normal condition for adult women and nothing to be hidden. Even today women automatically assume this position

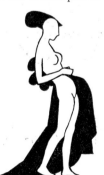

Posture in the Gothic period

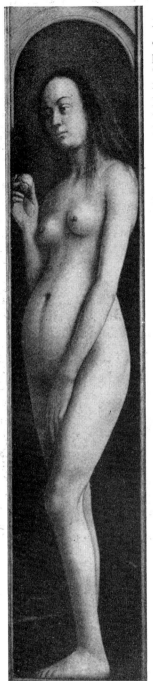

Eve, painted by Van Eyck, ca. 1425

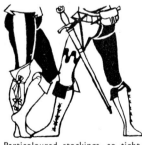

Particoloured stockings, so tight that it is clear the wearers have no need to bow and scrape

which may be the result of recent childbirth or possibly just fatigue. Chairs also played a part in creating the general posture. By this time, the chair was no longer a place of honour. Everyone had his or her own chair complete with back, so that huddling together on the floor was no longer necessary. Gothic frescoes show free-er, less restrained movements among artisan and peasant classes; moderate and restrained gestures, however, are represented as typifying the higher classes.

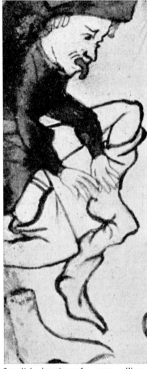

Swedish drawing of a man pulling on his stockings

Colourful Uniforms and Black Velvet.

The first uniform originated at court, where the various categories of courtier were denoted by clothes of different colours. In 1459, a troop of thirteen hundred cavalrymen was equipped by a Rhenish nobleman and

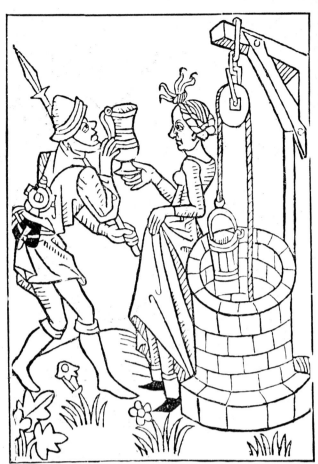

Gothic postures, a woodcut of the late Gothic period

went to battle in his personal colours of blue and white. This custom spread to such a degree that colourful dress came to be associated with soldiers and was, therefore, regarded as unsuitable for civilian wear. When the Emperor Frederick visited Rome in 1468, he and his retinue were dressed totally in black velvet. With this shift in fashion, only soldiers and women could be admired for their colourful clothes.

The Tailor's Craft.

Towards the end of the Middle Ages, fashionable clothes ceased to be made at home. A new profession, that of the tailor, came into being. The number of tailors in Paris increased between 1292 and 1300 from four hundred and eighty-two to seven hundred and two. By this time each catered either for men or women exclusively. An anonymous complainant in 1380 bewailed,

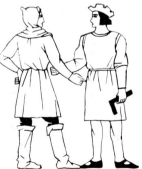

Artisans, 1475

'To be a good tailor yesterday is of no use today. Cut and fashions alter too quickly.'

Till this time, the art of tailoring and its influence on fashion had been the women's province. From now on it was a profession for men.

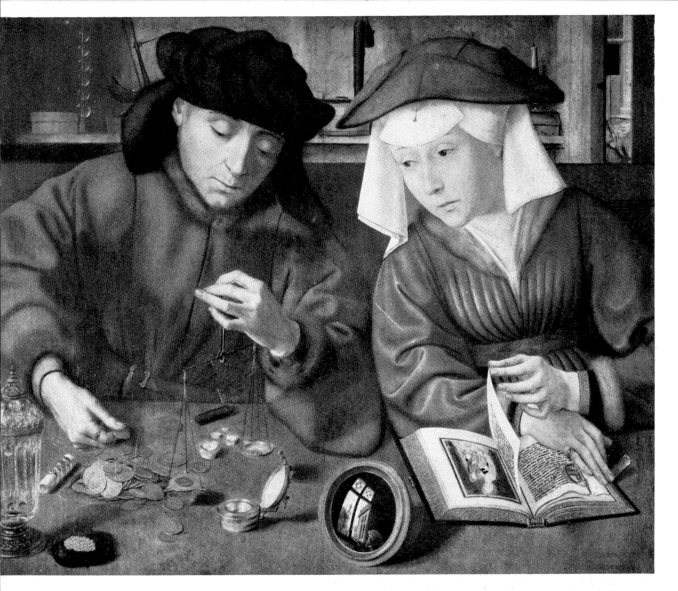

RENAISSANCE FASHION

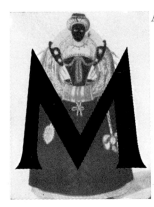**M**ANY examples of the new Renaissance style of dress were found in Scandinavia after 1490. But Renaissance architecture did not reach the Nordic countries until about 1550. Fashion reacted to new trends more quickly than architecture for the simple reason that it was easier and quicker to build a new dress than to build a new house.

The Renaissance affected people by making them more self-aware and extrovert. Clothes were taken very seriously. We read, for instance, of a merchant in

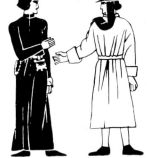

Merchants of about 1500

Augsburg who, throughout his life, commissioned a portrait of himself each time he acquired a new outfit.

The economic background of the Renaissance in Western Europe is the institution of a money economy. Commodities were produced far beyond daily requirements of the village or city. Consumer goods were now competing on the open market with recognized price levels and values.

Traders and financiers took the place of the feudal barons as rulers of society and formed a liaison with

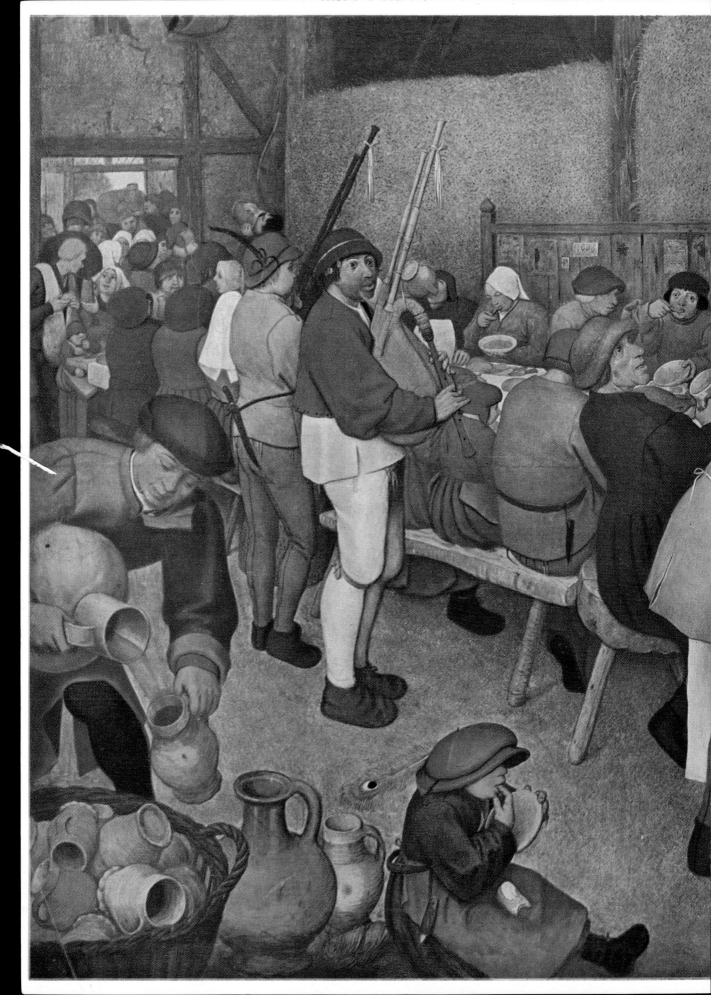

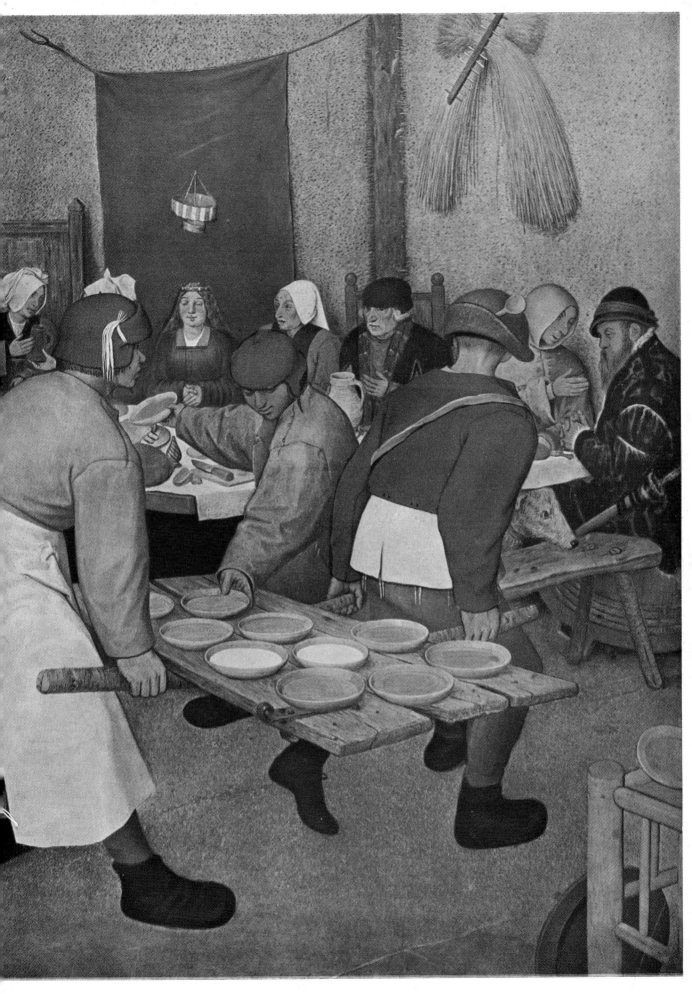

royalty to counter the power of the old ruling classes. A strong sense of freedom was abroad and ordinary citizens responded eagerly to the possibilities of progress in all spheres of life. Individuals previously restrict-

Peasant shoe from the beginning of the 16th century

ed by the conventions of village communities, guilds and monasteries were now liberated from their old ties and inhibitions. Horizons widened, limitless opportunities presented themselves. Christopher Columbus had discovered America, Vasco da Gama had opened up the sea route to India. The studies of the astronomer, Tycho Brahe, enabled Keppler to discover that the earth rotated on its own axis.

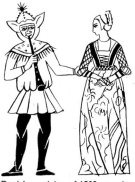

Danish musician of 1503, wearing a hood and cape with donkey's ears, and German lady of 1507 in a dress with skirt and bodice of different materials

New Directions of Thought.
Artists, such as Leonardo da Vinci and Michelangelo, and writers, such

as Shakespeare and Cervantes, opened up new perspectives. Whereas heaven and earth, in the old conception of the Universe, had been closely inter-related and the soul linked with eternity, the new world was felt to be limitless; the course of the soaring planets was vigorous, free and unconstrained by influence from above. No longer did men's sights stop at heaven above and hell below; now they took in the whole world, a world in which each man was unique, an individual standing alone in relation to all earthly circumstances.

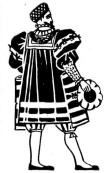

The Renaissance coat with sleeves

The earlier intense concentration on attaining heaven gave way to a broad critical awareness of this world. In a similar way the vertical emphasis of architecture and dress was replaced by an emphasis on the horizontal.

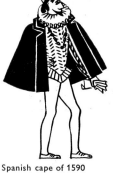

The individualism of the first half of the sixteenth century was a determining force in every aspect of life — religion, social organization and dress, all were affected by this disturbing and transforming energy.

It must be acknowledged that Spanish court dress with its expansive crinolines and wadded pantaloons, worn during the latter part of the sixteenth century in rigid court ceremonies,

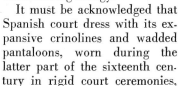

Spanish cape of 1590

was extremely uncomfortable. But this impressive style was intended to signify the alliance between the royal court and a new system of capitalism. Similar trends were to be seen in other countries during the Reformation, and new patterns were established in the forms of religious worship.

Propaganda and Expediency.
Religious worship during the Middle Ages related all human action to the Absolute — to God and eternity — but now religion gave way to worldly considerations. Machiavelli formulated the principles of practical politics. Falsehood and hypocrisy, previously regarded as sinful, were now considered praiseworthy, if they achieved the desired end.

The princes confiscated church property during the Reformation in order to save the souls of their

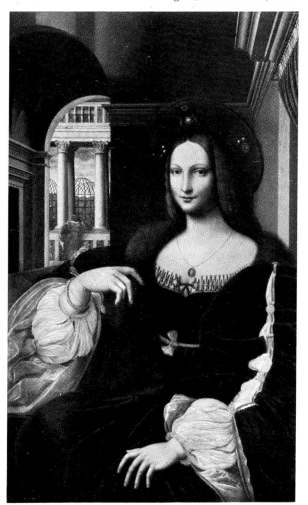

The wide sleeves of the early Renaissance. Painting ascribed to Leonardo da Vinci

The tight sleeve of the later Renaissance

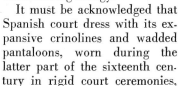

English burgher of 1517 and German vagrant of 1520

subjects. For a century, all wars were carried out

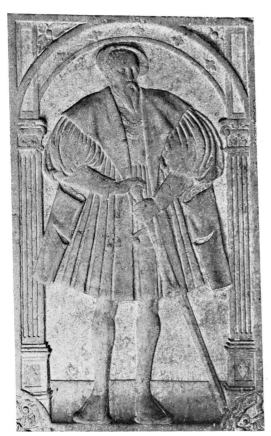

Danish tombstone, 1566. The free-hanging sleeves have slits for the arms to go through

'When Francis I came to Paris in 1521 he was attired in silver lamé. His retinue of noblemen were clad in golden material and white silk. His marshals were dressed in gold and silver brocade and his officers in golden material trimmed with crimson velvet. The knights were dressed in red or black velvet with golden appliqué and the archers in white velvet, embroidered with silver lilies. The leading citizens of Paris were dressed in black, scarlet or crimson velvet.'

The colourful uniforms of the Papal Guard, attributed to Michelangelo, bear witness to the violent outbursts of colour which occurred at this time and, indeed, continued to do so for as long as ostentation, bodily pleasures and sensuous delight were considered desirable and proper.

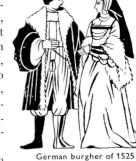

German burgher of 1525 and English noblewoman of 1530

Attitudes changed when the sober dress of the Spanish court became general. Colours became sombre and limited, with black as the principal colour. Armour was no longer worn because military conditions no longer required it, but its influence remained in the shape of starched linen and padded garments. Brilliant colours came to

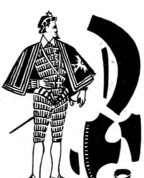

Spanish suit of 1551 with patterns of the facing of the collar, cape, jerkin, sleeves etc.

be associated more and more with military uniforms and a means of conveying rank.

in the name of God and religion. When the Netherlands fought Spain it was ostensibly for religion. But the real reason, safeguarding their flourishing trade, was never mentioned. Make-believe and pretence were admired greatly. Significantly, the modern theatre was born in this century.

Venice – Madrid Axis. The North Italian merchant cities, notably Venice, remained centres of European

Patterned velvet blocked in colour from the 16th century

fashion for as long as the Mediterranean trade route with the East was predominant. When gold started to flow into Europe from America, however, Spain assumed leadership.

The delight in rich colours and fabrics so alive in the Middle Ages continued throughout the first half of the sixteenth century. Silk, velvet, damask, brocade and gold and silver lamé were used for the clothes of both sexes. The favourite colours were scarlet, yellow, parrot green and sky blue. An historian relates,

Mobile Men and Immobile Women. Short clothes that exposed men's legs came in with the Renaissance and the Reformation. The male body eventually came to resemble a rectangular block supported on two slender poles, rather like a letter H. The great display of virility that this age witnessed is typified by the tight-fitting sleeves and hose, designed to show off strong limbs and muscles, and the padded shoulders that suggested a sturdy frame. Slits were cut at the elbows and knees to allow freedom of movement.

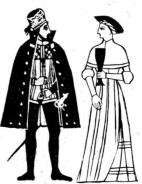

German gentleman of 1563 and Danish lady of 1576

While men looked like mobile beings on stilts, women still remained all muffled up in mountains of clothes. The more voluminous the dress, the more important was the person who had access to the woman within. The general outline of the woman looked like the letter X.

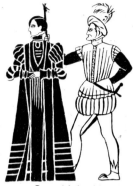

German lady of 1551 and Italian gentleman of 1552

The monumental crinoline, worn over layer upon layer of petticoats, was an expression of riches that proclaimed its wearer an obvious item of capital investment. The crinoline dress was like a cage; it guaranteed that the wearer could not indulge in any unbecoming escapades. (Women were not to apply the Renaissance slogans of freedom to themselves.) Men used it to provide tangible evidence of their wealth; they made the cage so big and so beautiful that woman's sole function was to move around in it, as if she were a covered wagon.

As women were treated more and more like decorative possessions, their own value became debased until they were eventually little more than objects for

sexual enjoyment. Endearments in the Middle Ages drew their metaphors from flowers; the Renaissance, on the other hand, expressed its affections in figures of speech borrowed from the animal world.

In both trade and politics, the spirit of this new era was evident in the accepted techniques of duplicity. This philosophy was reflected in a manner of dress which was misleading and, which departed entirely from the natural shape and curves of the body.

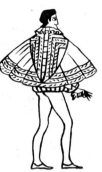

Spanish cape of 1590

Aesthetically Renaissance dress must be regarded in relation to current architecture which juxtaposed dramatic shapes and a great sense of space. The focus of architectural interest moved from churches to palaces. Consequently Renaissance dress was modified to match these new conditions.

The Spanish Cape and the Split Jerkin. The knee-length jerkin, worn under the coat at the beginning of

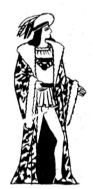

the sixteenth century, was plain at the top and cut like a skirt from the waist down. Towards the middle of the century, it started to resemble a sleeveless waistcoat and was worn over the long-sleeved undershirt. Even though male dress was so close-fitting, it was still felt that the underclothes should be seen; hence the slits found in the outer garments. Someone wrote in 1544,

'The tailor hacks, hews and cuts the material so that only narrow strips remain.'

English coat with long sleeves, ca. 1500

Laws, customs and social conditions were all undergoing drastic change. Fashion responded to the new spirit and developed accordingly.

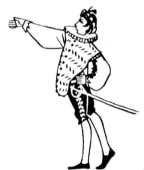

Soldiers needed more freedom to handle the heavy weapons now in use, without running the risk of bursting at the seams. Padding became more pronounced and waistlines dropped. From 1575 to 1600 a piece of material known as 'the goose's stomach' protruded in a point below the waist, sleeves were cut in the shape of a leg of mutton.

The goose's stomach

After 1600, the short coat was shaped rather like a corset fitting closely at the waist, the lower part grew in length, the shoulders became broader and the sleeves tighter.

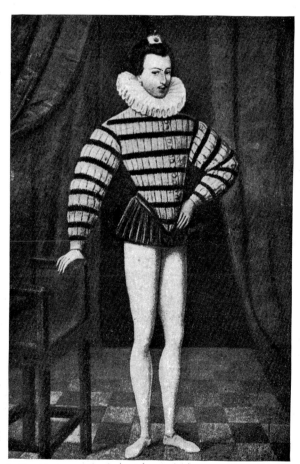

Fashionably-dressed Frenchman from the court of Henry III

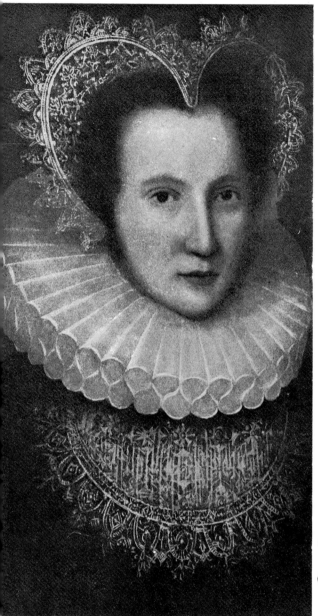

Mary Queen of Scots wearing a ruff which seems to offer the wearer's head on a platter. She was in fact decapitated, a form of execution reserved for persons of quality; commoners were hanged. It is interesting to note, incidentally, that women during the French Revolution wore red ribbons around their necks 'à la guillotine'

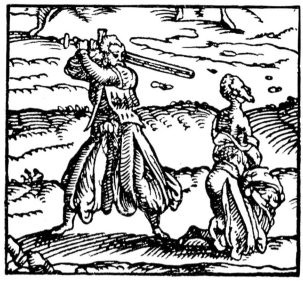

Execution of a brigand, 1564. Both executioner and victim wear trunk hose and the executioner's coat has slits. German woodcut by Jost Amman

Swiss soldier of fortune, his suit bedecked with ostrich feathers. Drawing by Urs Graf, 1523

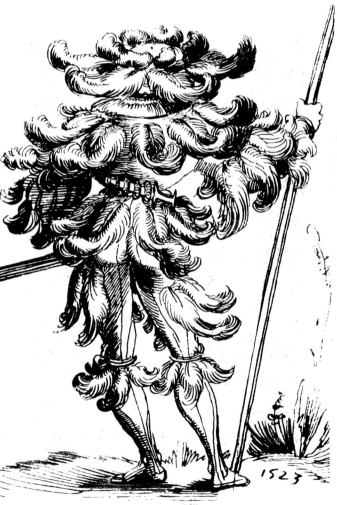

Millstones Round the Neck. At the beginning of the sixteenth century, the neck opening was large and square. Twenty-five years later, the neckline was

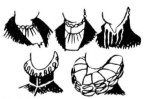

Neck fashions

gathered into fine pleats by a ribbon. From this time, necklines were cut very much higher and sometimes embroidered round the top. A piece of gathered material at the neck made its appearance at this time and the career of the ruff began. By 1550, the coat was built up over the chest, and tapered to the closely fitting neck. The gathered addition to the neckline gradually increased in size until, twenty years

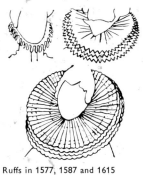

later, the neck was entirely surrounded by a ruff. Between 1580 and 1600, the ruff achieved such vast proportions that the head looked as if it were resting on a plate. This huge ruff features in the vestments of the Lutheran clergy of Denmark and Norway to this day. In 1630, an open lace collar took the place of the ruff, and matching lace was worn round the wrists. The latter were the forerunners of the shirt cuff.

Ruffs in 1577, 1587 and 1615

Voluminous Trousers. The general desire to show off masses of rich material received a welcome bonus

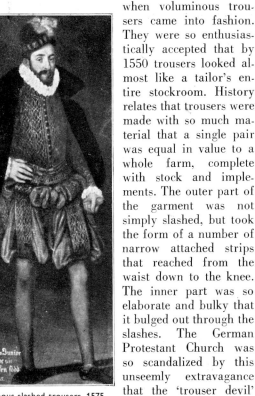

when voluminous trousers came into fashion. They were so enthusiastically accepted that by 1550 trousers looked almost like a tailor's entire stockroom. History relates that trousers were made with so much material that a single pair was equal in value to a whole farm, complete with stock and implements. The outer part of the garment was not simply slashed, but took the form of a number of narrow attached strips that reached from the waist down to the knee. The inner part was so elaborate and bulky that it bulged out through the slashes. The German Protestant Church was so scandalized by this unseemly extravagance that the 'trouser devil' was placed seventeenth in their list of the twenty devils.

Voluminous slashed trousers, 1575

The explorer, Andreas Musculus, asserted in a thesis written at this time that,

'Sinfulness and common misery have advanced so far because of a new and particularly malicious devil which just lately has emerged from Hell to enter into the trousers of our young men.

'The trunk hoses are a temptation to immorality and are contrary to the word of God, the Holy Baptism and the Fourth Commandment.

'They transgress against our customs, our religion and the image of God in which we are made.'

The Codpiece. Trousers were a development of the

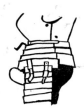

original hose and retained the codpiece. This had been in use from the end of the Late Gothic period but was gradually growing larger, until it eventually reached the size of a child's head. It was made from a different material than the trousers. The codpiece became necessary because of the close fit of the trousers, and was designed and made up with a disconcerting frankness. It was not until 1560, however, that it achieved its most provoking proportions. Rabelais' description of the codpiece of his hero, while slightly exaggerated, does illustrate the tendency of the period to enlarge and elaborate on an element of dress.

Codpiece

'For the codpiece sixteen yards of material was required. The shape was that of a triumphal arch, most elegant and

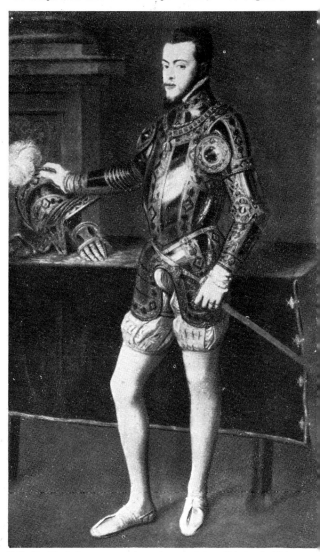

Philip II of Spain in armour and wearing a codpiece. Painting by Titian

Opposite Henry VIII of England's third wife, Jane Seymour, 1536. Her dress is in red velvet adorned with pearls and rubies. The sleeves and skirt are made of silver brocade. Painting by Holbein

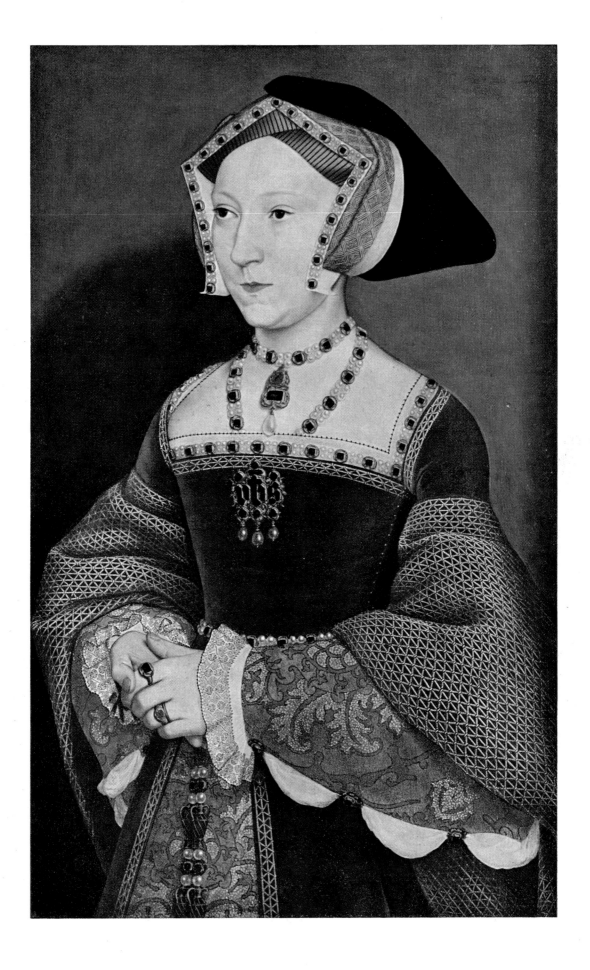

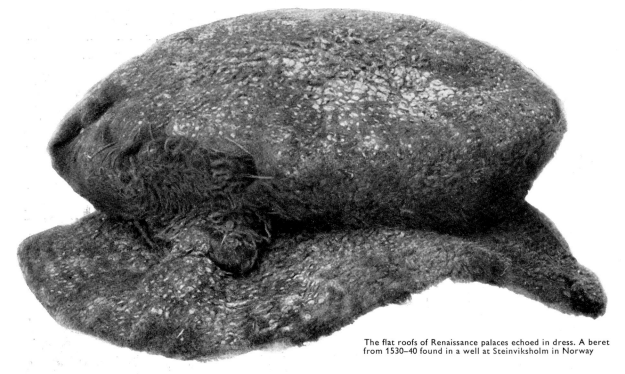

The flat roofs of Renaissance palaces echoed in dress. A beret from 1530–40 found in a well at Steinviksholm in Norway

secured by two golden rings fastened to enamelled buttons, each the size of an orange and set with heavy emeralds. The codpiece protruded forward as much as three feet and was grooved like the trousers and fitted with a loosely hanging front-piece made of blue damask.'

The French style of trousers was introduced into the Nordic countries about this time. They covered only the upper part of the thighs and

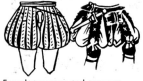

French trousers, and trousers with outer covering

were padded with horsehair, chaff or bran. They frequently had vertical slashes through which the lining could be seen and admired.

Toward the end of the seventeenth century, men began to wear knee breeches which were open at the bottom hem. Hose or stockings were worn on the lower part of the leg and were embroidered with a linen clock to cover the seam. In 1580, stockings

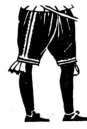

Knee breeches left wide at the hem

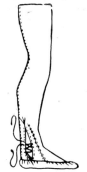

Linen stocking with lacing and stocking with clock ca. 1800

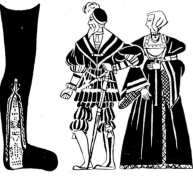

German mercenary of 1538, English noblewoman of 1539

were made from an elastic jersey-like material. Knitted stockings originated in France and Spain round about 1550 but did not reach the Nordic countries until after 1600.

Comfortable Shoes. With the disappearance of the old-fashioned hose with leather soles attached, boots

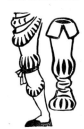

Slit stocking and boot

and shoes became a regular part of dress. After 1590 they acquired a new shape. The special fondness for ample line which existed during the Renaissance endowed footwear with good proportions and room for the toes to move. At first this new style of shoe looked like a duck's bill, but by 1510 it had come to resemble a bear's paw. The shoe was fastened by a strap over the instep, and the uppers covered the toes only. Some thirty years later, the uppers again enclosed the entire foot, and by 1560 the toe had again become slightly pointed.

Hat, Hair and Beards. Headwear, after the excesses of the fifteenth century, returned to a more simple shape, and the plain cap made a fresh appearance. A beret like the one worn by Martin Luther was common in Northern Europe from 1515 to 1530. During the subsequent twenty years, a flat beret made of velvet, silk or cloth was popular.

The beret then yield-

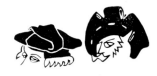

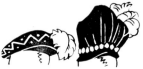

Headwear in 1525 above, and below in 1565

ed place to the tall hat. With its narrow brim and high crown, it looked like a sugar-loaf or a waste-paper basket upside down. The material most favoured for it was soft felt made of beaver hair. After 1600, the crown became even taller and the brim wider. The

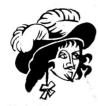

Man's plait, the cadenette

most common material was felt, and it was sometimes decorated with nodding feathers. In 1500, masculine fashion in hair style dictated a fringe cut straight across the forehead and hair falling to shoulder-length at the back and sides. The face itself was clean-shaven. A little later the trend was towards short hair and a very long beard. In 1535, the beard was divided, and from 1570 the moustache was brushed upwards in a sweep at either side. Short hair with side curls came into fashion; the hair at the back of the head was braided into a plait known as the cadenette, which was brought forward over the shoulder.

Décolleté. Until 1550, women's dresses normally comprised a bodice and skirt sewn together.

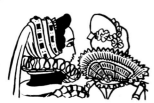

Collars of mid 16th and early 17th centuries

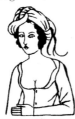

Sixteenth-century décolletage

The deep cut of the bodice went so far that the nipples were exposed. All through this period most of the bosom continued to be exposed. The bodice was laced so that the breasts were pressed upwards until they were said to look like a pair of turtle doves.

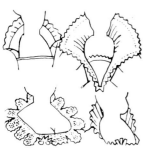

Collars in 1590, 1598, 1635 and 1778

After 1520, the bosom became again covered. The neckline was still cut on the same lines but a piece of pleated or embroidered linen was worn over the cleavage. A small frill was later sewn along the edge; by 1550, it had extended all round the neck, matching the ruff then worn by the men. At the turn of the seventeenth century, lace collars became fashionable for women. These were large and were supported on a wire frame worn over a décolleté bodice. The latter was laced so tightly that it was almost like a strait-jacket.

Skirt, bodice and sleeves were frequently made in different colours. Gold or silver belts were worn around the waist with a purse or the equivalent of a handbag attached.

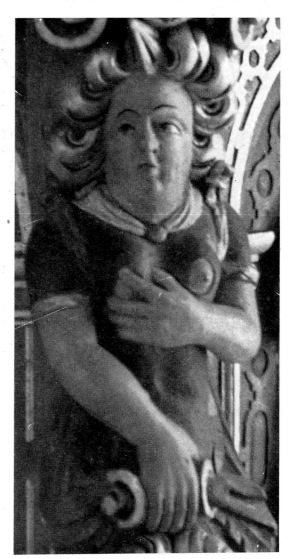

Dress with openings for the nipples, 1599. Carved figure from a Danish pulpit

Spanish and French Crinolines. Until this juncture, women favoured somewhat heavy materials, such as velvet, satin, taffeta and moirée. Their dresses were usually embroidered with pearls or diamanté which made them even heavier. But as this point, a rather different Spanish style was introduced. Here we find a dress seemingly consisting of two triangles of wadded material laced and so positioned that the points faced one another. The bodice and skirt were made in separate parts, but usually from the same material. The sleeves, however, were usually made of a different fabric and were slashed and puffed out.

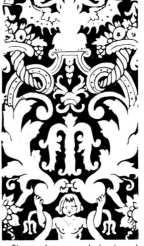

Sixteenth-century design in red, yellow and white on Italian silk

After 1550, the Spanish crinoline came in. This was made of felt or canvas built over a framework of wire

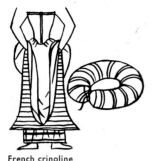

or whalebone and covered by a skirt and bell-shaped underskirt. The outer dress was made with an opening in the shape of an inverted V, which permitted the underskirt to show.

The French crinoline made its appearance about 1660. This had cushions sewn under it at the back

French crinoline

and front. An additional circular cushion, something like an inflated tyre, was suspended round the hips.

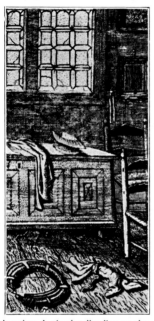

This had the effect of holding the dress out horizontally so that it looked like an enormous ruff. The material was not allowed to fall in natural folds but was stretched out taut and decorated with bows, ribbons and borders.

One thing that can be said for the crinoline is that it served to keep people at a distance. Nor did the wearer mind, of course, if lesser mortals got the impression that the mechanism of the woman of breeding was more delicate and she herself more complicated than the simple country girl!

Interior. A piped collar lies on the chest and on the floor, stockings garters and hip cushion

In 1550, women's sleeves puffed out and tapered off like pipe stems. Apparently female arms were thought to express too much sex-appeal in their natural shape and, therefore, had to be camouflaged.

Heads and Feet. At the start of the sixteenth century, the imaginative and stylish headgears previously sported by women disappeared. Their place was taken by the masculine beret with a close-fitting, pearl-embroidered cap underneath. Constant arguments took place as to whether or not the hair should be

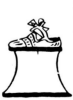

allowed to show. Italian fashion certainly never succeeded in making women hide their hair completely. At first, women took over the male fashion, on a smaller scale, but wore them at a jaunty angle. In this respect, women followed the lead of the men, albeit in humility and *en miniature*.

Venetian stilt shoe

Women also copied the male fashion

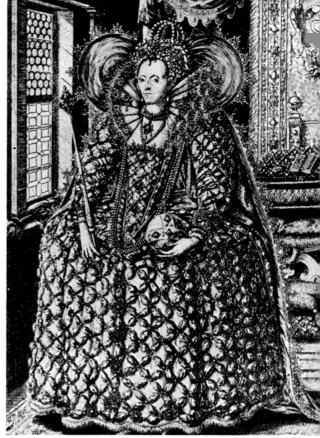

Elizabeth I of England dressed in crinoline, stiff collar and veil spread over wires. The dress is made of satin sewn with pearls and rubies

in shoes. The Venetian stilt shoe was so popular in Southern Europe that women were described in one proverb as being 'half flesh and half wood'. Society women, when out walking, had to be assisted by a servant; the present custom in which a male escort offers his arm to his female companion, is a relic of those early times when support was necessary.

The Position of Women. When considering woman's position in Renaissance society, we must go back to

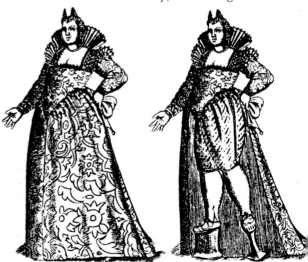

Venetian lady, 1592, with stilted shoes and trousers

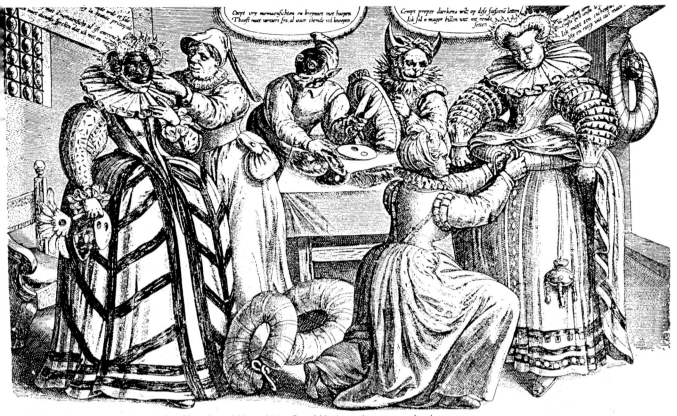

Flemish dress store, ca. 1580, which sold masks and hip cushions. Broad hips were in vogue at the time

the time when witches were persecuted. Witchcraft was not, as many people think, a phenomenon of the Middle Ages. Sanction for the prosecution of witches was not given by the Pope until 1484; the last trial of witches in Denmark took place in 1700. It should be noted, too, that witches were always female.

If, in the tradition of the Middle Ages, women were the black sheep of society, during the Renaissance, they dominated the sphere of social intercourse. Highly educated women, even women with scientific

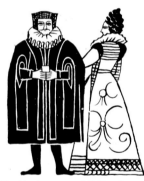

Danish clergyman of 1593 and German lady of 1594

training, were no longer uncommon. Erasmus, in one of his colloquies, permits an educated woman to defend herself vigorously against the criticism of a clergyman who suggested that she should stick to her spinning wheel instead of studying Latin. Martin Luther, on the other hand, often expressed the opinion that,

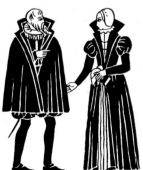

Danish husband and wife, 1610

'No dress or garment is less becoming to a woman than a show of intelligence.'

In Protestant countries, the wife would read from the Bible at mealtimes. Her sphere of influence was restricted to the Bible, the kitchen, housekeeping and household accounts. The high-born woman was represented on tombstones with folded hands and downcast eyes, and smaller in size than her husband.

Respectable Prostitutes. Women had more independence in the south than in other parts of Europe. The prostitutes of Venice issued a circular in 1509 which provided addresses, fees

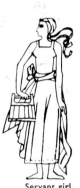

Servant girl, 16th century

and other detailed information. A visit to the beautiful Livia Azzolini, we read, would cost twenty-five scudi, whereas patronizing the less beautiful Veronica Franco would cost only two scudi.

These women could also be found in company considerably removed from their establishments: witness the following description of everyday life at the Papal Court given by a Papal master of ceremonies. An evening's entertainment in the Vatican on the last day of October 1501 would seem surely to have parallels with a modern strip club

'Fifty respectable prostitutes were present, so-called courtesans, who after dinner danced with the servants and with others present. At the beginning they were clothed but later

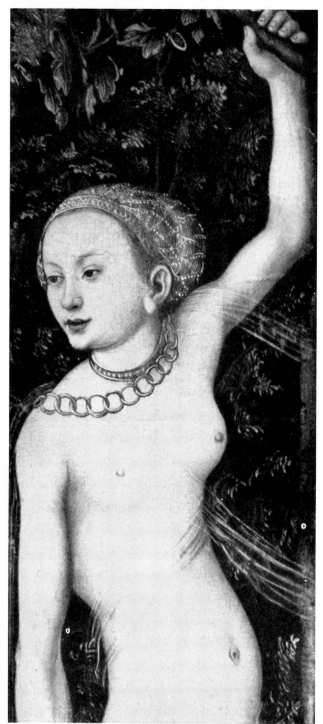

German Venus, 1528. Painting by Lucas Cranach

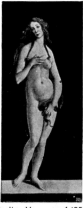

Italian Venus, c. 1485
Painting by Botticelli

of inquisitiveness and curiosity developed. Because the naked body was the principal subject-matter of art one can recognize the physical prototype of this period better than at any other time in history. The slender outlines of Botticelli's maidens reflect the aristocratic elegance of the Gothic period. The women in the paintings of Raphael, Michelangelo and Titian were the well-nurtured daughters of rich merchants. They give the impression of being women who expressed their personalities through an arrogant indolence; they evince a highly self-conscious sensuality and an erotic and monumental grandeur. Julius Lange wrote of Michelangelo's muscular youths,

'They were a revolutionary generation which one could fear, would some day refuse to work and lay down its tools.'

Beauty Culture. A considerable amount of make-up was used to improve the personal appearance. Blond hair was greatly prized in Venice and achieved by

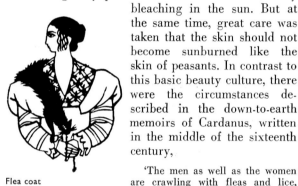

Flea coat

bleaching in the sun. But at the same time, great care was taken that the skin should not become sunburned like the skin of peasants. In contrast to this basic beauty culture, there were the circumstances described in the down-to-earth memoirs of Cardanus, written in the middle of the sixteenth century,

'The men as well as the women are crawling with fleas and lice, and the odour from their armpits, feet and mouths is quite terrible.'

The 'flea coat' existed, an item of party dress expressly designed to attract fleas into its fur. A nobleman of the time advised his son to wander about for a while in a cape lined with wolf's fur in order to divest himself of fleas before going to bed.

If modern underwear is intended to protect the body against any dust which might find its way through the outer garments, the function of underwear during the Renaissance appears to have been the direct opposite. The costly fabrics of the outer garments had to be protected from the dirt and perspiration emanating from the body.

Thick layers of paint covered over blemishes and other imperfections of the skin, and the use of heavy perfumes apparently disguised body odours. By this time the communal baths, which had formed such an important part of daily life during the Middle Ages, had been closed because of venereal disease which had spread over the whole of Europe after the discovery of America.

they were naked. After the table had been cleared, lighted candelabras were placed on the floor and chestnuts were scattered between them. The naked women crawled about on hands and knees between the lighted candles picking up the chestnuts while the Pope, his son and daughter, and the assembled gathering looked on.'

People of the Renaissance. People in the Middle Ages were modest and shy as far as their bodies were concerned, but during the Renaissance a strong sense

146

BAROQUE LACE AND FOOTWEAR

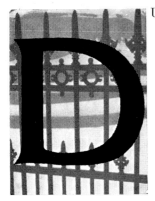

DURING the early part of the seventeenth century, the Spanish were driven out of Holland and the Dutch established their own republic. At this time, the ships of the Dutch mercantile fleet amounted in number to the total of all the other European fleets combined. When her naval supremacy and her stake in the New World was a thing of the past, Spain was forced to take an inferior position in European affairs. Amsterdam became the centre of European banking and finance. The first real capitalistic system, a cooperative effort on the part of industry, shipping and mercantile interests, was established by the Dutch in the seventeenth century. In France Louis XIV became the first absolute ruler in Europe, possessing dictatorial power. During the first half of the century, the main influence on manners, style

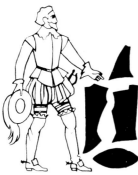

Gentleman of the early 17th century and the pattern for his clothes

and fashion came from the burghers of Holland but passed, in the latter part of the century, to the French Court at Versailles. Europe also gained a new perspective in geography: the Turks reached Vienna,

and European culture was introduced, willy-nilly into Russia by Peter the Great.

Galileo and Newton laid the foundations of modern physics. Spinoza propounded the philosophy of dialectic materialism. One of the most notable artistic innovations of the time was the musical drama; the first opera house was built in Venice in 1637. By 1650, performances were introduced by an orchestral overture. This transition from vocal to instrumental music parallels the advance made from handicrafts to industry, such as the manufacture of cloth, paper and glass. The first steam engine was built by Papin in 1688. Manners became more refined; the upper classes no longer ate with their fingers but used forks. Ice cream and mayonnaise were made for the first time, and people began to use tobacco and snuff.

Propaganda. Trade and industry became the driving forces of society and money became absolute dictator. A king had to ask his bankers for funds before embarking on a war, though since wars were almost always profitable money was usually forthcoming. The magnificent Baroque architecture of these times is evidenced by the castles, which were in fact aimed at impressing people with the wealth and importance of the castles' owners. The ruler had at all times to be sure of maintaining his power; he had always to display great dignity and pomp, his demeanour had always to inspire respect. The essence of the time was embodied in the qualities of splendour and reserve. Johann Sebastian Bach as no other expressed in his music the spirit of the age.

Spanish Cape and Polish Kassak. Spanish fashion had been, at the start of the seventeenth century, the

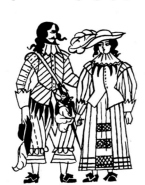

German husband and wife, 1629

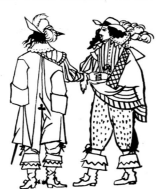

French cavaliers, 1629

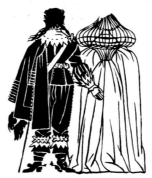

French cavalier with lace, 1635, and lady of 1633 with veil and collar in one

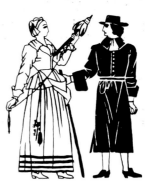

Frenchwoman with spindle,1680, and artisan, ca. 1700

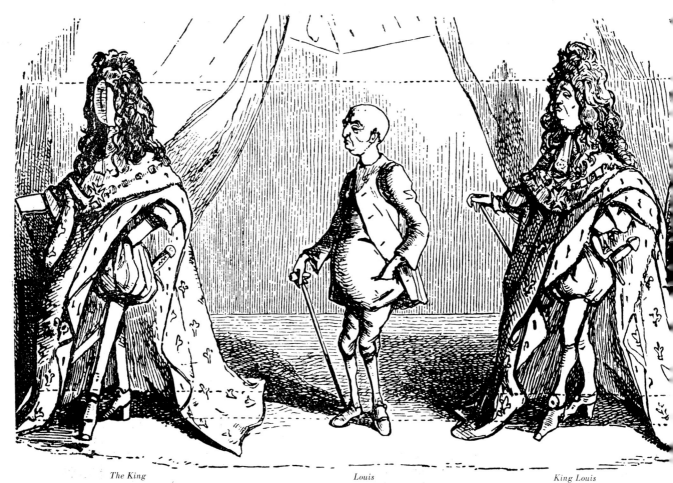

The King   *Louis*   *King Louis*

English caricature by W. M. Thackeray of the French painter Rigaud's portrait of Louis XIV

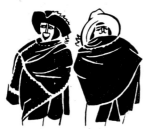

Two ways to drape the cape

dominating influence on European dress. With its sombre colours and severe lines, it produced a figure at once magnified by solemnity yet restricted by obligations of duty. By 1620, however, the initiative had passed to Holland, not because of any drastic reaction against Spanish fashion, but rather as a gradual change towards a looser cut and a more florid appearance. The circular cape became longer; it fell in graceful folds and was fastened on the shoulder by buttons. It could also be worn flung casually over the shoulders, or merely carried over the arm.

About the middle of the century, a challenger to the cape arrived from Poland. This newcomer eventually gained control of

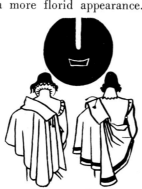

Two ways to hang the cape

the whole of Europe, and was indeed the forerunner of the jacket as we know it today. It originated in Asia, where it was known as the oriental caftan, and was renamed the kassak in Poland. The oldest surviving kassak may be seen in Rosenborg Castle in Copenhagen; this particular specimen is made with the slanted opening common in the East.

Spanish jacket

This early jacket started life with padded shoulders, a shaped waist and vents at the side and back. It was worn buttoned across the chest leaving uncovered a triangular area of shirt over the stomach. Gradually the shoulders became narrower and the waist wider. By 1650, the jacket was cut so short that a band of shirt could be seen all round the middle, so that it looked as if the wearer's trousers were falling down. When the knee-length overcoat came in,

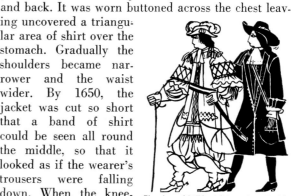

Fleming of 1676 with kassak and wide trousers, and Dutchman with overcoat, 1684

the jacket was also extended to the knee. This gave
the effect of two practically identical garments worn
one on top of the other, both with
capacious pockets. The inner coat had
shorter sleeves and turned into the
present-day waistcoat, while the outer
coat with its full-length sleeves and
cuffs developed into the modern jacket.
Both garments have remained true to
their origins. The waistcoat or vest
has remained buttoned up, the jacket,
like the caftan, is usually worn open.

Dutchman of 1670

The coats had vents in the back and
at the sides so that it could also serve
as a riding habit. Buttons were sewn
along the vents, as they also were on
the cuffs. The latter custom still survives in the useless
buttons on the cuffs of suit jackets. The coat could be
buttoned all the way down, but was usually worn
unbuttoned. The pocket flaps, too, had buttons.

Belts were not used, but between 1670 and 1690 a
sash was worn round the waist with the ends hanging
free. An opening was made for the sword when it was
not carried in a scabbard.

From Ruff to Neckcloth. By about 1620, the ruff
was no longer stiffened but fell loosely over the shoulders. About fifteen years
later, it was displaced by
the lace collar.

With the disappearance
of the ruff, short hair was
no longer necessary. And
as hair grew longer so the
lace collar grew smaller
until, by 1670, it was mer-

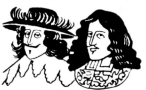

Dutch collars in 1630 and 1665

ely a narrow band with the ends resting on the chest.
This neckcloth is still retained today in Swedish
church vestments.

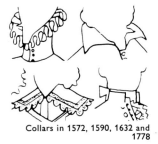

Hair style, 1650

Gathering at the wrist disappeared
at the same time as the ruff. But the
desire to show off linen sleeves remained, and broad linen cuffs edged
with lace became the fashion. Lace or
finely gathered material also appeared
on the front of the shirt, later developing into the cravat. The first cravat
appeared in 1636 in the uniform of a
Croation regiment in French service; here it took the

Collars in 1572, 1590, 1632 and
1778

form of a bow that could be either worn loose or be
tightly knotted.

Knee Breeches. From 1620 on, trousers were worn
just below the knee, their bottoms gathered with a

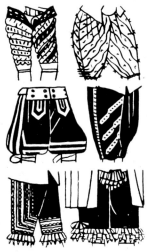

rosette or bow. Buttons
were sewn on the side,
some of which were de-
liberately left undone in
order to display the linen
underwear. Twenty years
later, trouser bottoms had
become wider and were
trimmed with a lace frill.
Ribbons also decorated
the breeches at the knee
and waist. These short
trousers gradually became
wider until they even-
tually resembled divided
skirts and had ribbons
and bows fluttering with
every step. Pepys tells in
his diary of a friend who
accidentally put both his
legs through one opening and went the day without

Trousers in 1560, 1578, 1609,
1630, 1640 and 1645

discovering his mistake!
Ribbons were used a great
deal at this time. Up to
six hundred bows could
be counted on a single
costume requiring some
two hundred yards of
trimming. By 1680, a
single bow on the shoul-
der was all that remained,
and from 1700 onwards
this was worn only by
liveried servants.

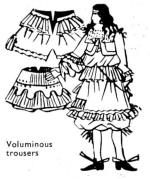

Voluminous
trousers

Shoes and Stockings. Silk stockings, with a ribbon
or garter below the knee, came into daily use. An

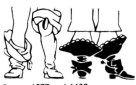

Boots, 1577 and 1638

additional heavier pair of
stockings was also worn.
These were trimmed with
lace which fell over the
top of the boot. The wider
the opening at the top of
the boot, the more lace
was used to fill the gap.

During the sixteenth century, boots had been
merely part of military uniform or hunting attire. But
during the following cen-
tury, when wars were fre-
quent, boots came into general fashion. From 1610
on, they were worn in-
doors, sometimes with an
overshoe. The leg of the
boot, made of soft leather,
fitted tightly but the top

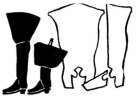

Swedish boots of 1639 and
their patterns

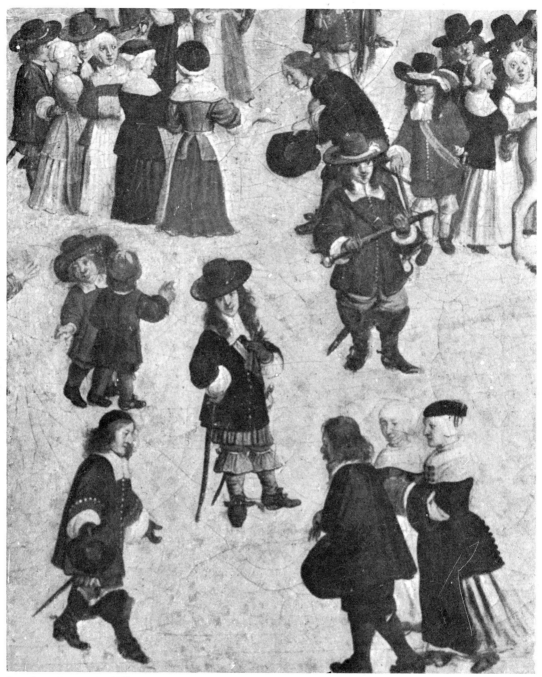

Copenhagen street scene, 1660

could be turned over. Later in the century the width of the leg increased once more and the toes got broader. While men's footwear broadened, women's shoes became narrower and slightly pointed.

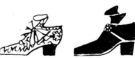

Shoe with overshoe

The price list of a Copenhagen shoemaker, dated 1605, makes the first mention in Scandinavia of shoes with heels. Presumably these were wedge-shaped pieces of leather laid into the sole of the shoe. The first example of a properly made heel comes from Persia, where it was used to give the rider a firm grip in the

Late 17th-century shoes with square, broad toes

stirrup. Heels were also worn during the Thirty Years' War, no doubt for the same reason, but heeled boots and shoes were not known in Northern Europe until about 1630. After peace was ratified in the Treaty of Westphalia in 1648, boots were no longer worn indoors, but heels persisted and grew in height. Shoes were built with uppers rising three inches above the instep. They had square toes decorated with rosettes or, by 1680, decorative metal buckles.

150

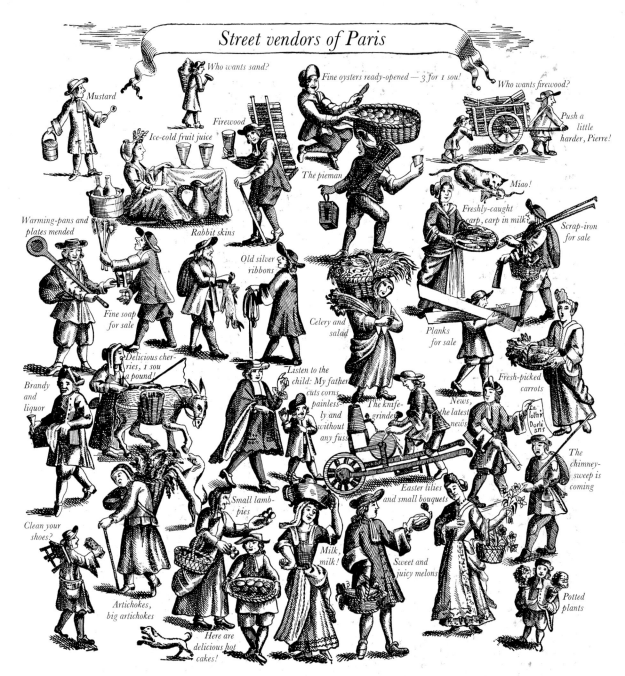

Street vendors of Paris

Mustard

Who wants sand?

Firewood

Ice-cold fruit juice

Fine oysters ready-opened — 3 for 1 sou!

The pieman

Who wants firewood?

Push a little harder, Pierre!

Miao!

Freshly-caught carp, carp in milk

Scrap-iron for sale

Warming-pans and plates mended

Rabbit skins

Old silver ribbons

Celery and salad

Planks for sale

Fresh-picked carrots

Brandy and liquor

Delicious cherries, 1 sou a pound!

Listen to the child: My father cuts corns painlessly and without any fuss

The knife-grinder

News, the latest news

The chimney-sweep is coming

Clean your shoes?

Fine soap for sale

Small lamb-pies

Easter lilies and small bouquets

Milk, milk!

Sweet and juicy melons

Potted plants

Artichokes, big artichokes

Here are delicious hot cakes!

Hats, Hair and Wigs. The new hair styles led to new types of headwear; the beret and tall conical hat gave way to a broad-brimmed soft felt hat decorated with ostrich feathers. After 1640, the brim almost disappeared, and ribbons took the place of feathers on men's hats. Within another twenty years, the crown had become lower and pieces of drapery were arranged round the brim. The next development was the three-cor-

Vagrants, ca. 1650

nered hat, known as the tricorn, which became the dominant fashion after 1690. Up to 1680, it was quite acceptable to wear a hat indoors, but after this time the hat was reserved solely for outdoor wear. Men greeted one another by sweeping their hats off with a grand gesture, at the same time bending the knee so that the feathers brushed the ground.

Not everyone could grow their hair long enough for the shoulder-length fashion; people in this unfortunate position

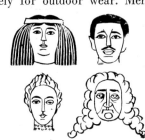

Egyptian woman wearing a wig and Egyptian man without one. A Baroque woman without a wig and Baroque man with a wig

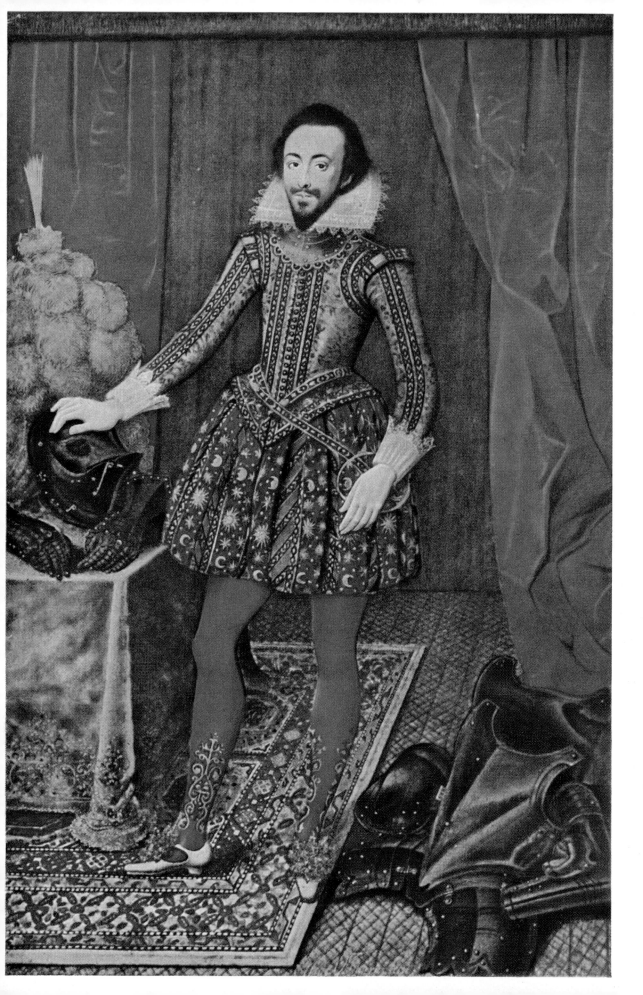

used artificial hair. Later, people shaved off what hair they had and wore wigs. The darker-haired French favoured blonde wigs, whereas the fair-haired Dutch preferred black wigs. The effect aimed at was that the face should shine out from below the wig 'as the sun shines through the clouds'. A night-cap was worn in bed to protect the bare head against the cold.

From 1630 on, the beard was reduced to a small tuft of hair on the chin, and the moustaches were brushed upwards in a sweep. Twenty years later, when wigs were the height of fashion, the beard disappeared entirely and men went clean-shaven.

Military Uniform. The Spanish style of uniform was in general use at the beginning of the Thirty Years' War. When the Swedes entered the war they introduced a somewhat different style. They carried light rifles and bandoliers of dummy cartridges, which in themselves gave the impression of military uniform. Different colours were employed to indicate various sections of the army; we read, for example, of the blue regiment and the yellow regiment. In 1645, during the English Civil War, the Parliamentarian forces were dressed in scarlet tunics. The French tunic was at first grey and then white with a brilliant lining in a contrasting colour which was repeated on collar and cuffs. The Swiss uniform was extremely colourful: it consisted of a scarlet jacket, blue waistcoat, blue trousers and white stockings. Blue was the principal colour of the Swedish uniform; Danish soldiers were clothed in red.

Baroque Women. Female fashion followed male fashion in the revolt against the severe Spanish style.

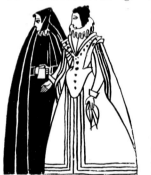

Swedish lady of 1625 and Spanish lady of 1630

In Spain the crinoline became larger and larger, while in the rest of Europe it completely disappeared between 1615 and 1620. In France, and in the rest of Europe, the skirt was allowed to hang in natural folds from the hips, sometimes caught up in such a way that the petticoat would show underneath. By the end of the century, as many as ten petticoats could be worn under the skirt. From 1680 onwards, the entire dress was festooned with ribbons and lace, and both skirt and petticoat were fitted with a train. The waistline was raised to just below the bust and emphasized by a narrow belt. The art historian, Carel van Mander, has described the tight lacing of this time,

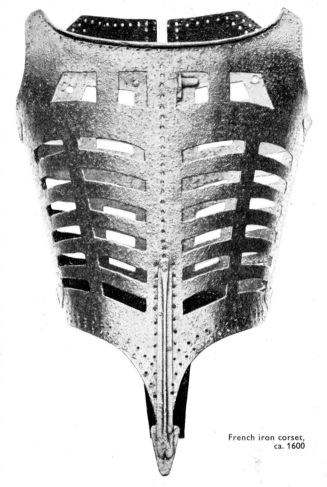

French iron corset, ca. 1600

'They lace and enclose their bosom so tightly that they can neither bend nor breathe.'

The bodice had a round neckline and a V-shaped opening which was laced together over a piece of embroidered material. Collars were fan-shaped and supported on wire, but this style gave way in the 1630's to flat lace collars. Lace cuffs, similar to those worn by men, also featured largely at this time. Sleeves became shorter and by 1660 were elbow-length. Thirty years later, padding had disappeared entirely from sleeves.

A sort of draped mantilla with long ends was worn outside the house. Sometimes a small cap which tied beneath the chin was worn, but usually women went

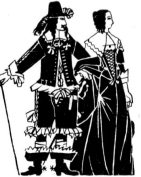
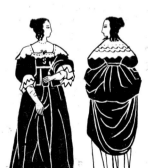
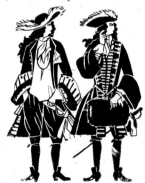

English gentleman, 1648, and ladies, 1640–54. Frenchman in summer clothes, 1693, and in winter clothes – with a muff – 1694

Opposite English portrait in miniature by Isaac Oliver from the beginning of the 17th century. It is reproduced in the original size

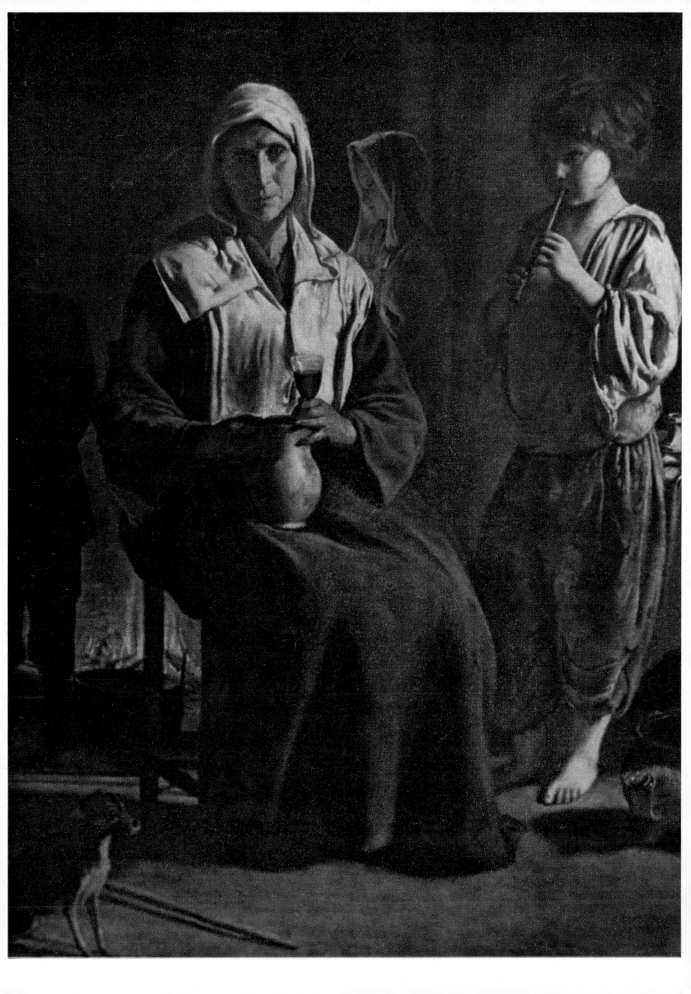

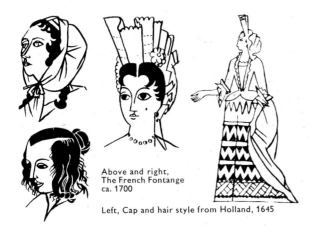

Above and right,
The French Fontange
ca. 1700

Left, Cap and hair style from Holland, 1645

bareheaded. For riding, broad-brimmed hats like those worn by men were used and the hair was tied up with ribbons. This later developed into the Fontange style which sat high on top of the head. By 1700, the height of the hair was greater than that of the head itself. With high

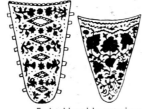

Embroidered breast-pieces,
1670 and 18th century

Shoes, ca. 1675

hair styles came longer trains. From 1660 on, women also wore high heels; their shoes, made of satin or brocade, had very pointed toes.

Puritan Dress. This period was characterized by the rich burghers' growing self-esteem, and by the triumph of the monarchy when absolute power was introduced. Wherever the bourgeoisie remained adamant in the face of the monarch's demands, fashion assumed a more practical and sober look. This was very evident in Holland and even more so among the Puritans in England. The new capitalist class which had sprung up in England had nothing but contempt for the idleness of the old aristocracy. Their adoption of the simple and practical Puritan style of dress expressed this view unambiguously. These people

Puritan hat

were businesslike even in private life. The cut of their clothes was simple and economical. Colours were black or grey. No ribbons and bows were worn, no provocative display of underwear was made. The men's close-cropped heads demonstrated their repudiation of worldliness, as expressed by long flowing locks and tresses.

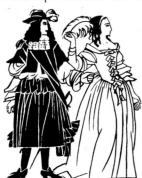

Dutch husband and wife of 1660

All over Europe elaborate forms of dress were disappearing. Once again the vertical line became sig-

nificant, though there was still a tendency to be less severe than in the Gothic period. Outlines became fuller and more pleasing to the eye; once again we find material hanging loose in folds or frills.

Dressed in Silk and Lace.
A list of the various materials used in the dresses — which date between 1625 and 1695 — in the Rosenborg Palace Collection gives a good impression of the dazzling beauty and enormous value of clothes of the Baroque period,

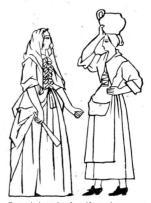

French burgher's wife and peasant
girl, ca. 1670

'White silk with silver, violet silk with gold, flowered material of silver and gold, brocaded silk in black, ivory satin with red sheen, light brown cloth lined with golden brown velvet embroidered with silver thread, pale blue satin with silver cords, black silk with lace borders, grey-brown cloth, green silk, yellow silk damask, rose damask, gold brocade, yellow silk, wine red velvet, salmon pink silk damask, scarlet silk velvet lined with white silk damask, pale blue silver cloth ...'

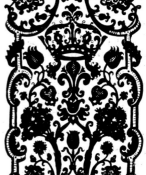

Seventeenth-century Italian velvet,
wine on a blue background

This list certainly illustrates the variety of materials and colours used for court dress by men and women alike. At the start of the century, clothes were made up on a cool refined colour scale with gentle nuances of pale blues, pinks, pale greys and yellows. As the century progressed, colours became stronger and more pronounced. The kassak, jerkin and trousers at this time were all made in the same colour, so as to obtain the greatest effect possible.

Delicate multicoloured patterns, often in overall designs of small flowers, were superseded by large patterns of leafed garlands in a colour contrasting with the background, or by stripes of harmonizing colours.

The story of lace illustrates, more than that of any other material, the

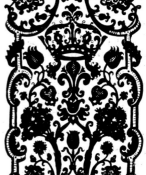

Silk velvet from Lyons
17th century

pains people would take to obtain the finished product. The Marquis de Dangeau relates most charming-

Opposite   French peasant woman, 1625–50. Painting by Le Nain

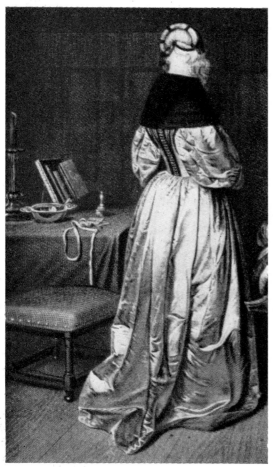

Rear view of dress ca. 1650. Painting by Gerard Terborch.

in which a style that began as a practical measure is gradually transformed into high fashion. The high heel was first designed to hold the riding boot securely in the stirrup. Then it was discovered that the same high heel gave the wearer a distinctive walk which denoted unmistakably the exalted nature of his profession.

The extra height imparted a pleasing sense of superiority which the wearer attempted to impress on other people. Further dignity was achieved by lifting the heel slightly from the ground when walking which

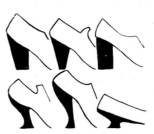

Above, Baroque heels, 17th century. Below, Rococo heels, 18th century

gave a rather pompous effect. And so a new man was created, a man referred to by Swift as 'the fork-shaped individual with narrow legs'. The normal gentle rhythm was replaced by a mincing gait, and it became fashionable to point the toes outwards. The out-turned foot, a

necessity in the time of the long Gothic shoe, now became accepted fashion and was adopted enthusiastically by dancing masters.

Thick hair was regarded as a sign of masculinity, but nature did not always allocate this endowment according to social standing. Wigs were the solution. What could be easier than to use hair of others to cover deficiencies of one's own. We come into the world with a certain amount of dignity, but not with wigs. Even for children of tender age, wigs were provided; a certain Danish nobleman, Christian Gyldenlöve, acquired his first wig in 1682, when he was only eight years old.

ly how the French army ran out of lace when surrounded by the Spaniards. A message was dispatched to the Spanish commander, the Marquis de Castagnaga, explaining the French predicament and requesting that a lace-merchant be allowed through the lines. The request was granted and when the bill was called for the merchant said there was nothing to pay as the Spanish commander had

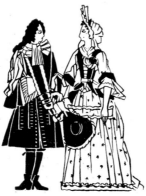

French nobleman with neckcloth and tricorn hat, 1689, and lady with Fontange, 1693

personally defrayed the cost of the transaction. There was an understanding, based on the fact that both officers knew and appreciated the value of lace (though it is doubtful if the Spanish commander showed similar consideration toward his own rank and file).

Heels and Wigs. Like lace, high heels and wigs were symbols of elevated social status. The heel, in particular, can also illustrate one principle of fashion

Erotic Aspects. Dress of this nature was intended clearly to demonstrate social and financial status rather than the person as he or she was. It hid more than it revealed. On the other hand, erotic interest was centred frequently on the clothing worn next to the body. The shirt had to show in certain places, primarily to prove that the individual possessed a shirt at all. The lace on the undergarments showed at the wrist and knee. Things did become a bit difficult when the custom of letting the shirt show all round the waist coincided with the newer custom of a low-cut shift.

Women also started to reveal more; for the first time in a thousand years arms were exposed. Spanish fashions had aimed at disguising the natural

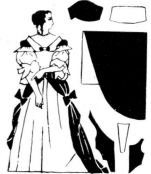

Female dress, ca. 1650 and patterns for its components

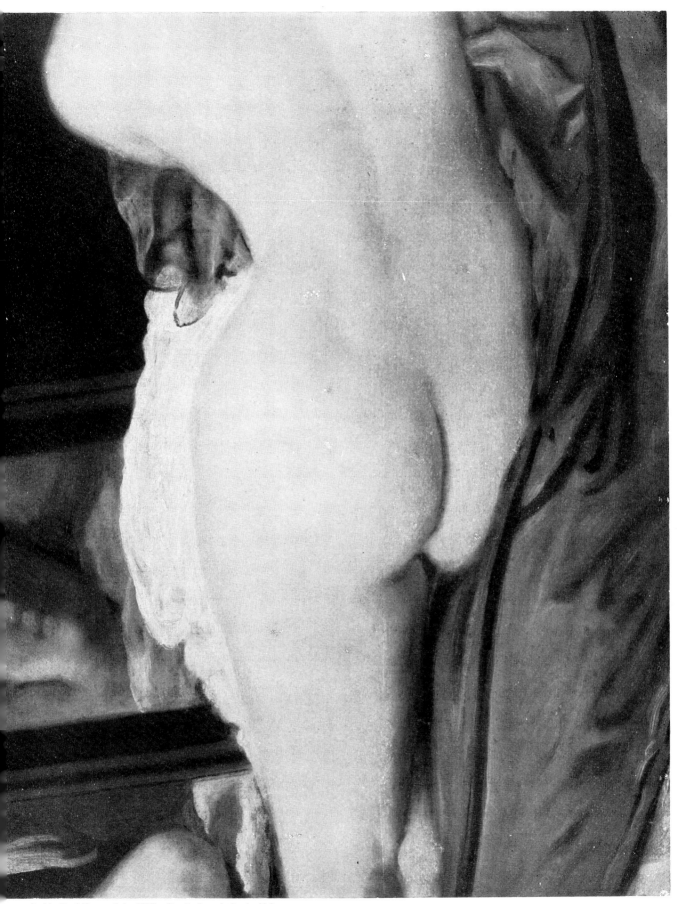
An idealized Venus of the 1650's. Detail of a painting by Velasquez

shape of the arms; this new trend represented a deliberate breakaway from the old tradition and an attempt at a more natural appearance. Now that women had arms once more, the neck, shoulders and back began to emerge. The bosom remained concealed, but the many covering layers of material disappeared one by one. The Spanish endeavoured to counteract this trend by introducing a thin sheet of lead to be worn over the bosom, but elsewhere in the world it was coming more and more into evidence. Instead of walking with the stomach thrust forward as in Gothic times, women now pushed their breasts forward. This posture was initially the result of high-heeled shoes, but the effect was clearly not unpopular: we hear at this time of 'falsies' — small bags filled with chaff — being worn.

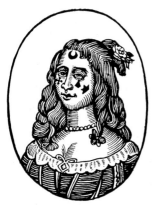

Beauty-spots or patches

A special feature of beauty culture was the artificial beauty-spot or patch suitably positioned on the face or neck. These were small silhouettes sometimes in the shape of ships, carriages or stars.

North African sun glasses, mask of 1650 and modern sun glasses

Weak Men and Strong Women. After the Renaissance and until the mid-seventeenth century, the focal point of female dress was not the waist but the bosom, a sure sign of women's increasing self-assertion. At the same time, a distinctly effeminate trend manifested itself in male dress which had appropriated the lace, ribbons, bows and rosettes of the women.

Women were no longer to appear as the eternally pregnant Gothic girl with her bashful look and downcast eyes. The Baroque women threw their heads back and thrust their chests forward.

The paintings of Rem-

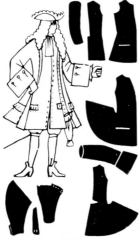

Male attire, ca. 1799

brandt and Rubens provide ample evidence that the ideal woman had literally grown in stature and proportion. Were not Rubens' women so vital and alive, they might almost be called flabby; but their fresh lips, healthy colour, bright eyes and luxuriant blonde hair reveal tremendous energy and charm. The aristocratic woman, as portrayed by Velasquez and Van Dyck, clearly knew her own mind.

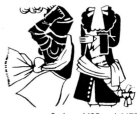

Sashes, 1625 and 1675

Gloves were made with fingers lengthened to suggest the extreme slimness of the hand, and seams along the back of the glove assisted the effect. They were worn by slender hands, hands made to be kissed and to carry many splendid rings, but also able to command without any unseemly gesture. The term 'mistress' assumed a new meaning, implying a woman who asserted herself through her lover to influence laws and fill high positions of state. In France, the whole court was permeated by the power of such women, a power which asserted itself as subtly and sweetly as ether, leaving the men drugged and helpless. Montesquieu wrote,

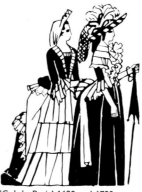

'Cul de Paris' 1690 and 1790

'Anyone who has seen the ministers, high civil servants and clergy at work at the court at Paris without discovering that it is the women who rule, is like a man who looks at an engine without being conscious of the power which drives it.'

These women came to positions of power and influence through the back door. Other women regarded themselves in quite a different light. A woman who had ample time for contemplation expressed the following view in the year 1670,

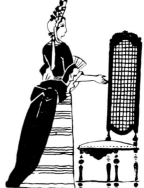

Lady with chair, ca. 1700

'The soul is without sex and will not be changed by exterior appearance or dress ... Not all who call themselves men behave as such in reality, but often women do brave deeds albeit they carry the name of woman. How often is not the weakness of woman found in the hearts of man, and manly strength in weak vessels.'

These words are not to be dismissed as nonsense. They were written by Leonora Ulfeldt, sister of the king of Denmark, and one of the most courageous women of her time.

Opposite   Interior of Dutch burgher's home, ca. 1650. Painting by Gabriel Metsu
Following pages   French Baroque costume in 1600 and Italian military uniform in 1966

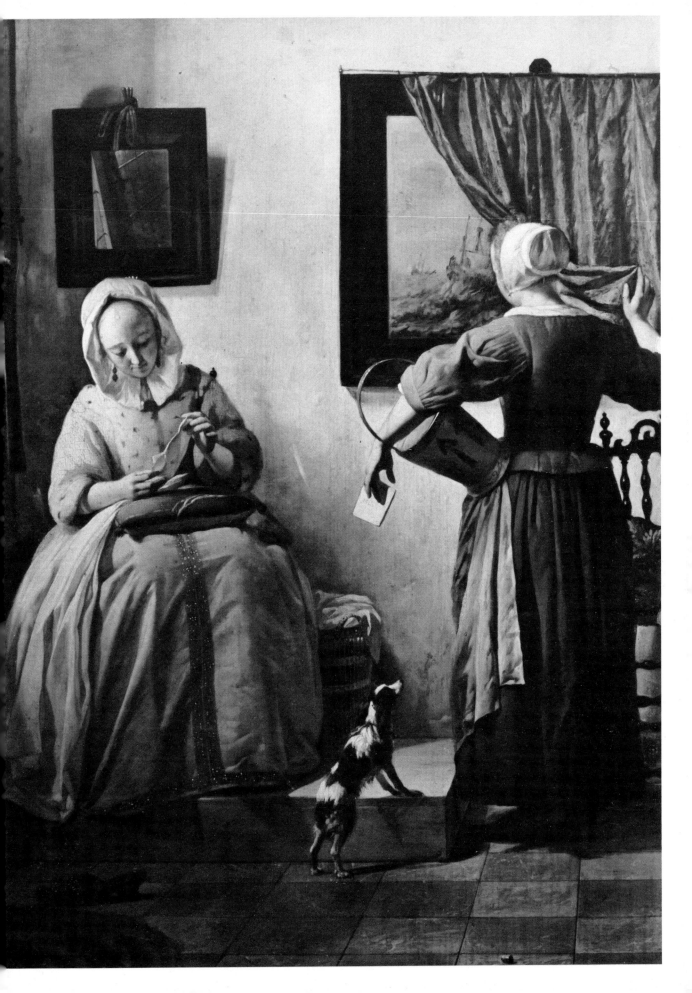

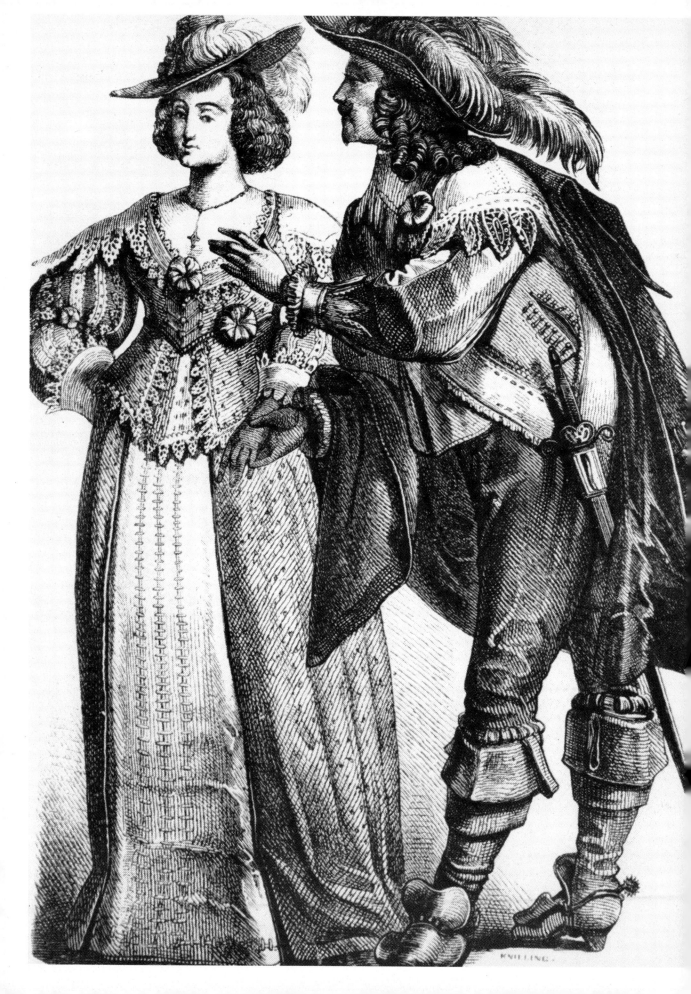

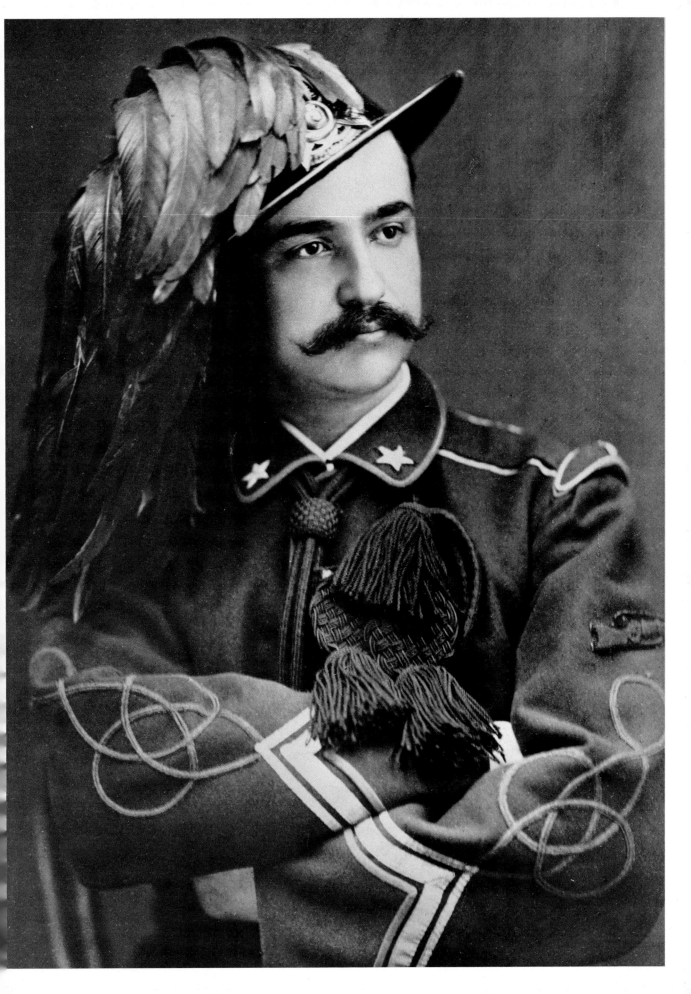

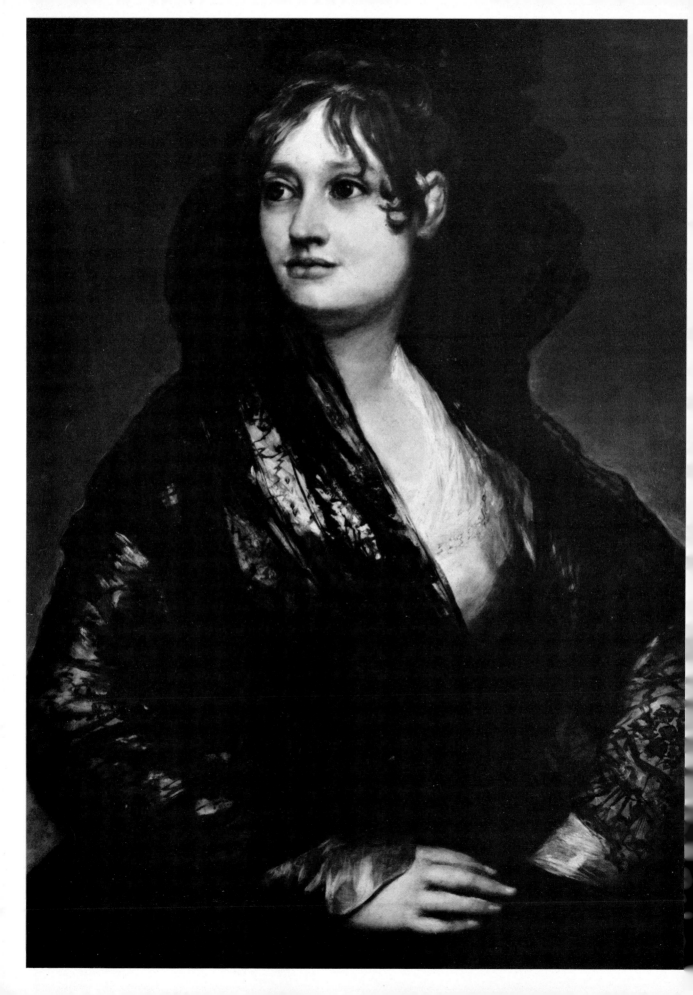

ROCOCO FASHION AND POWDERED WIGS

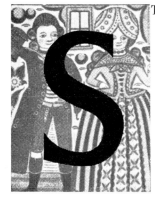

STYLES changed little during the early eighteenth century. Both dress design and the arts in general continued to follow Baroque fashions. Peter the Great had absolute power in Russia and Charles XII ruled in Sweden. In the 1770's, however, the War of Independence burst out in America and by the end of the century the French Revolution was under way. Open rebellion against the old class system was rife and the close of the century saw the end of the absolute power of ruling princes.

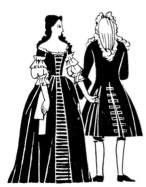

English couple of 1710

During this period, known as the Age of Enlightenment, Holberg was writing in Denmark; Voltaire and the Encyclopaedists were leading intellectual lights in France. Rousseau produced his sentimental work on nature which exercised a tremendous influence on thought. Education became available to all classes of society in Prussia, and compulsory enlistment for military or naval service was introduced.

Machinery was designed and produced for spinning and weaving. Porcelain was also introduced. A large number of novelties were made, such as the lightning conductor, the thermometer and boxing-gloves. The first typewriter was patented by an English inventor, and in the same year the last witch was executed.

The spirit of the age found expression in the music of Bach at the beginning of the century and of Mozart at the end. The waltz was introduced in about 1770 and its unrestrained movements, branded as licentious, gave rise to much concern.

The Boned Skirt. The crinoline reappeared in Europe, after having remained in fashion in Spain for over a hundred years. This revival supposedly came about through a theatrical performance in Paris in 1719 where the appearance of a crinoline caused a great sensation and no little scandal. This notoriety ensured its immediate success, and for the next forty years a dress without a crinoline was quite unthinkable.

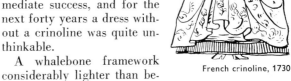

French crinoline, 1730

A whalebone framework considerably lighter than before, was devised. This consisted of five hoops connected first by oilcloth material and later by silk or cotton. In the 1720's the skirt was bell-shaped and up to six feet in diameter. It was later flattened at the front and back; this trend continued until, by 1740, all the width was at the sides. Cushions that were large enough to use as arm-rests were tied on the hips. In the 1760's, the crinoline became narrow again; twenty years

French crinoline, 1744

later all the fullness was at the back, forming the 'cul de Paris', better known as the bustle.

The Laced Bodice. Although the crinoline varied in size from time to time, the bodice retained its original shape. It was fastened over a wire or whalebone

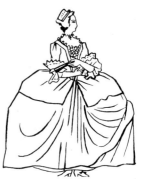

English crinoline of 1759 with hip cushions

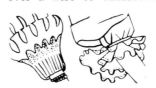

Sleeves of women's dresses with cuffs, 1615 and 1725

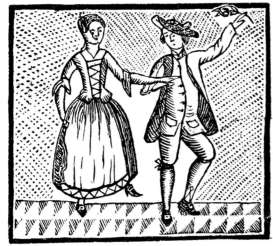

A young man and his girl, 1775. Danish woodcut

Opposite Spanish beauty wearing a black silk mantilla. Painting by Goya

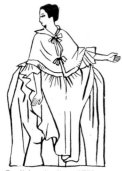

English crinoline, 1759

frame that was covered with coarse linen. The waist remained narrow and tightly laced. The neckline plunged so much that the breasts were only half covered. A scarf could be tucked into the neck if desired, but more often than not this was not done. The lower arms were normally uncovered.

Two garments were worn on top of the bodice and crinoline. The outermost had a V-shaped opening that displayed the garment underneath. The latter had a round neck; it was usually in a contrasting colour and profusely decorated with gathered borders, ribbons and pompons. The skirt of the outer garment came in time to be caught up at three points at the hem to permit the skirt to be lifted and raised at the back so that the feet were seen.

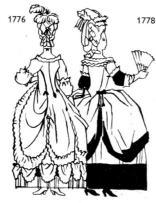

1776   1778

Négligé. All dresses, other than those worn on formal occasions, were referred to as 'négligé'; when at home, in the street, or travelling, négligé was the normal attire. From 1720 onwards, it was designed as a bodice with an attached skirt that hung loosely from the waist giving a tapered effect. The original cut of this so-called adrienne was on the lines of the tunic but it later acquired long sleeves and a front opening. This would have been a very comfortable garment were it not for the fact that the laced bodice was worn underneath. A new fashion in négligé came in about 1770 which was a copy of the kassak or caraco worn by men. The design changed frequently, sometimes falling loose and straight, at other times built upon the hips, sometimes with short tails at the back, at others with tails so long that they became a train. From 1740 on, lace edging or cuffs appeared on the elbow-length sleeves. Ten years later these gave way to elbow-length gloves of silk or soft leather.

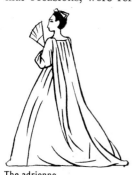

The adrienne

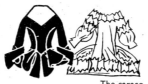

The caraco

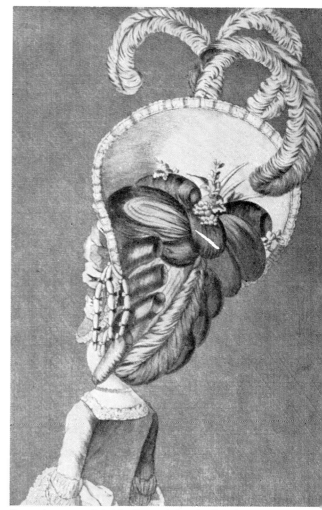

How to increase one's height: Rococo hair style of the 1770's

Hair Styles for the Crinoline. Tall piled-up hair styles went out in 1714, when hair began to be worn low over the forehead and close to the head, and was surmounted by a small lace cap. With the wide crinoline, hair styles were moderate, but with the smaller crinoline of the 1760's and 1770's the tall hair styles came back. The hair was combed back from the forehead and sides and fell in ringlets over the shoulders. During this period, hair styles reached enormous proportions and fantastic tableau-like decorations appeared on them, some representing, for instance, a farm complete with farmer, shepherd, cows and sheep. There was a saying in France at this time that the finest ships in the French navy were to be found in Marie Antoinette's hair. Hair was worn so high that the chin was half-way between the top of the head and the feet. Women had to be careful in ballrooms not to get their hair caught in the chandeliers. More than one head of hair, and ballroom too, went up in flames for this

Lace cap, 1725

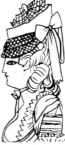

French lady of 1779

very reason. The roof of the main entrance to St. Pauls Cathedral had to be raised four feet in 1776 so that ladies of the court could enter without disarranging their hair.

Hours could be spent arranging hair over wire frames and rollers. This was done usually about once a week, or once a fortnight at least, by society women, and perhaps once a month by ordinary people. In between these sessions the hair could be neither brushed nor combed; elegant 'scratchers' of gold, silver or ivory, had to be employed if the itch got too unbearable. Wigs, which rested on the top of the head and allowed the natural hair to fall loosely down the back, became fashionable in 1775.

Satin Shoes. Women's shoes, which were usually made of silk or linen and were decorated with bows or buckles, had high heels and pointed toes. The heel

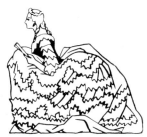
Rococo lady sitting on a tabouret or low stool

slanted forward and at one time achieved such an angle that the supporting point was mid-way between heel and toe. A woman laced up in a corset and encumbered by a crinoline had to move with even greater care when wearing these shoes. She seldom ventured out of doors and had to move slowly and deliberately within the house. Casanova described the action of some of the court ladies when they wanted to move quickly; they apparently hoisted their crinolines up to their chins, bent their knees and leapt like kangaroos.

Half-way through the eighteenth century, heels be-

came lower and toes less pointed. In the 1780's, heels became even lower, and ten years later flat sandals were adopted.

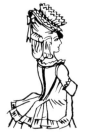
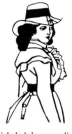
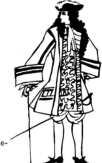
Caraco à la Polonaise, English lady's masculine-style coat of 1784, gentleman's attire

The Rococo Women's Deportment. The following instructions were given in 1734 by a dancing master of the Spanish court as to how a lady of quality should deport herself,

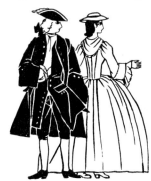
Frenchman in 1744 and English lady in 1749

'She must carry herself tall and straight so that people may say "that is a fine looking lady". She may not move her head when she walks, otherwise she would look nonchalant. The shoulders must be drawn downwards and the elbows carried well back so that they shall not rest on the hips. When she curtsies she may not bend her head and must place her feet in the fourth position. When bending the knees they must turn outwards as it is most improper for the knees to be seen through the dress.'

Norwegian bridal shoes from the Rococo period

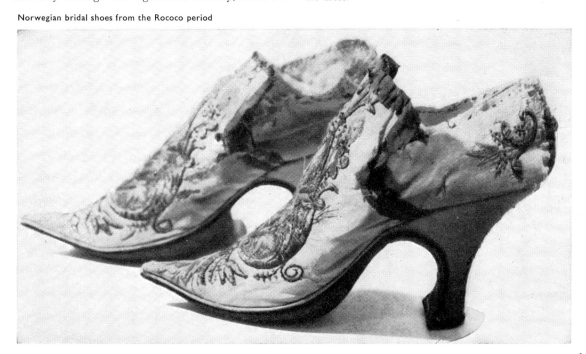

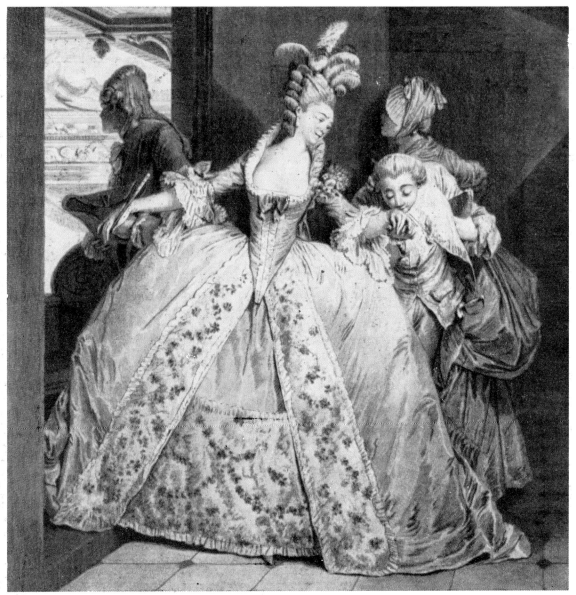

Parisian lady in *grande toilette* leaving the opera – sideways in order to get through the door. After a painting by Moreau, 1777

Just as the man carried his dress sword, so the woman carried her fan, 'with which she can at times achieve even greater deeds'. This contemporary writer continues,

'The fan is a safeguard to modesty, reveals what one wants to show and conceals what is not to be seen. It prevents the rays of the sun from burning the face of the princess as indelicately as the face of the peasant girl. It shields the eyes from the heat of the fire in the grate, hides bad teeth, the cynical smile and the frowning countenance ... Should a woman feel depressed she should push her chest forward, open her fan to full size and wave it vigorously in front of her face so that

French lady of 1762 and patterns of her costume

the small click-clack can be heard ... If there is something interesting to be said the fan should flutter like a pigeon's wings and fall closed at the end of each sentence.'

Male Dress. While female dress altered completely in style after the death of Louis XIV in 1715, male fashion remained much as before, except that the jackets fitted more tightly at the back, giving a much neater effect.

The outer garment was a knee-length dress-coat with tails which hid most of the long silk waistcoat underneath. The tails of the dress-coat and the vest were stiffened with a lining of oilcloth or paper, and the cuffs were smaller

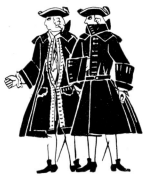

French redingote, 1730

166

Opposite   Rococo woman, about 1715. Painting by Watteau

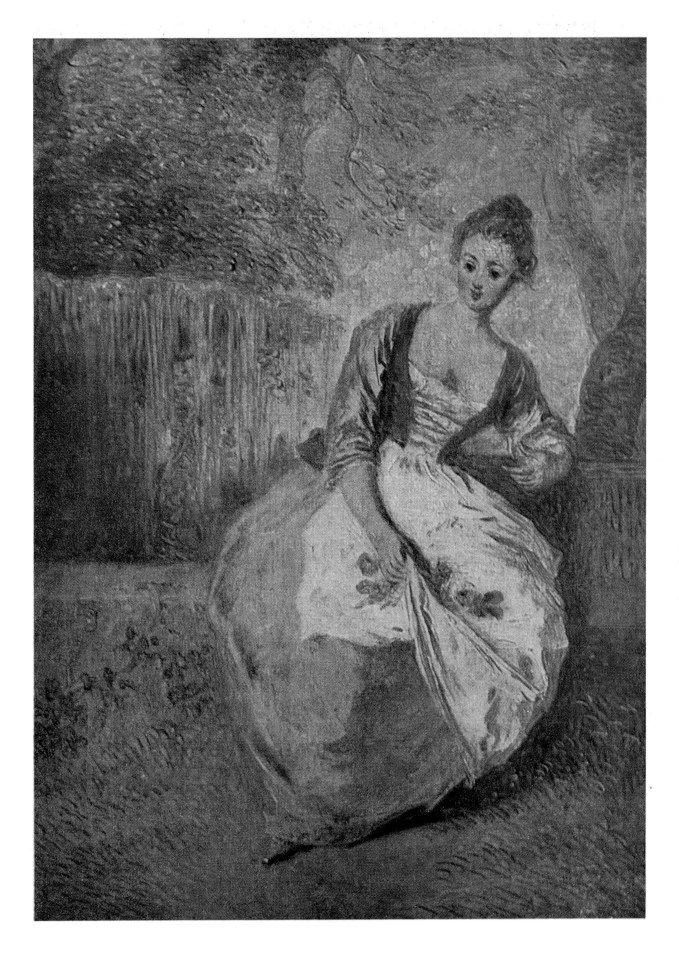

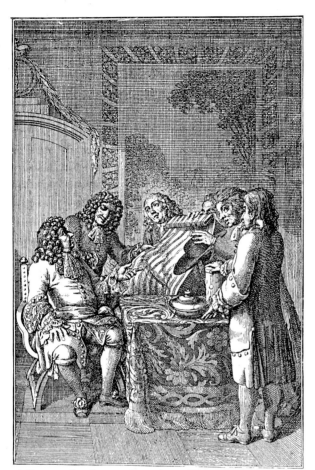

A German prince inspects the products of French immigrant weavers. Engraving by Chodowiecki. The Germans are wearing allonge wigs and lace collars

the tails disappeared and the coat became double breasted.

The sleeveless linen waistcoat with a half-belt that was worn under the dress-coat was now regarded as underwear. The top buttons were left open to show the frilled shirt underneath. The cravat was no longer tied so that the ends hung loose, but was passed round the neck and fastened under the shirt collar.

Between 1725 and 1760 trousers, although close-fitting, had a roomy seat. Later they were tight all over, and it was difficult for a fashionable man to sit

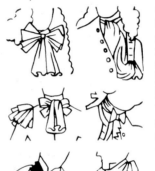

Man of fashion, 1780

down without bursting at the seams. The original flap opening in front was replaced by fly buttons at the same time. Trouser legs were tucked inside light coloured stockings until 1730. Later, the trousers were worn over the stockings and fastened with a buckle.

After 1750, men's shoes had lower heels and more pointed toes and, later still, acquired large buckles. In 1770, the top-boot was introduced; it resembled

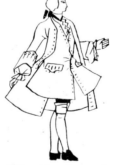

Cravats in 1678, 1695, 1678, 1745, 1830 and 1830

closely the riding boot of today in style. Until 1730, men of rank carried their swords, but later they bore only walking sticks, symbolic swords, whose handles were decorated with gilt, amber or ivory.

In the home, men wore coloured dressing-gowns, perhaps green with a red lining; scholars and artists were pictured in this attire with a night-cap instead of a wig.

The ideal male figure was no longer thick-set, but had now become slim, neat and elegant.

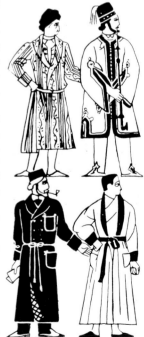

Robes in 1770, 1840, 1879 and 1950

than before. As the stiffening was not practical for military uniforms, the coat was cut away in front. This fashion was later adopted in civilian dress. The cut-away front on the military uniform was accompanied by an upright collar which first appeared in the 1730's. This collar grew taller as time went by and eventually became separated from the lapels and was folded over.

When cuffs became smaller, flaps were no longer fitted to the pockets, and the coat acquired a more slender line.

By 1760, the coat was cut away in such a broad curve that only the top three or four buttons could be done up, although buttons and buttonholes were still fitted all the way down. The function of the others was purely decorative, just like the buttonholes on jacket lapels today. Twenty years later

Stiffened French coat-tails, 1745

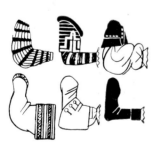

Men's coat sleeves in 1580, 1615, 1663, 1689, 1725 and 1778

Hats and Wigs. Beards at this time were out of fashion and were associated merely with stage villains. Holberg says,

'We do not see beards any more except on old Norwegian peasants and goats.'

Wig styles altered around 1730, becoming flat on top, curled at the sides and gathered at the back into a bag or pouch of silk or other material that was tied with a large ribbon. The wig of this period was designed to frame the face in fine white powdered hair.

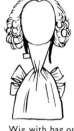
Wig with bag or pouch, 1771

Wigs were always powdered, usually with flour and considerable care had to be taken so that it was spread evenly. In large houses a special room was set aside for this purpose; the normal procedure was to blow the powder up at the ceiling and then allow it to fall and settle evenly on the wig.

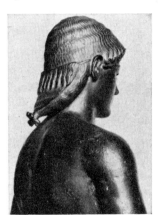
Pigtail, 1778

In smaller houses this performance usually took place in the stairway. A vast quantity of flour was expended in this way, giving the poor just cause to complain about the price of bread. The white, powdered wig had the effect of making everyone look very much the same age.

After 1760, the wig went out of fashion. The natural hair was combed back from the forehead, raised over the top of the head and tied at the nape of the neck like a pony tail. A little later the hair was plaited at the back.

The tall Quaker hat had been everyday wear since 1700, but the three-cornered hat was considered more stylish. This had started life with three equal sides but later became 'two-sided', taller at the front. This hat was carried under the arm. In fact, for some time to come, hats were never actually placed on the head, not even out of doors.

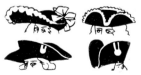
Pigtail from Greece, about 600 B.C.

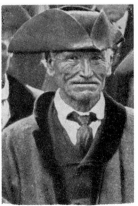
Tricorn hats of 1675, 1700, 1782 and 1789

The peasants of Andorra still wear the tricorn today

Uniforms. Prussia's victories during the Seven Years' War made her army a model for the rest of the world. The new military strategy that resulted called for a high degree of discipline.

Military dress became trimmer. Sleeves and trouser legs grew narrower. A high collar, worn with a black neckcloth, bore the regimental colours. Officers' uniforms were embroidered with silver and gold thread, and shoulder epaulettes were introduced in about 1800. Gaiters were added, and the tricorn hat was replaced by the flat two-sided hat on which the initials of the ruler appeared.

Colours and Material. The ordinary man in the street in 1780 looked something like this: blue topcoat, lilac waistcoat, yellow trousers and white stockings, or perhaps nut brown topcoat with black velvet collar, cherry-red waistcoat with gold braiding, black velvet trousers and grey silk stockings.

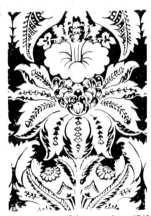
Crimson velvet, 1769

The waistcoat was always embroidered with pictures, for example, of scenes from well-known plays. Its buttons were highly decorative and carried miniature paintings placed under glass.

The clothes of the rich were made of silk, damask and brocade, while poorer people wore printed cotton. Fortunes were spent on lace for decorating collars and cuffs which accompanied their owners to the grave.

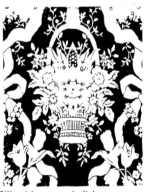
Silk with pattern in light green, brown and white, ca. 1775

Notwithstanding the passion for fine lace, the general tendency of the period was in favour of moderation. Colours became more delicate and refined than they had been in later Baroque times; soft pastel shades were appreciated, like pale blue, lilac, silver grey, rose and apricot. Curious improbable terms came into use in the world of fashion to describe the various shades of brown, such as flea's head, flea's back, flea with milk-fever, street dirt, nymph's thighs, nun's belly and poisoned monkey.

The heavy patterns popular in late Baroque times gave way to regular undulating lines and faint horizontal stripes which were woven into the material.

169

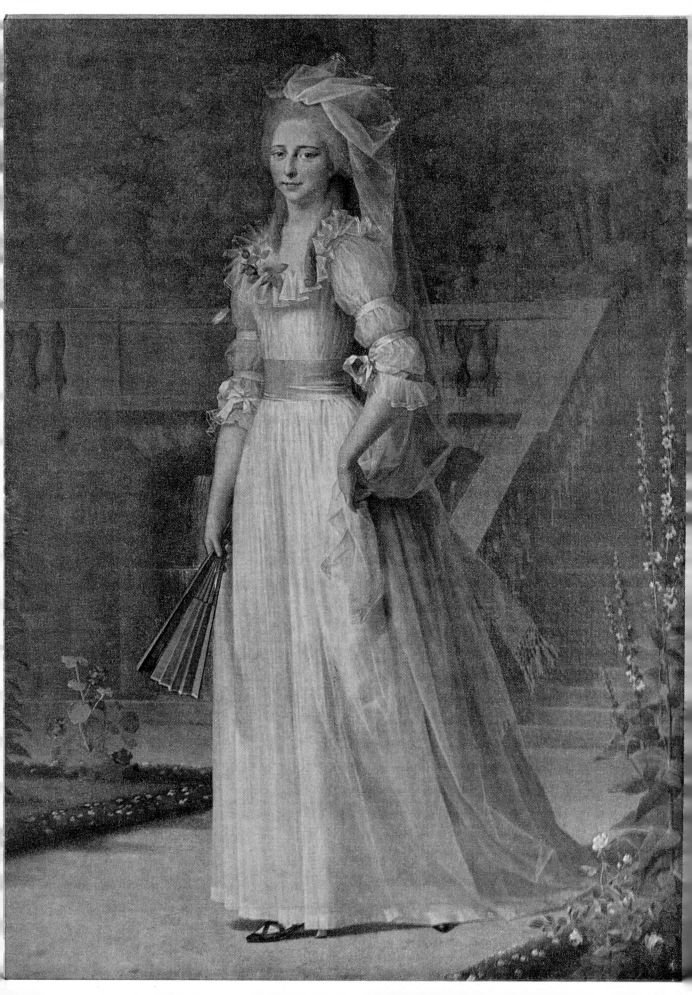

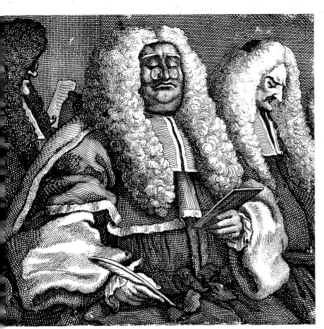
Allonge wigs. Engraving by Hogarth

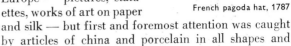
French pagoda hat, 1787

Ribbons, tassels and bows continued to appear on women's clothes so long as the crinoline remained in fashion. Men's dress became plainer, and in the 1770's embroidered edges dwindled away until they finally disappeared completely.

Make-up. Make-up was used to counteract the excessively pallid complexion which the powdered wigs could produce. The eyebrows were first emphasized with a black pencil. Then the face was covered with a white foundation, the veins were picked out with blue paint and the cheeks were rouged. The rouge was intended to look like rouge. No attempt was made to make it look like natural colouring. The only people to appear with naturally rosy cheeks were ladies of easy virtue.

The culminating point in applying make-up was reached with the patches or beauty-spots. These had become smaller but more numerous and were named according to their position on the face. On the forehead was 'the majestic', on the nose 'the insolent', next to the eye 'the passionate', at the side of the mouth 'the kissable'. We also hear of beauty-spots on parts of the body normally covered by clothes.

Poisonous elements in cosmetics resulted in all sorts of skin trouble and eye infection. The powdered wig was also most unhealthy for the natural hair and scalp. Headaches were accepted suffering among well-to-do women, and anaemia was regarded as the unavoidable concomitant of tightly-laced stays.

Chinese Influence and Nature-Worship. The first examples of applied asymmetry in art and decoration were seen during the Rococo period. This system was called the rocaille. It played its part in, among much else, the positioning of beauty-spots. In Rococo gar-

den architecture, asymmetrical layouts were considered the most beautiful. This was connected with a general enthusiasm for Chinese art. Examples of chinoiserie were flooding Europe — pictures, statuettes, works of art on paper and silk — but first and foremost attention was caught by articles of china and porcelain in all shapes and sizes. Chinese pagodas,

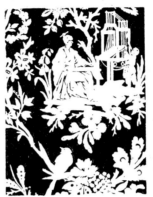
Chinoiserie on French textile

teahouses, pavilions and bamboo bridges appeared in the gardens of European stately homes. The Asian peacock and goldfish then introduced were living images of the Orient. Everything that was small and elegant in Europe during what Voltaire called 'this century of trinkets and knickknacks' reflected the Chinese influence. This passion for the oriental extended even to behaviour; Goethe writes, talking about the time of his youth,

'As I had to be made up in such a fanciful way and powdered since early morning, and had to be careful not to spoil it by excitement or large gestures, this discipline compelled me to behave in a more restrained and quieter way.'

The fashionable world was still regarded as a stage, but the old style was no longer acceptable. The weighty seriousness expressed in slow, measured movement and solidity of person gave way to a spirit of graceful hedonism. People no longer felt a moral duty to act out their parts for the edification of onlookers. They played their fresh roles only for themselves,

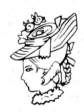
Straw hat, 1778

for their personal pleasure and for sheer delight in the play in which they were all involved.

This trend, defined by Rousseau as a 'return to nature', went side by side with the new atmosphere in court circles. It seemed futile to try to preserve customs and conditions of the past. The view prevailed rather, 'Après nous le déluge, so let us enjoy the pleasures of paradise while they are yet ours'.

These people lived for the present. They were in love with nature and with spontaneous feelings un-

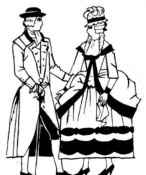
Gentleman and lady of 1780

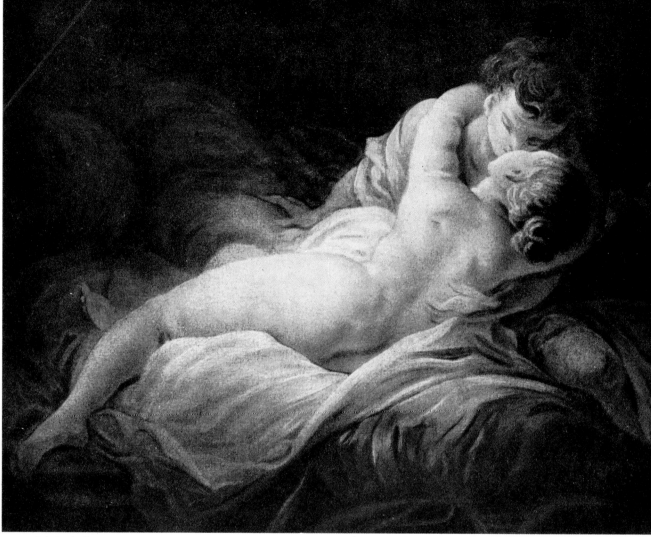

Painting by Fragonard

restricted by reflection and recrimination. Pleasure had never before been so well-organized. The desire for enjoyment and for sensation, whether great or small, unsophisticated or highly refined, had never been so developed. The pleasures of the table and the bed were appreciated no less than beautiful colours and elegant shapes were admired.

The first really comfortable chairs since the attempts of the Greeks, were designed and produced in the Rococo period. Curves were moulded to the shape of the body and gave adequate support to the back. A person could sit at ease with crossed legs and feel completely relaxed.

Rococo chair and chair pictured on antique Greek vase

The Ideal Woman.
The women sought to attract admirers either by a piquant display of feminine charm or by the reverse process of tantalizing restraint. So one crinoline might have had a low and seductive cut while another was extremely modest in design, all according to the wearer's mood and intention. (Of course, we must remember that an artificial bust is better hidden.) Jewellery round the neck and on the bosom had largely gone out of fashion. Ear-rings were still worn, also ornaments in the hair and brooches on laced bodices.

The response to female nakedness was both chivalrous and erotic. Paintings of the time display a light-hearted insouciance to the intimacies of the human body. Indolent coquettes appear with skin like mother of pearl, full breasts, dimpled

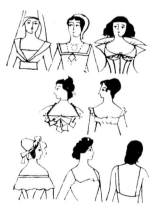

Décolleté necklines in 1460, 1550, 1640, 1760, 1790, 1840, 1900, 1931

172

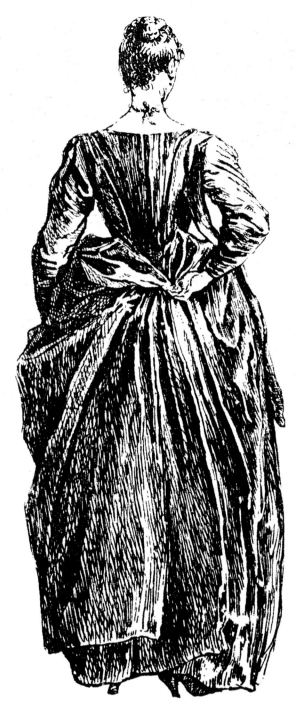

Venus Kallipygos fully clothed. Study by Watteau

The differing nature of the two sexes was expressed to some extent in Rococo dress: male attire conveyed a more rational commonsense attitude to life, while female dress expressed sentiment and depth of feeling.

The Salons. This was a time of extraordinary contradictions, a time in which reason and emotion could exercise equal sway over the same human being. Both the natural and the artificial were revered. And while class consciousness reached an ultimate sophistication just at this time, its overthrow was simultaneously heralded in the principles of liberty, equality and fraternity.

What were the sources of this insurrection of the spirit whose climax was the French Revolution? In going through letters and memoirs of the time, we become increasingly aware of the salons and their role.

Leading society women took great pride in surrounding themselves with thinkers, men of wit and devotees of art and literature. The very word 'salon' suggests a gathering of artists and intellectuals. The word was later employed by the Louvre to denote the rooms housing its art collection.

It is typical of this period of contradictions that ideals encompassed finally by guns and the guillotine should have been conceived in the amiable atmosphere of the grande salon, the results of conversations, exchange of ideas and discussions about the new philosophy.

Women employed a new strategy for gaining position and power. This they achieved not by rejecting their femininity but rather by claiming full recognition and liberty in their relationships with the opposite sex. This new outlook was reflected in their choice of colours. Spirit and colour have been closely connected throughout the ages; the sombre colours of the Baroque period were succeeded by the light pastel shades of the Rococo, which gave way to the white and gold, greyish blue and lemon of Neo-Classical times.

The World at Large. Outside the pleasures of the Rococo court and the sophistry of the salon lay a larger world, governed by different ideals. The modes of dress proscribed by high society indicated the extent to which this very hierarchy was threatened. At one time, middle-class women were not permitted to dress like noblewomen. Later, wives of workmen were not permitted to dress like wives of masters of trades or crafts. In 1790, servant girls in Prussia were forbidden to wear embroidery or lace.

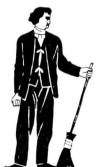

French street-sweeper, 1778

When one handles clothes from the Rococo period, one can see how worn they became. The surface was of good quality but the material underneath was poor. The linings of the most elegant garments were frequently as rough as sacking.

elbows and pink nails at the tips of slender white fingers. But what their souls were like was evident in their misty blue eyes and the supercilious curl of their lips. They were untroubled by deep thoughts or by turbulent emotions. Affairs were begun and ended as elegantly as a bow was untied on their bodices. Nothing could be more deliberately feminine then the Rococo woman. She would swoon, not because of tight lacing or even for dramatic effect, but simply because swooning was a womanly act. Men in their own way adopted similar attitudes, and their whole appearance acquired a distinctly effeminate effect.

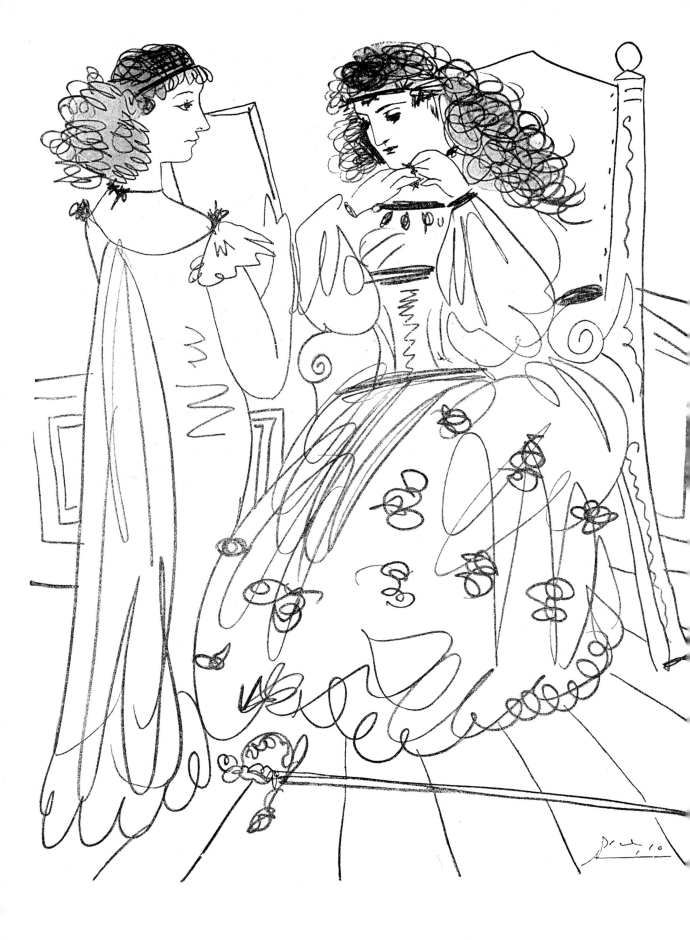

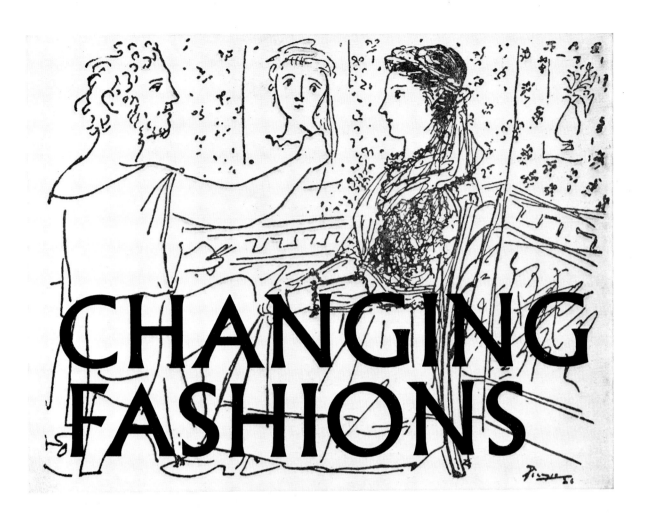

CHANGING FASHIONS

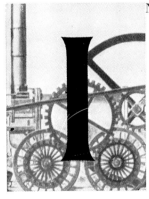

I N THE nineteenth and twentieth centuries rapid change, one feels, occurred in the world of fashion. This impression partly comes, of course, from the fact that we are so close to this period in time. Small details tend to become obscured in a large general survey, and so it is with fashion. It is clear, however, that the general tempo has quickened, particularly in the realm of female fashion. Men's fashions, on the other hand, have become more established and settled than they were before.

A change in style of dress is one way in which a person or a group of persons can express their individuality and independence. On the world stage, the actor has a voice in determining his costume. Any new fashion is a break with tradition and an expression of spiritual liberation, even though it may cause personal discomfort, and to follow it evidence of a degree of self-confidence. All new fashions are regarded with suspicion and dislike at first by all except their creators.

The changes which have taken place in women's clothing over the past hundred and fifty years can be likened to the gradual shedding of shackles, even though each chain might be replaced by another of a different kind. It is significant that as women have come more and more to follow occupations regarded hitherto as specifically masculine, they have also adopted various features of male clothing.

Various theories, usually erroneous, have been applied to try and explain fashion. Some have suggested, for instance, a connection between the broad shoe and the fact that a certain prince was supposed to have a broad foot. Similarly it has been put forward that the crinoline was originally designed for an empress who was pregnant. Nevertheless, the instinct of imitation, however ridiculous a form it may take, has always played a strong part in fashion. The power of the magical mask dissolves as soon as it is seen as nothing but a mask.

It must not be thought that women embarked on a deliberate process of emancipation. Men have always been convinced that the female acceptance of inferiority must arise from a related awareness that they lack male sex organs. This belief is gradually losing ground, perhaps because men themselves have become aware of their own inability to bear children.

Opposite Drawing by Picasso

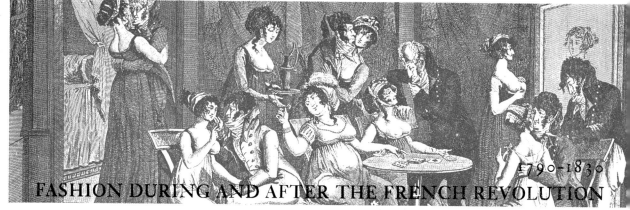

FASHION DURING AND AFTER THE FRENCH REVOLUTION

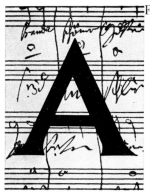

AFTER the French Revolution of 1789, came a period, ending with the July Revolution of 1830, in which all the signs were manifest of a political awakening in France. This led not only to the birth of a new regime in France and in other countries, but also to a new era. The bourgeoisie which, because of its economic strength, had long played a leading part in the social sphere, now acquired power in the political sphere. An ideal of freedom, based on the ancient patterns of democratic Greece and Republican Rome stormed the imagination. The power of turbulent emotions was reflected in the music of Beethoven. The gavotte and minuet were replaced by the sweeping rhythms of the waltz.

Industrial development forged quickly ahead. In 1794, the ball-bearing was invented; in 1807, the first steamship was afloat. The ship's propeller was invented in 1812, and the first locomotive was running in 1814. Gas lighting, electromagnetism, sterilization and vaccination came into being. The first

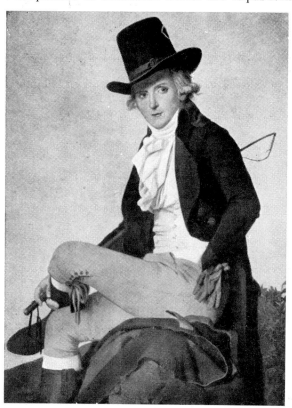

Pin-maker, 1824

Portrait by David

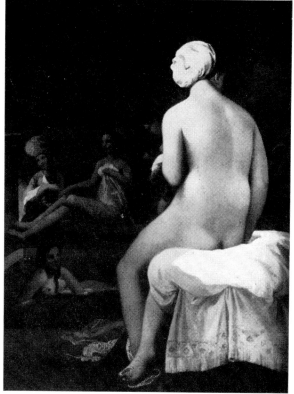

Nude by Ingres

usable lead pencil was made in 1790 and the first steel pen in 1828. Industrial production developed so rapidly in England in particular that a law had to be passed limiting the working day to twelve hours.

The Statuesque Dress. The world had been conquered by the Neo-Classical fashion of the Revolution even before Napoleon helped complete the process. The sharp break with the earlier past made itself felt both in politics and in fashion. The changes it entailed seemed unanticipated. Aristocratic women adopted classical poses and moved in a classical manner. Goethe wrote from Naples, in 1787, that for two consecutive evenings he had watched tableaux in which he had recognized all the statues of antiquity, the beautiful profiles from Sicilian coins, even the grace of Apollo.

The Shift. Hippolyte Taine stated that, in his view, the greatest civilizing event in European history was

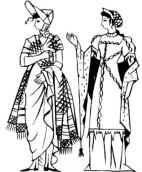

the introduction of trousers. And it cannot be denied that the introduction of knickers was an epoch-making event in the realm of women's dress. The escape from tight stays and whaleboned skirts was a further relief; a foreign correspondent described the Parisian woman of the 1790's,

French tunic dress with shawls, 1796 and English, 1812

'Flesh-coloured knickers in silk tricot with lilac inserts

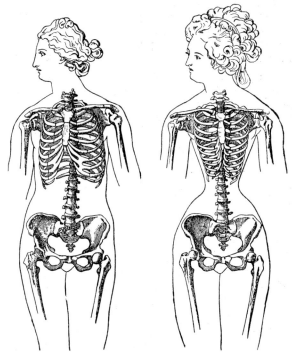

Not until the corset was no longer in fashion did doctors discover its harmful effects. This drawing, which dates from 1793, shows the difference between a normal chest and one deformed by tight lacing The 'normal woman' is drawn with the head of Venus de Milo

and bands round the knees. Over the knickers a straight linen shift was suspended from the two bands over the shoulders, leaving virtually the whole of the upper part of the body uncovered.'

This situation developed even further. Knickers and stockings were discarded for a time and the dress made so finely in tulle, organdy, muslin or batiste that it could be

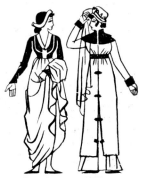

French outfits, 1799 and 1803

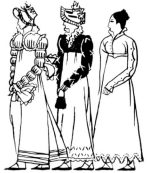

1811, 1814 and 1817

pale colours such as lavender, beige, pink or powder blue were chosen. Contrasting colours were introduced in the ribbon on the hat or a bright red scarf. Unlike Rococo fashion, which employed colours that were not too far apart, the new style selected its colours from opposite ends of the spectrum, providing emphatic contrasts such as red and blue.

Borders were embroidered with palmetto leaves, vases and lyres; after Napoleon's victories in Egypt, Egyptian motifs appeared.

drawn through a woman's ring. Madame Tallien was reputed to have attended a ball wearing a dress which weighed only 150 grams (approximately five ounces), including the common accessories of Roman sandals, anklets and toe-rings.

This 'antique' gown was usually white, reminiscent of marble. If the dress was not plain white or ivory,

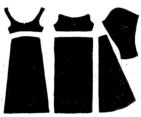

Dress pattern of 1805 showing the parts of which the dress was made

The Draped Garment. The light décolleté tunic with its simple short sleeves was a welcome change. Arms and legs now met the light of day after their long incarceration. Shawls and stoles on classical lines

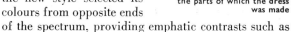

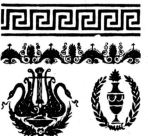

Neo-Classical motifs in fabric

were imported from the East and formed an important part of female dress. The criterion for the well-dressed woman was not so much the clothes she wore but how she carried them and how the material was draped.

Hats acquired crowns like chimney-pots and brims that flanked the face like blinkers; they were

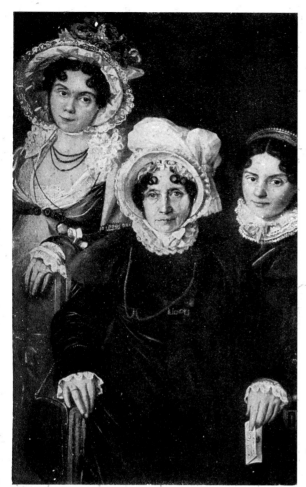

The ideal at the height of the Neo-Classical period. Three ladies painted by David in 1819

nude. During the Rococo period, various parts of the body were admired, but it was never admired as an entity. The rediscovery of the beauty of the entire human frame was a new and exciting experience. The ideal of physical beauty postulated a general impression of grace and harmony, such as Madame Récamier gave, with her

'boyish waist, long slender hands and feet, dazzling white teeth, eyes with a glint of gold and skin like cream with floating rose petals.'

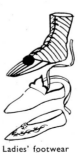

The proportions of the Neo-Classical body

Character and personality previously hidden behind a flirtatious façade now became important elements of female power. The sensuous appeal of womanly charm gave way to the attractions of the free spirit, the ardent lively eye and the smooth intellectual forehead. Virtue became more attractive than coquetry.

The long slender figure was synonymous with high ideals, so legs were made to look longer by raising the waistline. The breasts were pressed upwards and exposed by the low neck. The gossamer scarf, known as the fichu, did more to attract attention to the breasts than to conceal them. Motherhood was much admired as being in keeping with the spirit of the time. When Madame de Staël asked Napoleon what type of woman he most admired, he replied simply, 'the one who has borne the most children.'

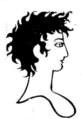

Short Hair and Small Fans. Short hair became fashionable once more at the start of the nineteenth century. Hair had been worn shoulder-length for some time previously and had often looked very bedraggled. Now the hair, left unpowdered, was cut short, with small curls 'à la Titus'.

Hair 'à la Titus'

Fans, though never discarded, became smaller. A woman of the time explained,

'Previously when we blushed so frequently, and wished to hide our embarrassment and timidity, we used a large fan. Now we seldom blush and no longer feel timid. There is no longer any inclination to hide oneself, therefore, the fan has become smaller.'

Reticule

Other feminine accessories also became smaller including the reticule, or handbag as it is now.

tied under the chin with a ribbon. They were usually made of plaited straw, or alternatively, of material built over a wire frame. In Denmark this hat, known there as 'Kiss-me-if-you-can', remained in fashion till 1850. The main purpose of the hat was to give protection against the sun. A pale complexion and hands as white as marble were the signs of a highborn lady who had little cause to be in the open; outdoor clothes were seldom worn.

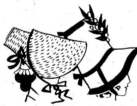

Straw hat of 1797 and cloth hat of 1813

Long-Limbed Graces. The aftermath of the French Revolution brought hard times and people were forced to concentrate mainly on essentials. Underwear made in flesh-coloured materials exemplified the veneration of nudity. A German poet of this time, Novalis, wrote,

'Only one true temple exists in the world and that is in the form of the human body. When we place our hands on the human body we are touching heaven.'

Marble sculptures made of Napoleon and his beautiful sister, Pauline Borghese, showed them in the

Daughters of the Revolution. Side by side with the flimsy dresses, which so unconcernedly revealed the curves of the wearer, came a growing sense of freedom and self-assertion. When all is said and done, sun and air are the natural elements for the human body.

One of the many women intellectuals who came to the fore during the French Revolution was Olympe de

Ladies' footwear

Opposite A son of the Revolution. Painting by David, 1793

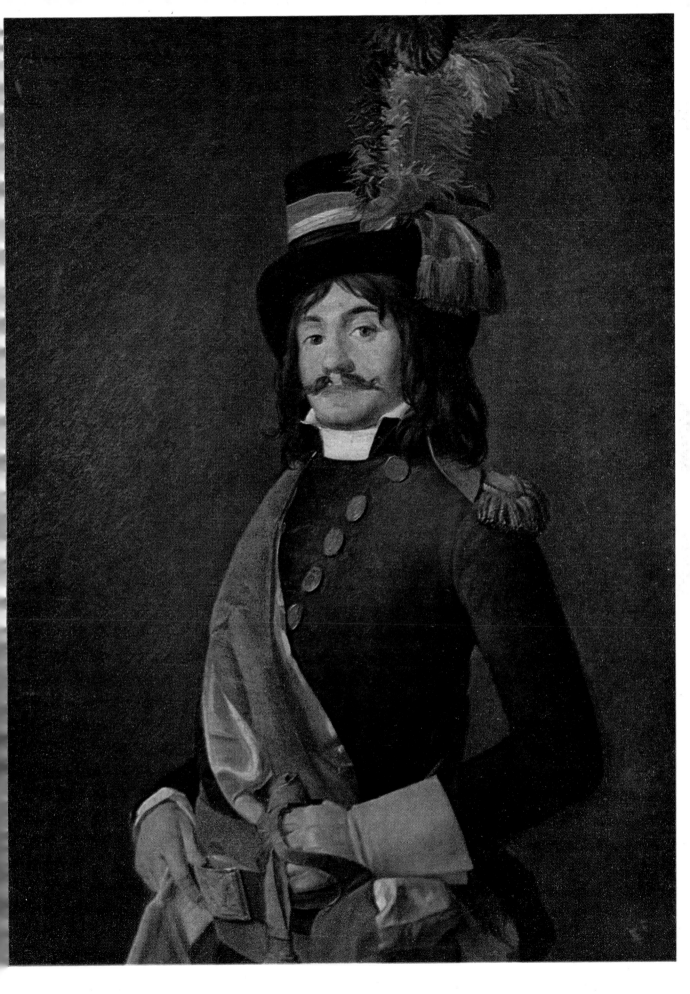

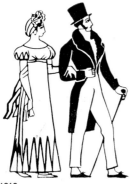

1818

Gouge. Her remarkable essay of 1789 was virtually a counterpart to *The Declaration of the Rights of Man*. In it she wrote,

'Women are born free with equal rights with men, and these include an equal share in freedom, progress, security and the right to fight oppression. The State rests equally on men and on women and the law must acknowledge its collaboration. Women citizens, like all other citizens, must take part in the framing of laws whether personally or through their elected representatives. All official appointments, promotions and professions must be open equally to men and to women. A woman has the right to be executed but she also has the right to become a Minister of State. Because women contribute to the nation's wealth equally with men, they must also decide how the money is expended.'

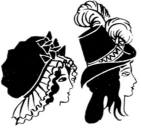

French headwear of 1789 and 1797

The Return of the Crinoline. The 'Grecian' dress was a definite step towards freedom of movement. At the same time, it was, however, still bound by ideas of the past and by incidental limitations. For instance, the shift was not draped on the body as it had been with the Greeks, but was shaped and sewn together. Although shoes continued to have flat soles without heels, their shape was pointed. The

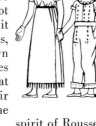

Women's hair styles of 1795, 1802 and 1817

leon, the source of inspiration changed from being Greek democracy to Imperial Rome. Here it was not the classical world in itself which exerted a fascination; the selfconscious monumentality and grandeur of Rome constituted a mirror image of Napoleonic times. Powdering the face came back into fashion, in emulation of the white marble of the statues of Ancient Rome.

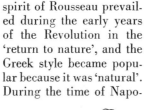

Children, 1815

spirit of Rousseau prevailed during the early years of the Revolution in the 'return to nature', and the Greek style became popular because it was 'natural'. During the time of Napo-

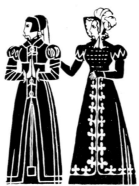

Reactionary fashions: dresses of 1558 and 1822

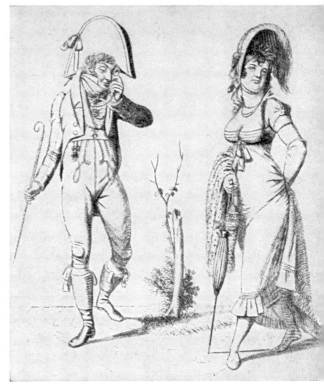

The height of fashion in Copenhagen, ca. 1807. Engraving by Senn

A period of reaction followed the Congress of Vienna and Vienna became the city of traditional fashions, competing with Paris, the city of eternal revolution. In 1820, the waist returned to its natural position, and the tightly-laced bodice also reappeared. The body was once again divided into two distinct

Broad lapels, ca. 1800

parts. Colour came back at the same time, first as a coloured bodice worn with a white skirt and then a complete dress in colour-

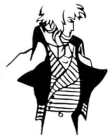

Men's hair styles of 1804, 1809 and 1810

ed material. The dress, which gradually became fuller and fuller, was held out, at first by one stiff petticoat and later by several. A short jacket with narrow sleeves, known as the spencer, became usual outdoor wear; like the dress, it gradually became wider and puffed out to increase the effect of the wasp-waist. These changes in fashion were restricted to the outer garments.

Children with pantalets, ca. 1830

On young girls, the legs of the knickers, or pantalets, were allowed to peep below the skirt. Children of well-to-do parents had, up till then, been dressed in the same style as their parents, but now simple loose-fitting play clothes, modelled on workmen's smocks, appeared.

Opposite Madame Récamier. Painting by David, 1785

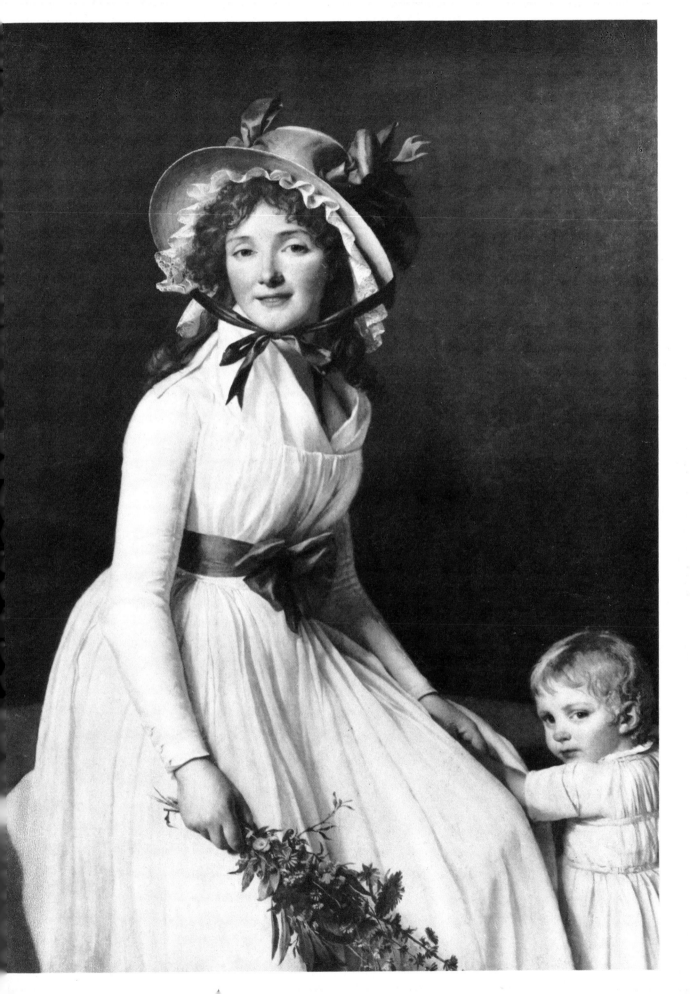

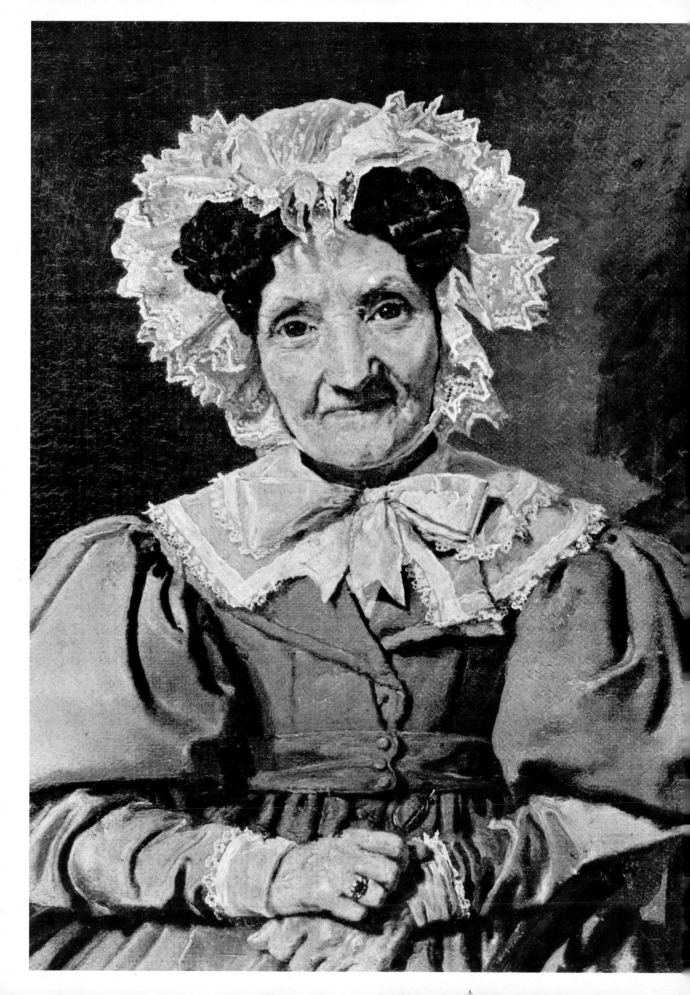

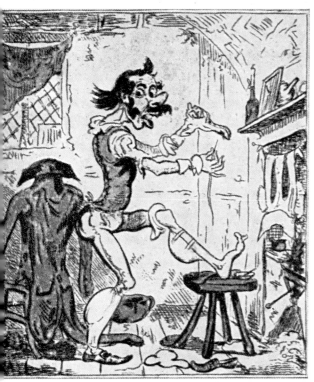

Artificial calves. When long trousers were introduced skinny calves were ridiculed. This English caricature drawn in 1800 by Lewis Marks shows a dandy of the old aristocratic school getting dressed to comply with new fashions

Sons of the Revolution. The first few years of the French Revolution saw change and excess in all spheres, not excepting the realm of fashion. The dandies of the Revolution wore tight trousers, so long that their tops came up almost to the chest. Having declared war on the whole established world, they felt justified in breaking into new fields themselves. A new style of coat was introduced which had a high collar and wide lapel, and was worn with a large hat,

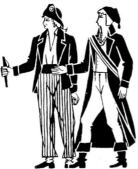

Male dress during the French Revolution

later called the Napoleon. A heavy walking stick completed the ensemble of these liberated gentlemen.

One of the great painters of the Revolution, Jacques-Louis David, designed new fashions based on Classical traditions, but these were worn only for parties or as stage costume and not adopted generally.

The revolution in fashion in general had begun before the political upheaval. Goethe's *The Sufferings of Young Werther* was written fifteen years before the start of the French Revolution, but in it he describes the same fashions,

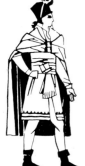

David's sketch for the suit of a 'revolutionary'

'It was a heavy decision for me to give up the simple blue coat which I had worn for the first time when I danced with Lotte, but it was quite worn out. I have had another made for me just like the old one with collar, lapels, waistcoat and trousers in yellow.'

New colours came in. Blue, yellow and brown took the place of pink, violet and pale green. Men's and women's clothes had previously

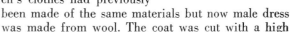

Frenchman in 1790 and in 1792 with the hat à la Napoleon

been made of the same materials but now male dress was made from wool. The coat was cut with a high collar, broad lapels and a double row of buttons down the front. The bottom of the coat was cut away in front to show the thighs. Trousers were close-fitting and in a lighter colour than the coat. In the Rococo period trousers had always been in a darker shade. Top-boots were worn in place of buckled shoes, and a circular hat replaced the tricorn.

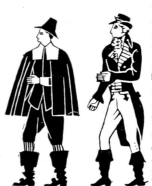

A Puritan of 1650, and Werther, 1775

Puritans and Long Trousers. The Puritan style of dress originated in America. From there it travelled to England and then to France and Germany. The seventeenth-century Cromwellian coat had a cutaway front and was worn with close-fitting top-boots. This garment reached the Continent as the redingote, or riding coat. Anything English was held in high regard at the time, because of the much admired English parliamentary sy-

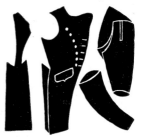

Pattern for the redingote, 1800

stem; England was regarded as the land of freedom. English hunting attire made a great impact in France, but the French preferred the Napoleonic hat to the tall hat usually worn in England. The long wide-bottomed trousers which were worn by sailors in the English Navy were quickly adopted as a general fashion for men.

And so the dress of the proletariat appeared in the grande salon. There one

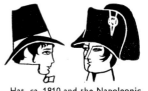

Hat, ca. 1810 and the Napoleonic hat

now saw the high boots previously reserved for coachmen and grooms and the bell-bottomed trousers previously associated with sailors.

Opposite Elderly lady with lace headgear and collar, leg-of-mutton sleeves and high waist. Painting by Købke, 1835

Revolutionary Behaviour. With the new style of dress came a new conception of manners and behaviour. Men no longer appeared decorated, as it were, with powdered wigs, silken jackets and buckled shoes. Their figures came to assume a tall, slender line which gave the impression of youth and agility.

The vigorous ideal of the French Revolution stood in sharp contrast to the Rococo dandy who had minced along on a real or imaginary parquet floor to join his carriage or sedan chair waiting at the door. This new man was above all a man of action. He strode along purposefully and sat firm in the saddle. There was no special form of outdoor clothing

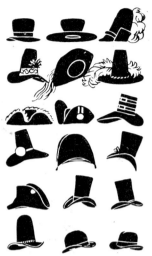

The battle between the crown and the brim:

1400	1435	1564
1606	1630	1660
1700	1786	1787
1791	1795	1800
1812	1845	1853
1853	1930	1930

but the coat collar could be turned up and knee-boots gave protection in bad weather.

The highest admiration was reserved for the heroic type whose countenance was calm, gaze was level and stance upright. Always aware of himself, his movements were positive but restrained. Napoleon made the large head a desirable characteristic, and this was enhanced by the large Napoleonic hat worn diagonally.

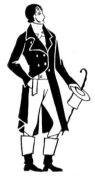

French coat of 1799

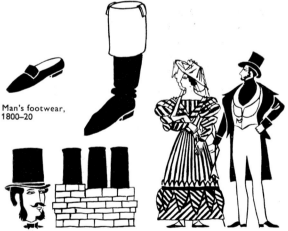

Man's footwear, 1800–20

Stovepipe hat and tall chimneys

1827 and 1828

Fancy Waistcoats and Puritan Hats. The waistcoat now became short and sleeveless. A light material was used for the back and the front could be either fancy or plain. As many as three sets of lapels were added at the neck. These could be in contrasting colours and thus gave the effect of three waistcoats being worn at the same time. The long neckcloth came in at this time; this was wrapped several times around the neck and came up to the chin. After 1800, it assumed reasonable proportions, and the shirt collar made its first appearance with points so tall that they were nicknamed 'the parricides'.

The Puritan high felt hat, long popular in England, now became the sign of the steady, reliable citizen and remained fashionable. The crown was sometimes cylindrical, sometimes tapering towards the brim. The silk hat made its first appearance at the beginning of the nineteenth century and gradually became taller. By the middle of the century, it had become the status symbol of all decent citizens.

Neckcloth

The Dress of the Commoners. The new style of dress involved politics as well as fashion.

When the Estates General met in 1789, the Master of Ceremonies specified various forms of dress. People of the Third Estate were not permitted to wear any colour in their dress or carry any form of ornament. Mirabeau criticized this veto in one of his very first speeches and asserted the right of the individual to dress as he pleased, a view which gradually gained general approval. The mode of dress should be an expression of liberty, equality and fraternity. Since not all could aspire to equal beauty and aristocratic elegance of attire, a different standard form of dress, a democratic mean, came to be accepted. The higher ranks of society sacrificed their old elegance and the lower classes had the satisfaction both of retaining their original style and finding it in general use. A simple coat with velvet collar and bright buttons now became the usual wear of all orders of society. Discreet colours such as olive, chocolate and dark blue remained in fashion for some time. The overt splendour of bright colours and silver and gold embroidery was restricted to military uniforms.

After 1800, the purpose of civilian dress was no longer to indicate what a man was, but what he had: figure, taste and money.

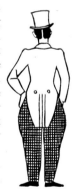

English suit, ca. 1825

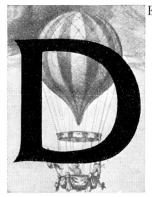

DEFINITION was given to the new industrial world by myriad developments. By 1840, many important things had become part of life — the telegraph, photography, postage stamps, shorthand writing. The first sewing-machine was devised in the 1840's, the oil lamp and analine dye in the 1850's, dynamite, the typewriter and the rotary printing press in the 1860's. The dramatic and romantic spirit of the time was expressed in the music of Wagner and Berlioz.

The Romantic Woman. It has been said, not without reason, that whereas man was liberated during the Renaissance, woman had to wait for Romantic litera-

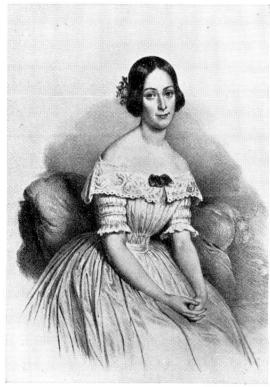

Sloping shoulders and wasp-waist

ture; and even then, she was merely discovered, not liberated. Self-assertion was not encouraged in a well brought up woman of that time. Factory and business life were beyond her province; she was not concerned with politics. The duty of a young woman was to marry and then to look after her home. A woman's life was dictated to her as a series of attitudes; her passive role was exemplified by her humility — be it the resigned dignity of the mature matron, or the languishing romantic pose of the unmarried girl, her hair parted demurely in the middle, and covered by a shawl, her sloping shoulders again draped in shawls, her eyes cast downward. Everything betokened a shy, unassuming outlook on life. Her restricted social life was expressed in tight

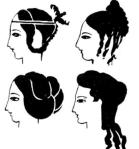

Hair styles in 1834, 1840, 1850 and 1870

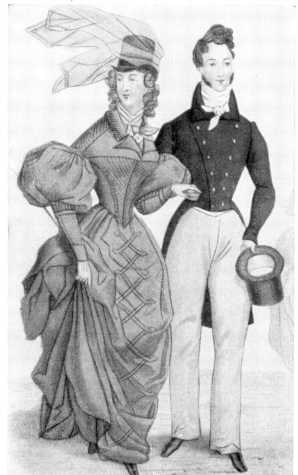

Plate in a fashion magazine of the correct outfit in which to go riding, 1831. The lady wears a tall hat with a veil and a long skirt which hides her legs even when on horseback

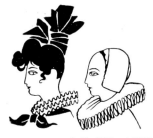

Ruffs, 1830 and 1580

15*

lacing up to the armpits and sleeves so narrow that she could not even raise her hand up to her hair. Just as middle-class women were separated from the industrial and commercial world by barriers of convention, so were they separated from their immediate surroundings by the half a dozen petticoats they wore beneath their skirts.

Souls without Bodies. The body was covered up. The poets Robert and Elizabeth Browning, who spent a lifetime of marriage together and whose love poems occupy an important place in English literature, apparently never saw each other naked.

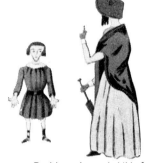

Danish mother and child of the 1840's

As long as marriage was regarded as the only possible career for a respectable woman she had, of necessity, to cultivate her outward attractions rather than develop her particular talents. She concealed herself cunningly under an armour of flat panels and straight lines that bore no connection to the soft curves of her body. Heavy petticoats and corsets made natural movement irksome. Anaemia was an interesting malady and swooning was evidence of a sensitive soul.

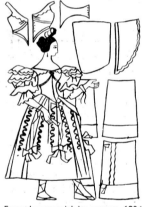

Formal gown with its pattern, 1834

The design of evening dress in particular was absurd. Heavy and voluminous, and laced tightly round a wasp-waist, it made the body look quite out of proportion. These dresses were made in floating, frothy effervescent materials that were suffused with a play of softly harmonizing colours — lavender, leather brown, pale blue, grey-green, silver grey — and made the wearer look like an unsubstantial dream! A man displayed his wealth by showering great masses of expensive materials on his closely-bound wife and daughters.

The industrialization of cotton production in 1830 and of wool ten years later made full dresses even more a practical possibility.

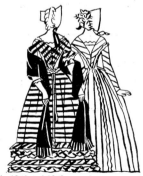

In 1841 and 1842 women wore seven or eight skirts though the climate was the same as it had been in 1800 when they wore only one

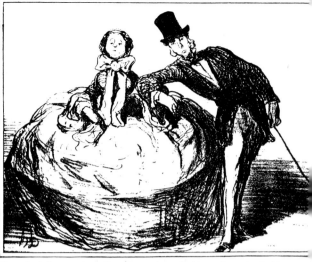

'Since the ladies wear iron skirts, the gentlemen had better be made of rubber so that they can lead them by the arm.' Lithograph by Honore Daumier, ca. 1855

The Harbingers of Emancipation. A low angry growl could be heard in the political world of 1847; it emanated from the very cellars of society and took printed form in *The Communist Manifesto*.

In February 1848, fighting broke out again in the streets of Paris. A political thunderstorm engulfed Germany, culminating in the March Revolution and a demand for constitutional law and individual liberty.

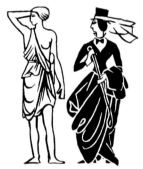

Greek Amazon, and French amazon, ca. 1850

While this was going on another rumbling could be heard. It was the first positive move toward the emancipation of women. Many a middle-class girl had woven fantasies of gaining the power and influence of a Lola Montez, the raven-haired, blue-eyed toast of the 1850's, whose power lay solely in her charm and intelligence. Through her influence, rulers could be unseated or reinstated. Worthy matrons secretly read the writings of George Sand behind drawn blinds decorated with wild mountain scenery and romantic castles. Fiery claims were made by George Sand and others to women's right to share freely in sexual pleasure, previously the undisputed province of the men.

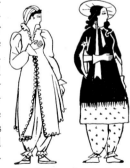

Trousers for the theatre and Bloomer outfit, 1850

In 1849, Mrs. Bloomer introduced trousers for women in America and England, and at about the same time women adopted the men's leather-soled shoe.

How great an impression was made on their gentler sisters by these courageous women is difficult to

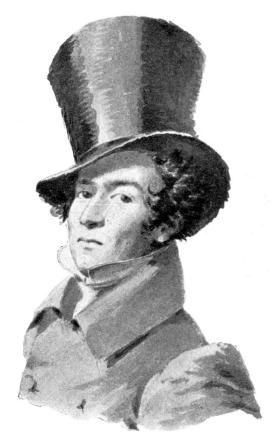
Tall stovepipe hat of the 1840's. Self-portrait by the Danish painter, Louis Aumont

Court Crinoline. The crinoline was originally designed for court wear. It was truly a dress fit for a queen, only the grand ballrooms of palaces and castles could provide an adequate background. Descriptions of the dresses worn by the reigning queens of the time read like a fashion article. The beautiful Empress Eugénie of France spoke of her 'political dresses', five hundred of which she took with her for the opening of the Suez Canal. The romantic Elizabeth of Austria disassociated herself from her banal surroundings by the extravagant splendour of her wardrobe which included many beautiful crinolines. Queen Victoria with her tea-cosy figure was the cornerstone of the British Empire.

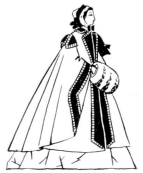
Correct dress for taking a promenade, 1860

A vast quantity of material was used to make all these dresses. When Lyon silk was made popular by the Empress Eugénie, the number of looms employed in production increased from fifty-seven thousand to one hundred and twenty thousand. The steel industry also expanded, as ninety million kilograms of wire were

estimate; certainly at first the doctrine of female equality made slow progress.

Clothed in Steel.

Increasing quantities of horsehair were woven into petticoat material in order to obtain the necessary degree of size and stiffness, until eventually the weight became unbearable. In 1857, the machine age produced a solution which liberated women from this torture; following the Great Exhibition of 1851

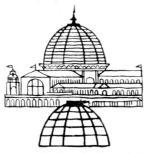
The Crystal Palace and the crinoline

which took place at Crystal Palace in London, a light steel cage appeared which was to replace the cumbersome horse-hair petticoat. Inside this steel framework, women could now move easily. It is interesting to see how its rather bulbous shape was echoed in the dome of the Crystal Palace itself.

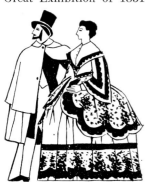
Male attire of 1855 and crinoline, 1858

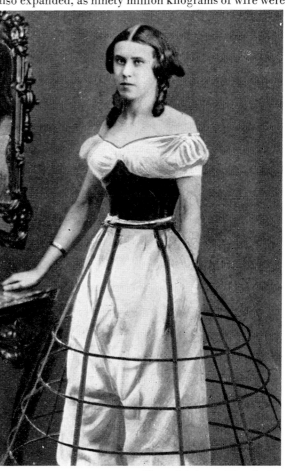
The steel skeleton of the crinoline

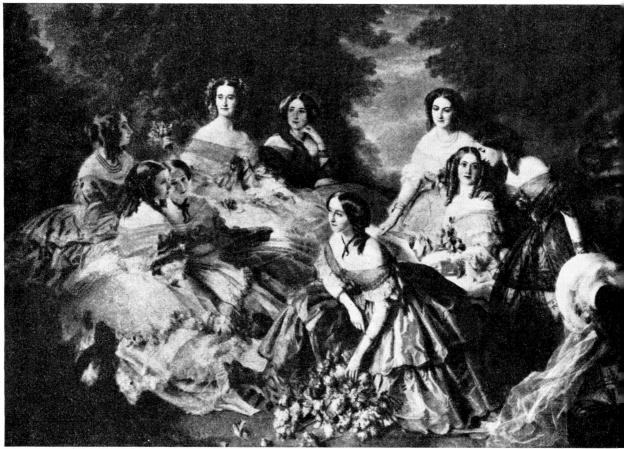

Empress Eugénie, the beauty queen of Europe, surrounded by her ladies-in-waiting. The group forms a pattern reminiscent itself of a crinoline. Painting by Winterhalter

used for crinoline frames between 1854 and 1866. During this time a single factory turned out a total of nine hundred thousand frames.

These crinolines were enormous. An ordinary room could accommodate only one crinoline and a large ballroom looked like an encampment. As the size of the crinoline increased, the sleeves became larger until they too had to be supported by steel springs. The crinoline had to be a certain size to indicate the necessary degree of importance; importance being a line of demarcation between the social classes. Status was denoted by the design and perfection of the dress rather than by the dress itself. The crinoline could be worn by a peasant girl, but the standard of workmanship and size made sure that she would not be mistaken for a countess. Crinolines and jewellery went well together, and ear-rings, cameos, necklaces and diamonds were worn in abundance. The Empress Eugénie wore a ball-dress of tulle embroidered with diamonds worth a fortune. Everything connected with dress spoke of splendour both in the materials themselves and in the ornamentation. The cont-

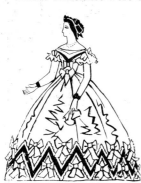

Wide crinoline of 1861

rast between the crinoline and the shift dress of the previous period was similar to the contrast between the Romantic conception of art and the severe outlines admired by the Neo-Classical period.

Restricted Muscles. The striking colour combinations of the Orient came to Europe from Turkey after the Crimean War in the mid-nineteenth century. Strong clear colours now competed with the soft shades which had previously been the vogue. The impact made by contrasting colour schemes was to become more pronounced later on, but even at first a contemporary writer expressed the opinion that the general effect was 'characteristic of the disharmony of the time'.

The picturesque effect of these colour combinations was also found in Impressionist paintings which employed all the colours of the rainbow and which made such a great impact on European art at this time. Colour was first let loose in fashion, and afterwards in painting.

It is possible to associate colour contrast with the latent discontent of the time. If women could have exchanged their heavy garments for dresses of an airy lightness they would have emerged like lilies from the suffocating flower-bed of the crinoline. But they were imprisoned,

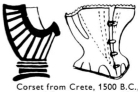

Corset from Crete, 1500 B.C., and European corset, 1862

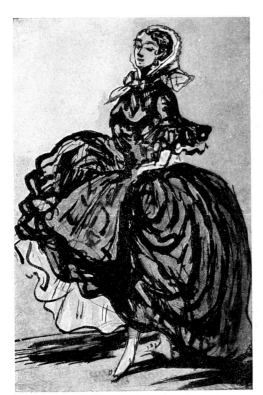

Crinoline drawn by Constantin Guys

Reigning queens could outdo their subjects in the beauty and value of their jewellery. The same could not be said, however, about daring in the cut of a dress. It was the demi-monde who set the pace in this fashion.

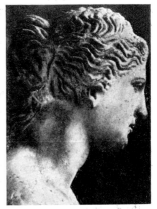

Greek chignon, ca. 450 B.C.

The narrow decorous life led by the well-bred married woman resulted in the husband inhabiting two separate worlds. One was at home with his wife and children, the other was with his mistress. The two worlds met in the opera house and at the gaming table where a nobleman's wife and mistress might sit side by side.

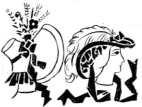

1836 and 1856

The demi-monde occupied a recognized place in society and was celebrated in the literature of the period. *The Lady of the Camelias* was written by Alexander Dumas the Younger in 1852.

their souls were enclosed in a straitjacket. The woman of this period laid a heroic sacrifice on the altar of fashion; she had to pay dearly for her wasp-waist.

Décolleté and Gloves. Somehow people had to see that within all that pyramid of clothing there was a human body. The neck was therefore exposed and the neckline cut very low. The décolletage terminated in a horizontal line, as if to say, 'so far and no further'.

No well-dressed woman was ever seen out of doors without her gloves. The shawl was still regarded as indispensable both inside and outside the house.

Bonnets

Knickers were worn under the crinoline. Originally these terminated at the knee but they later were extended by a lace frill. White cotton stockings were worn and also booties with Rococo heels laced on the inner side.

Bonnets were tied under the chin with broad ribbons. The hair had a demure centre parting, and either

Chignons in 1630, 1690, 1830 and 1860

fell in long ringlets at the sides or was wound in coils over the ears. The bun, or chignon, appeared after 1850.

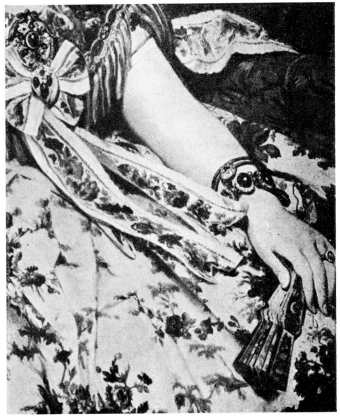

Dress with floral pattern, bracelets and fan. Detail of painting by Ingres

189

That high fashion in dress was made such an unassailable bastion by 'la grande cocotte' surely exposes the hypocrisy of human nature — or, perhaps, the innocence of human nature: every little middle-class girl carefully kept to the rules in her mode of dress if she had the means to do so. Not everyone could afford to take her daily bath in milk, although we know for a fact that the milk was afterwards returned to the dairyman for re-sale.

In 1859, the hemline was raised a few inches so that the tip of the shoe was occasionally seen. No one could have convinced the scandalized public that this was the first protest against the tyranny of the cocotte; indeed it was clear to them that young

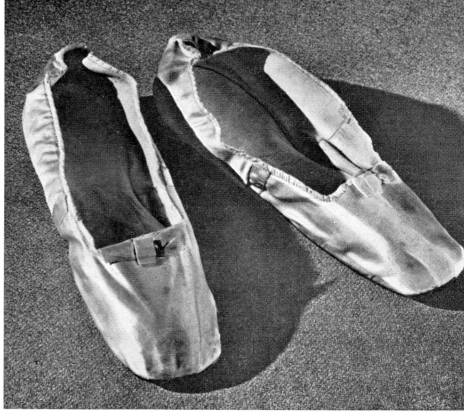

Satin bridal slippers

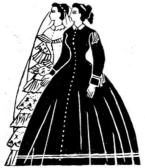

'Tea-cosy' crinolines of 1857 and 1867

Layered dress of 1865

girls shortened their skirts merely in order to throw themselves wholeheartedly into the new fashionable game of croquet, a pastime which offered so many opportunities for the daring to show a dainty satin-shoed foot!

Woman's and man's shoes, 1850

New Rococo and New Revolution. As dresses became shorter so necklines plunged deeper. The crinoline no longer concealed the hips but assumed an oval shape from which the body appeared to emerge like a figurehead at the front. Seen from the side, the outline was that of a right-angled triangle.

Crinolines, 1858 and 1863

190

Opposite Putting on the bridal head-dress, 1859. Painting by H. Olrik

The crinoline suddenly disappeared in 1868. The deciding factor, which would have been ignored had the garment not already lost favour, was the risk that the crinoline entailed. Many people talked of accidents. The diaphanous material frequently caught fire, and one incident occurred in which a woman in a crinoline was blown into the sea and drowned. But the main reason for rejecting it lay in its shape which was considered undemocratic; the greatly improved education of women made the splendid isolation of the crinoline no longer appropriate.

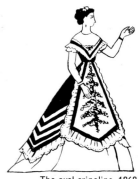

The oval crinoline, 1868

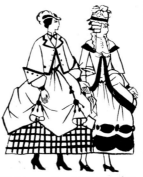

Walking outfits of 1860 and 1780

Hat with ostrich feathers, 1847

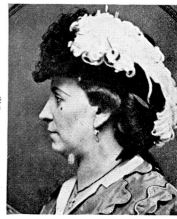

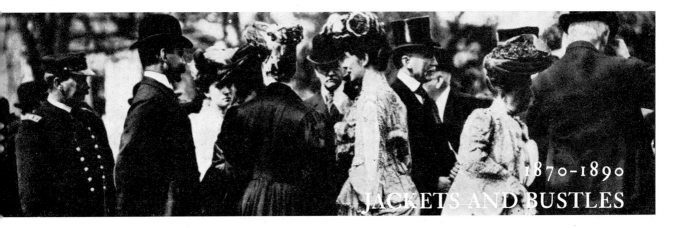

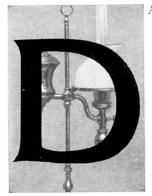

DANGERS experienced in Africa led Stanley to some striking conclusions. When he returned to England in 1877, he gave an address to the Manchester Chamber of Commerce in which he spoke about the large Negro population in the Congo who went about completely naked. He pointed out a duty to convert these unhappy natives to the Christian faith and to teach them to dress. If, he said, these people could be persuaded to wear clothes, even if only on Sundays, three hundred and twenty million yards of Manchester cotton would be needed for the purpose. This announcement was greeted with great enthusiasm and loud applause. The race for colonization by the great nations of the world was speeded up. Instead of developing out of free competition and private enterprise, power in the industrial market fell into the hands of large public companies in which the shareholders had virtually no say.

This was what the Germans termed the 'Gründe Jahre'. The world-wide feeling of triumph was expressed in the Toreador's Song in *Carmen*, composed by Bizet in 1875. The air hummed with turning wheels. Everyday life ran on ball-bearings. The

centrifugal pump, the rotary printing press, the typewriter, roller skates and bicycles came into general use. The fast tempo of whirling machinery was exciting, no less the advent of the new brilliant lighting.

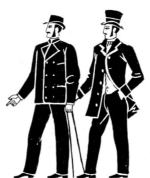

The suit in 1874 and 1885 . . .

'Let there be light!' was the excited cry of men of progress. But Henrik Ibsen lit up all the murky corners of society in *A Doll's House*. The lower classes were provided the opportunity of public libraries. The radical writings of Georg Brandes formed the vanguard in the tempestuous demands for female emancipation.

Male Accessories. The style of male clothing gradually changed from being ponderous to possessing a degree of elegance and perfection. The figure was divided in two by the V-shaped openings: the top opening of the jacket which allowed the shirt to be seen, and the points in which the waistcoat ended. The morning coat remained a symbol of respectability but the ordinary jacket was in everyday use. A stiff shirt collar was worn either with the points folded down or upright with an opening for the Adam's apple. A crossover cravat made of stiffened silk was worn round the neck or, alternatively, a machine-

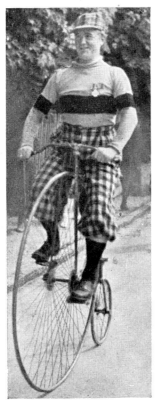

Penny-farthing of the 1880's

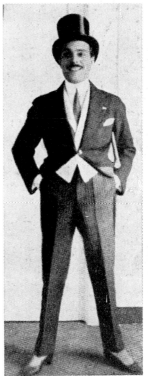

. . . and how it had changed by 1914

Opposite   Sunday promenade in Paris, 1866. Painting by Seurat

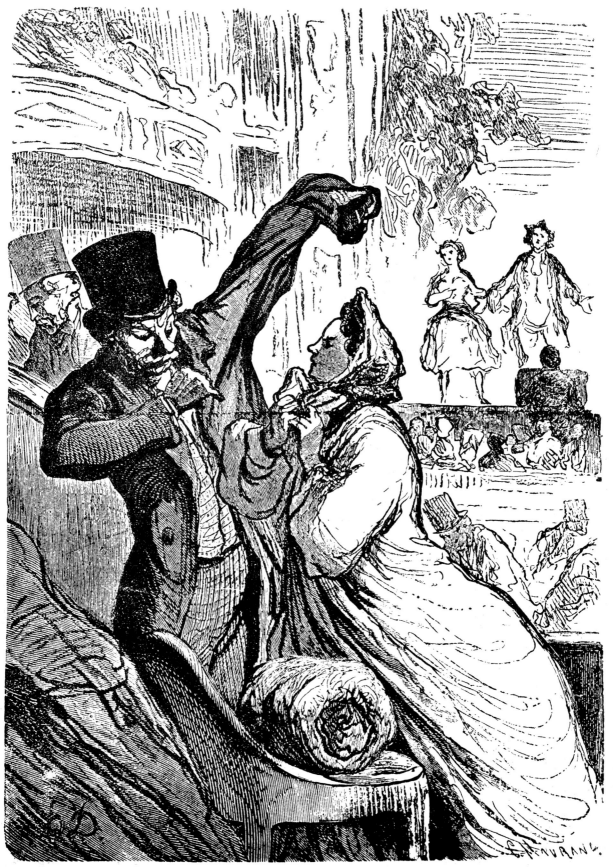

'The top hat has a flat crown. On a certain level – the upper middle classes – every one is equal.' Woodcut by Honore Daumier

knitted tie was hooked in at the back. The cuffs and the shirt-front were starched, and the latter was fixed to the main shirt with buttons.

The Chignon and the Bustle. It is interesting to note that more attention was paid to the woman's head than had been before. The hair was gathered behind with padding, and false hair was added to form a chignon. At this point the crinoline reappeared, in the form of a bustle. We now also find a modified crinoline known as the crinolette.

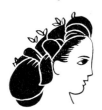
Chignon

This was arranged over a semicircular wire frame open in front or over a horsehair foundation supported by bamboo canes.

In 1867, a walking dress was designed in Paris which had a polonaise that was tied up with a scarf at the back and finished in a bow. The typical bustle dress consisted of this polonaise, a

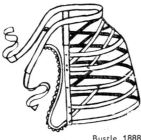
Bustle, 1888

Shoes at an exhibition in Copenhagen in 1888

short overdress draped extravagantly over the bustle behind. It was tied with bows down the sides and cut away in front to give the impression of an apron. The polonaise was worn over a full-length underdress with train attached for party wear. The elegance and chic of this fashion lay in the close fit of the front panel, that emphasized the basic female shape. For this reason, close-fitting underwear was introduced for the very first time.

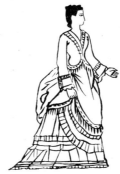
Polonaise with bustle, 1817

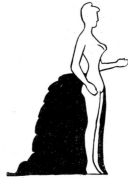
Ideal shape for wearing a bustle

A Curious Fashion. It was difficult to stand upright in this kind of dress, awkward to walk and positively dangerous to sit down. It is tempting to

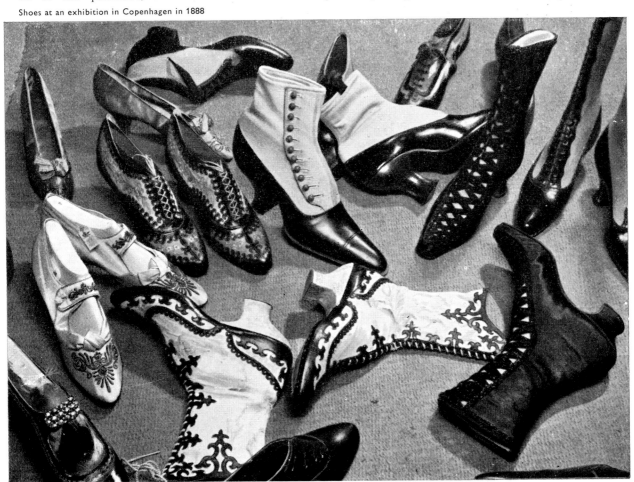

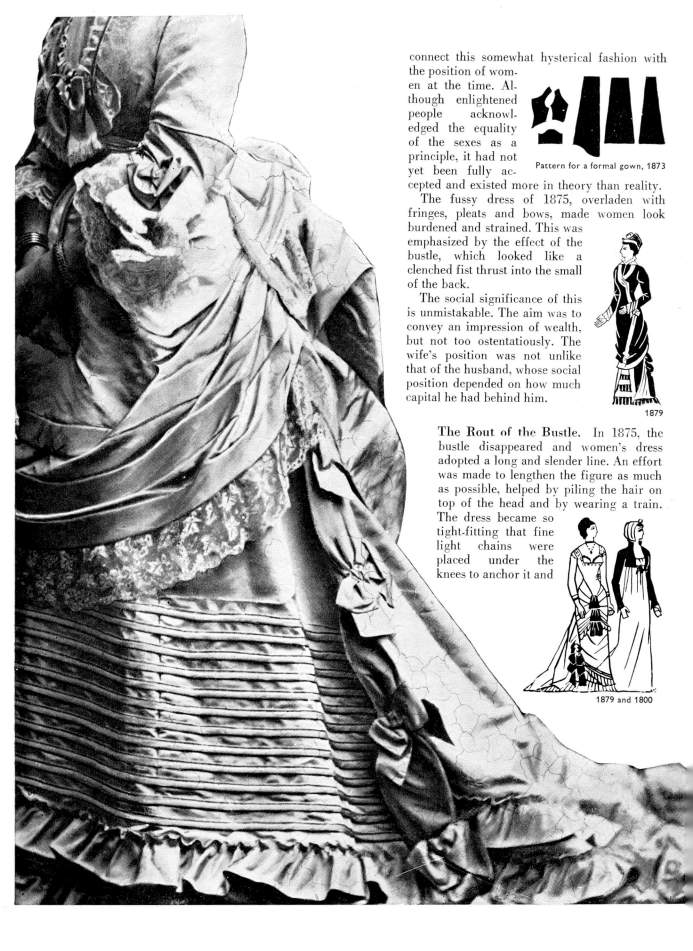

connect this somewhat hysterical fashion with the position of women at the time. Although enlightened people acknowledged the equality of the sexes as a principle, it had not yet been fully accepted and existed more in theory than reality.

Pattern for a formal gown, 1873

The fussy dress of 1875, overladen with fringes, pleats and bows, made women look burdened and strained. This was emphasized by the effect of the bustle, which looked like a clenched fist thrust into the small of the back.

The social significance of this is unmistakable. The aim was to convey an impression of wealth, but not too ostentatiously. The wife's position was not unlike that of the husband, whose social position depended on how much capital he had behind him.

1879

The Rout of the Bustle. In 1875, the bustle disappeared and women's dress adopted a long and slender line. An effort was made to lengthen the figure as much as possible, helped by piling the hair on top of the head and by wearing a train.

The dress became so tight-fitting that fine light chains were placed under the knees to anchor it and

1879 and 1800

prevent it from splitting. This new use of chains signified a kind of voluntary slavery which must indeed have intrigued the opposite sex. But, first and foremost, the aim of the slender, tightly fitting dress was to show off the voluptuous shapes and curves of the body. The woman of this time was fully conscious of her female attributes, though in a different way from her bashful sisters of previous times. She now appeared as if she were clad in only corset and petticoat, and the ballroom came to resemble a boudoir; tiny fanciful aprons were worn, known as 'fig leaves'!

When the long cotton gloves were peeled off with an affected and deliberate gesture, the response must have been something like the excite-

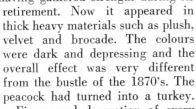

The enormous bustle

ment generated by the modern strip-tease act.

Some women are known to have had on occasions a rather disquieting inclination to step out of the part of a dressed doll and appear *in natura*.

The Return of the Bustle. The bustle returned to fashion in 1882, having gathered strength during its retirement. Now it appeared in thick heavy materials such as plush, velvet and brocade. The colours were dark and depressing and the overall effect was very different from the bustle of the 1870's. The peacock had turned into a turkey.

Finery and decoration of every variety became the keynotes of the day and extravagant dress was vied by ornate knick-knacks in the drawing-room. Strident and fantastic hues chanced upon by artists in their experiments permeated fashion. A constant competition existed between the quiet colours produced by the old organic dyes and the sharp colours made possible by the new aniline dyes. As soon as primary colours could be produced cheaply they were regarded as vulgar; the original soft harmonious shades were considered dull because they were old-fashioned.

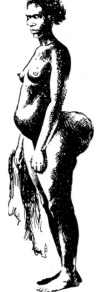

Hottentot woman with huge buttocks

Fashion at this time became very unsettled, and pattern and cut changed frequently. Dress was no longer a class privilege. Serving-girl and manservant could dress as they wished within their means. Social position could only be established by being ahead in style. Not only had the tempo of fashion change quickened but fashions had become gaudy and this period had a number of different standards and ideals.

The Buxom Woman. The impression aimed at was a Rubens type, with full bust, broad hips and large behind. This also appealed to the men who built themselves pseudo-Renaissance palaces, making a great display of their wealth and property. Advertisements for methods to gain weight were just as persuasive as those of the present day which make claims in the opposite direction. The stomach was pushed forward provokingly and the bust was pressed upwards in a most inviting manner. An innovation which was characteristic of this time was the padded brassiere.

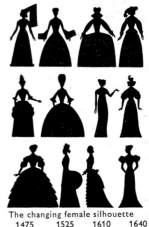

The changing female silhouette

1475	1525	1610	1640
1700	1770	1800	1825
1850	1872	1885	1890

The desire for enhanced femininity was demonstrated very clearly in women's footwear. No consideration was

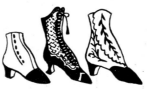

Ladies' boots in 1871, 1883 and 1890

given to the natural shape of the foot and no distinction made between left and right. This suited the boot and shoe factories very well, who had just begun to turn out ready-made footwear in comparatively large quantities. Self-respecting women always wore boots, but with high French heels. The effect sought after was the grace of the ballet dancer's pointed foot, the front of the leg and the instep extending in one straight line.

The natural habitat of this pouter pigeon-like lady was the over-furnished home, an artificial retreat where, behind drawn curtains, time stood still. Double curtains subdued the sunlight and hushed the noise from without. These noiseless rooms were galleries of still-life, funeral-halls of dead

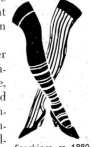

Stockings, ca. 1880

nature exhibited in mysterious, fantastic, complicated and meaningless forms: a thistle cast in bronze from the living plant and mounted under glass, artificial flowers, lacquered bullrushes and dyed feathers. The cosy, hermetically-sealed home, abrim with possessions, provided a place of refuge from the threatening chaos of the outside world.

People became accustomed to a faster tempo after 1890, but during the previous decades a certain anxiety was present with regard to a world in a rapid process of change. Even flourishing world trade, which had hitherto been regarded as a guarantee of security, became a victim of depression, and this was something no one could understand. Did industry nurture a serpent within its bosom, in the form of the workers organizing themselves specifically to overthrow the established order?

The Willowy Type. A new philosophy of art now developed in order to counter the general trend of industrial development and its effect on the arts and crafts. Among the artists who fought this battle was William Morris. He hoped to effect a revival of the crafts, drowned at that

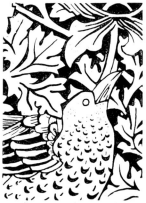

Fabric designed by William Morris

time in a torrent of spurious imitations such as carved wood simulated in plaster of Paris, imitation stained glass made from printed wax-paper, plants and flowers cut from coloured zinc plate, made possible by the machine age.

In the eyes of those idealists, the perfect woman was to be a dreamer and not of this world, and possess the physical characteristics of the women of late Gothic and early Renaissance paintings. The model who sat for the artist, Dante Gabriel Rossetti, when he painted his greatly admired 'Beata Beatrix' was a salesgirl in a London milliner's. One glance at her delicate features, her slender neck and golden red hair, convinced him that he had found the most perfect example of womanhood in all the world, and the woman who must become his wife. Gradually, slender girls with long limbs were seen moving in

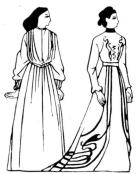

English gown of the 1870's and German dress of 1900 in Art Nouveau style

the highest social circles side by side with ample women with generous busts. These girls wore no corsets and were clothed in long, wide-sleeved dresses with long trains. These dresses, made from soft light materials, fell in natural folds, and were decorated with stylized flat patterns in delicate colours. The Morris Movement in art did not reach a very wide circle during the early stages, but other trends eventually came to support the same broad principles which at length gained general acceptance. At the same time, Japanese art started to influence Western Europe.

Japanese woodcuts delighted western artists, and Japanese industrial art became very fashionable. Several generations later, European architecture came under strong Japanese influence and moved toward the functional in design.

Meantime, the kimono was greeted enthusiastically by women in Europe. Its simple cut and natural folds were in themselves a rebuke to the complicated draperies of the bustle. The female posterior was now regarded as comical rather than seductive, so the large bow on the back of the Japanese kimono did not accompany it to Europe.

The Emancipated Woman. Finally, we have the third type of woman who played an increasingly important part during the latter part of the last century. This was the woman who endeavoured to set the final seal on equality between the sexes. Such women entered the professional world by graduating from university and becoming doctors, teachers and librarians. A woman from the middle classes

Hat, ca. 1875

who failed to get married had previously resigned herself to becoming a piece of furniture in the house of relatives more fortunately placed. Now she could establish herself individually, stand on her own two feet and earn her own living.

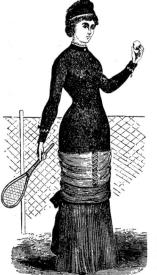

Tennis-dress of the 1870's

Once women had been emancipated, they wished to make clear, by their style of dress, that they had other objects in life beyond merely attracting men. To avoid receiving the mixture of respect and contempt which was normally meted out to unmarried females, these self-supporting women assumed a somewhat masculine style of dress. Tailor-made suits were adopted, made from the worsted fabrics which previously had been exclusively reserved for men.

The hat was regarded as a symbol of emancipation and in the 1880's it knocked the bonnet completely off its perch. At this juncture, men promptly changed their allegiance from the hat to the cap.

Notwithstanding all the influences brought to bear on women's fashion by emancipation, the bustle received its death-blow from a totally different quarter. The bicycle came on the scene during the 1890's and killed the bustle stone-dead.

CORSETTED WAIST AND WING COLLAR

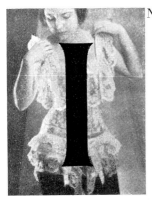

IN THE 1890's, both wireless telegraphy, known to most of us as the radio, and the X-ray were invented, and at the same time the principles of radioactivity were discovered. The miraculous weapons which were employed by women in the sex war were not so invisible, but they had properties as remarkable as those of electricity.

Women had by now stormed a new bastion. They had obtained the freedom to express their own personality, something regarded hitherto as a rather unladylike thing to do. More than this, female psychology became a subject for examination and free discussion. Even the main battleground of the constant conflict between the two sexes shifted from the conscious to the subconscious. Sigmund Freud's treatise on dreams and the magical power of sex symbols had appeared in the last year of the nineteenth century.

New Weapons. The dress, from 1892 on, was long and had a train which was worn even outdoors. The upper part of the body was unnaturally stiffened by the corset. High heels, combined with the tall hair style achieved by back combing, completed the imposing picture. The hat was really something to look up to, because it exhibited so much decoration. The light blouse gradually replaced the stiffened bodice as standard wear and brought with it the advantage that it could be changed independently of the skirt. Women wished to express their equal rights with men by an increased freedom of bodily movement.

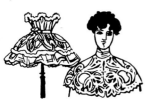

Lamp-shade and dress top, ca. 1905

A certain amount of reaction set in, directed against the mannish appearance of the modern emancipated woman. This feeling expressed itself in bell-shaped skirts, puffed leg-of-mutton sleeves, lace collars and over-trimmed hats — all those things, in fact, cited by protagonists of female emancipation as tokens of the old inferiority. But when all is said and done, the generation which produced the fashions of the late nineteenth century certainly enjoyed much greater freedom than the generation they followed. Brilliant colours intro-

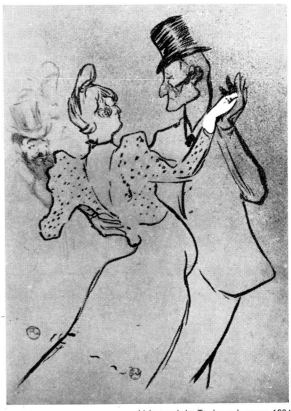

Lithograph by Toulouse-Lautrec, 1894

duced a gay, festive atmosphere. Lace borders, no longer restricted to outer garments, gave an air of amorous intrigue and underwear became more decorative and attractive. A certain type of undergarment made of tricot and shaped like combinations, became very popular. When we look at old lace panta-

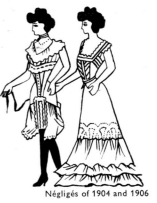

Négligés of 1904 and 1906

loons in museums now, it is perhaps difficult to see them as either romantic or seductive, but there is absolutely no doubt that they were made with both these impressions in mind. The French can-can provides a good example of this new conception of feminine attractiveness, even though it shocked a good many people at the time.

At least one of the underskirts beneath the party dress was usually made in heavy silk which rustled in a most tantalizing manner whenever the wearer mo-

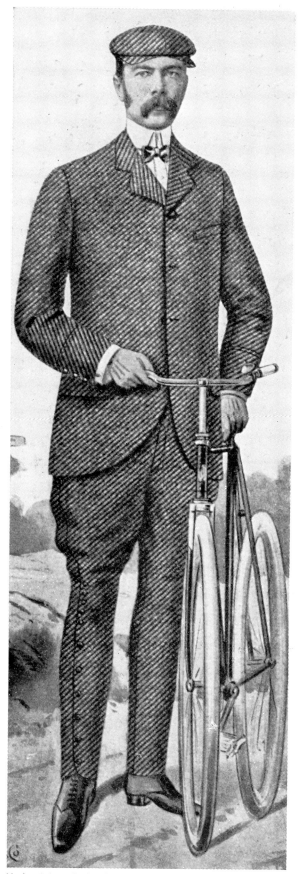

Man's suit in an English fashion magazine, 1899

ved. The effect of that whispering sound, known to the French as the frou-frou, was quite electrifying.

The emancipated female had proved herself able to meet man on his own ground. The subsequent generation, however, employed a different weapon in the fight for freedom, that of being essentially feminine. The secret weapon, which had been so discreetly used just after the French Revolution, was now part of open combat. The hunter and the hunted were in the process of exchanging roles.

The New Woman. Women who fail to make a matrimonial killing prefer on the whole, a succession of short-term victories to a lifetime of being *hors du combat.* At this point a new energetic woman arrived on the scene. In the early 1890's everything was still in a state of chaos. Picturesqueness was the most prominent feature in dress; inside the house a studied disorder was the aim, with perhaps an easel stuck in the corner for effect.

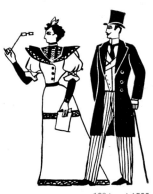

1894 and 1899

The ideal woman was tall and slender. Dried-up spinsters consequently sought to transform themselves into supple seductive females.

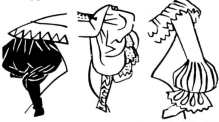

Sleeves in 1833, 1894 and 1901

Sleeves had been rather attractive at the end of the 1880's, but the slightly puffed shoulders developed into epaulettes and then into something looking like small bags until, by 1895, they were rather like a pair of large balloons quivering on the shoulders. After this apogee, they decreased in size year by year. By the beginning of this century, all the fullness was on the forearms; after 1906 sleeves were relatively tight-fitting. The big sleeves were certainly useful for a woman who could use her elbows with effect. They also served to distract attention from those features more attractive to man's primitive instincts. Apart from this, full sleeves made the waist look beautifully slender. The gown undulated as gracefully as a wave when the wearer moved, and the gossamer ball-dress was light as thistledown.

Sporting Dress. Two distinct categories of clothing existed, one for day wear and one for the evening. It was hence officially accepted that women could at

Opposite Parisian lady with powder-puff. Painting by Seurat
Following pages German butcher's apprentice and woman's walking dress in blue flannel. The National Museum, Copenhagen

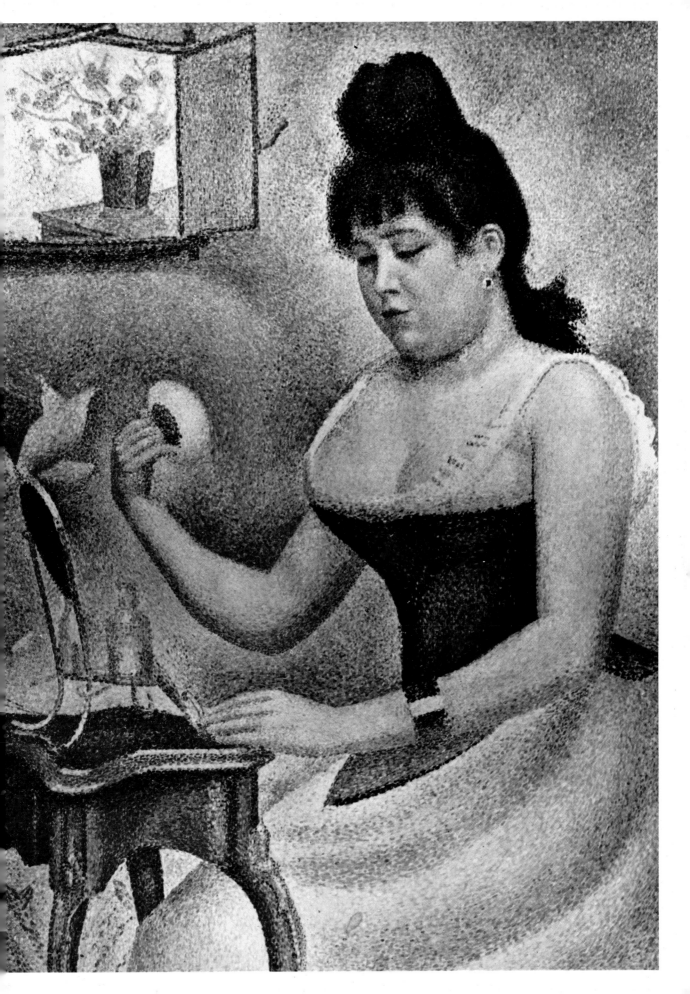

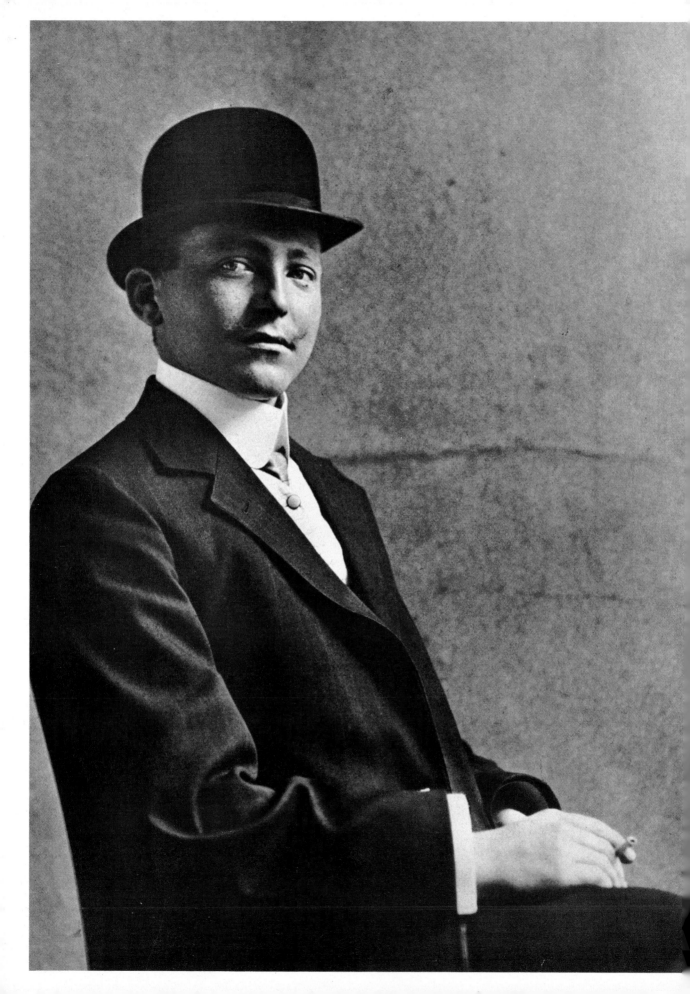

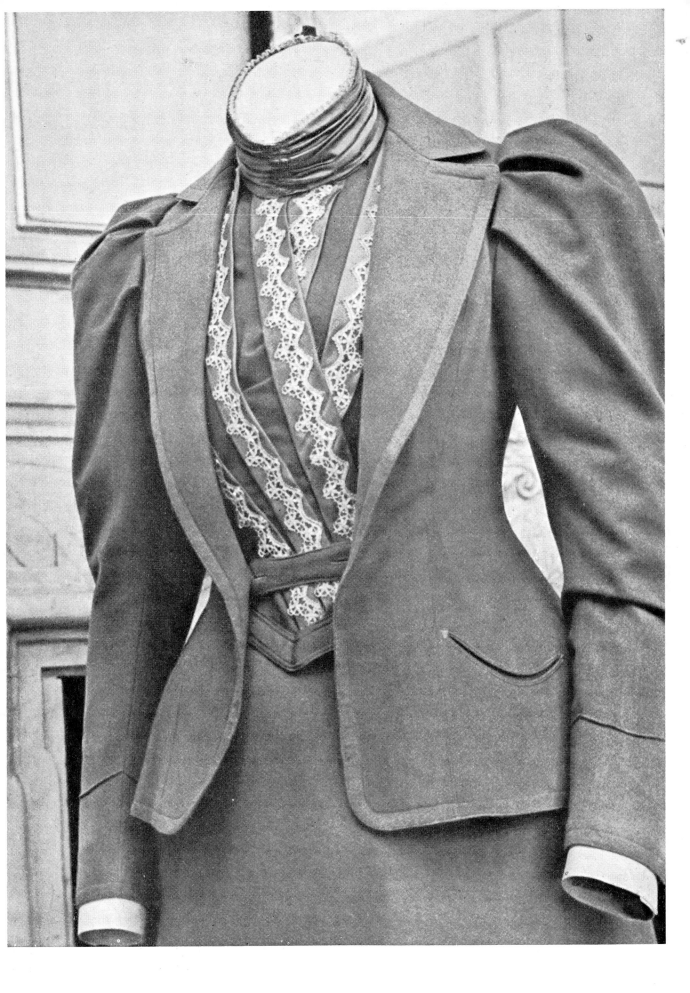

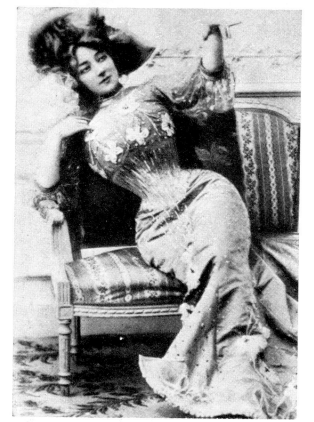

The corsetted waist can be achieved – as in the picture above – by having the bottom rib removed

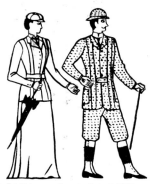

English sporting clothes of 1891

times turn their attention from men for a moment or two. The tailor-made costume came from England and was a product of the same trend towards emancipation. The industrial character of the modern world also affected fashion in so far as it created new environments such as office and factory. Formal dress was usually rather uncomfortable so that it should not be mistaken for 'working clothes'.

It was quite in order, however, to exert oneself, provided this was done for pleasure. Riding had

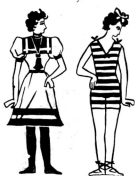

Bathing suits of 1900 and 1911

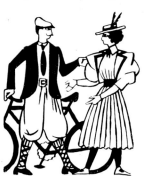

Cycling dress of 1898

hitherto been the only sport considered suitable for women and even so had been almost entirely the prerogative of the aristocracy. Public bathing or swimming were not yet considered quite proper for women and the bathing costume was really a modified version of normal dress, complete with ribbons, flounces and long sleeves. Golf and tennis were played in an ordinary coat and skirt.

When the bicycle achieved a practical shape and was set on pneumatic tyres a number of new fashions evolved. The male monopoly of trousers was seriously and successfully challenged. Wide trousers were worn by women for the first time for cycling; riding and fencing breeches followed, even pyjamas.

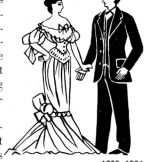

1903, 1906

In the evening, the practical blouse, skirt and jacket were exchanged for a dress made of chiffon, tulle, crepe or artificial silk. The décolleté was several inches lower than was considered proper for day wear, a strategic variation already well

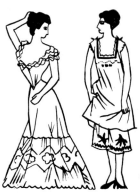

Négligés of 1907 and 1911

established. During the day women looked like an army in close formation dressed in the drab uniform of an industrial society. At night, however, they became individualistic partisans engaged in hand-to-hand combat. Cunning ambushes were set and reckless assaults carried out. Full advantage was taken of dazzling colours in the attack, and subtle weapons, developed over a thousand years of guerrilla warfare, were employed.

The Turn of the Century. Great technical advances had been made by the turn of the century which made a strong impact on everyday life. The gramophone, for instance, the vacuum cleaner and the cinema were introduced. Education, in all classes of society, was bearing fruit. The general principle of evolution was generally accepted after science and religion had agreed that bourgeois morality was grounded in natural law. Certain accepted humanitarian ideals, monogamy, care of the poor, free competition, came to be seen not only as Christian virtues but also as arrangements implicit in the very nature of things.

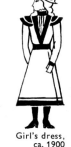

Girl's dress, ca. 1900

A deep sense of security prevailed, and the menacing march of the workers' movement did in time merge harmlessly into the bourgeois system.

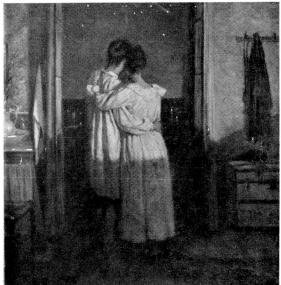

Night-dresses in a painting by Irminger

Bust and Skirts. The new female figure was an outstanding example of the modern undulating line. The stiffened corset pressed the stomach in to such an extent that it became known as 'sans ventre', without stomach. In profile, a woman looked as if she were divided in the middle. The upper part of the body, bedecked with embroidery, lace and crochet-work, gave the impression of a mature and very feminine woman while the hips displayed the slenderness of a young girl. For the first time the skirt was

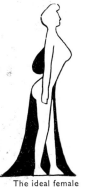

The ideal female figure 1900

Art Nouveau. Art Nouveau was launched when Germany first showed signs of becoming a world power. Naturally enough, it was Paris that first displayed the style at the 1900 Exhibition. It is fairly certain, however, that this fashion of excessive interwoven ornamental design originated in Germany. Van der Welde was the prophet of industrial art as William Morris had been of handicrafts. Europe was flooded with a whole host of German ornaments depicting subjects as diverse as laburnum blossom, poppies, chestnuts, swans and scantily clothed girls. These were really more than mere ornaments as they were representative of the German outlook on industrial art. The music of Rachmaninoff and the paintings of Edvard Munch were also influenced by the Art Nouveau period.

Art Nouveau jewellery, 1903

Ladies' stockings advertised in a 1902 catalogue

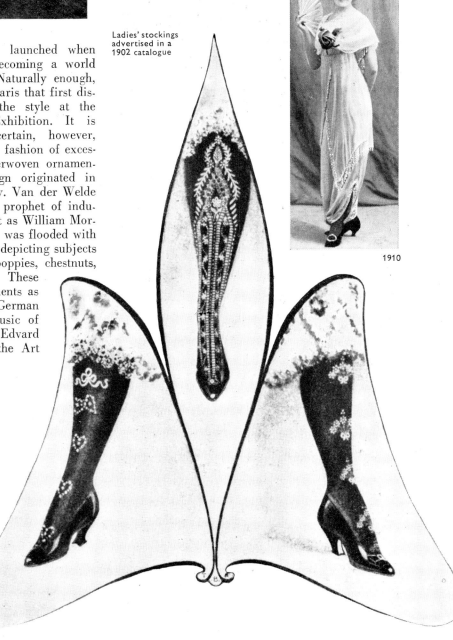

1910

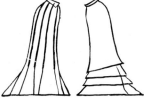

Bell-bottomed skirt, 1902

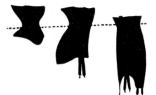

Corsets in 1894, 1904 and 1914

16*

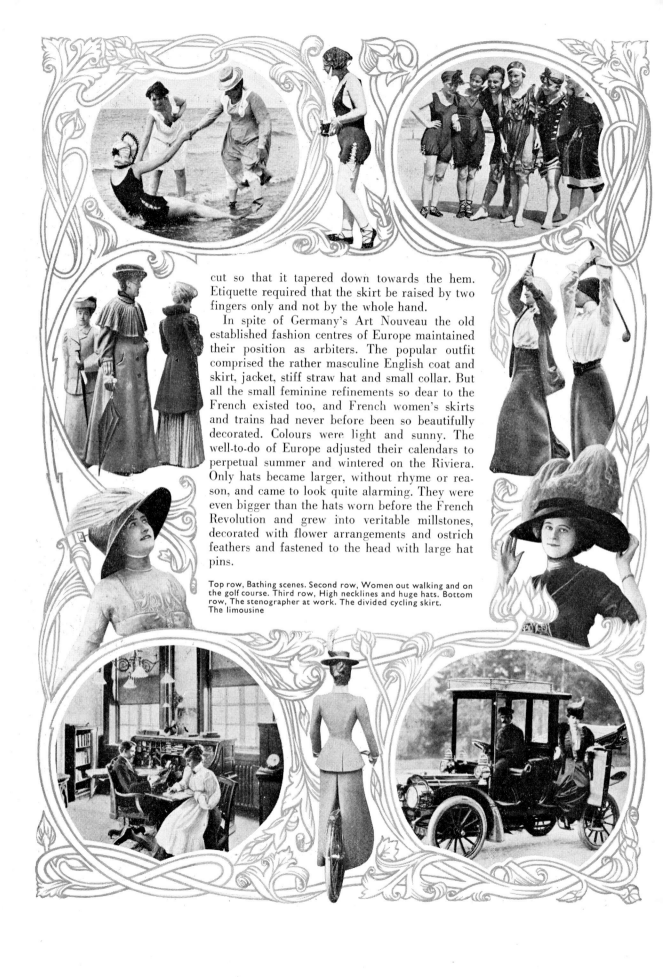

cut so that it tapered down towards the hem. Etiquette required that the skirt be raised by two fingers only and not by the whole hand.

In spite of Germany's Art Nouveau the old established fashion centres of Europe maintained their position as arbiters. The popular outfit comprised the rather masculine English coat and skirt, jacket, stiff straw hat and small collar. But all the small feminine refinements so dear to the French existed too, and French women's skirts and trains had never before been so beautifully decorated. Colours were light and sunny. The well-to-do of Europe adjusted their calendars to perpetual summer and wintered on the Riviera. Only hats became larger, without rhyme or reason, and came to look quite alarming. They were even bigger than the hats worn before the French Revolution and grew into veritable millstones, decorated with flower arrangements and ostrich feathers and fastened to the head with large hat pins.

Top row, Bathing scenes. Second row, Women out walking and on the golf course. Third row, High necklines and huge hats. Bottom row, The stenographer at work. The divided cycling skirt. The limousine

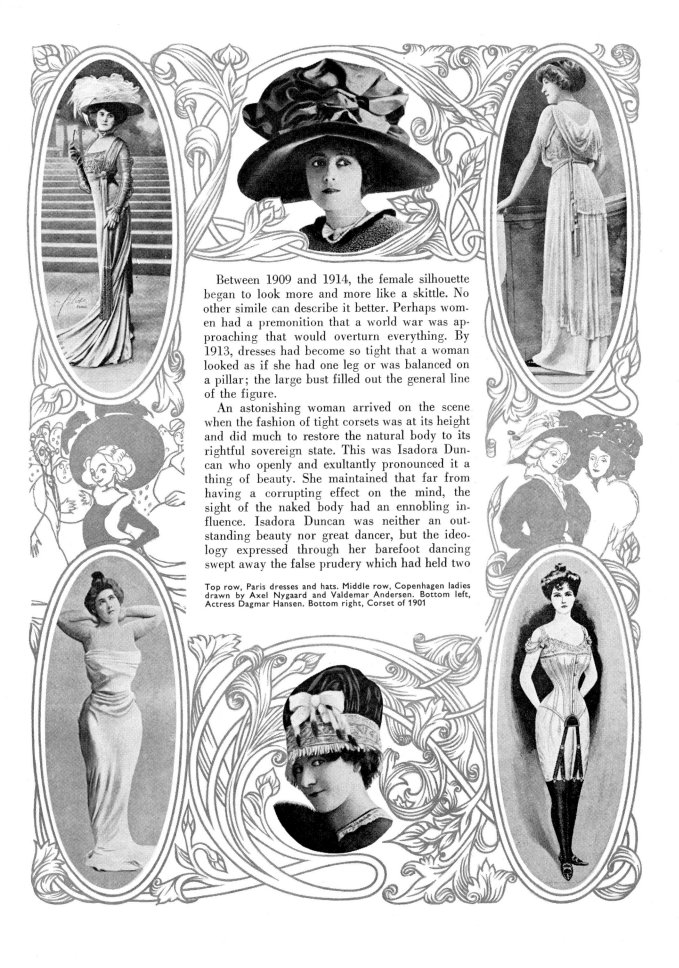

Between 1909 and 1914, the female silhouette began to look more and more like a skittle. No other simile can describe it better. Perhaps women had a premonition that a world war was approaching that would overturn everything. By 1913, dresses had become so tight that a woman looked as if she had one leg or was balanced on a pillar; the large bust filled out the general line of the figure.

An astonishing woman arrived on the scene when the fashion of tight corsets was at its height and did much to restore the natural body to its rightful sovereign state. This was Isadora Duncan who openly and exultantly pronounced it a thing of beauty. She maintained that far from having a corrupting effect on the mind, the sight of the naked body had an ennobling influence. Isadora Duncan was neither an outstanding beauty nor great dancer, but the ideology expressed through her barefoot dancing swept away the false prudery which had held two

Top row, Paris dresses and hats. Middle row, Copenhagen ladies drawn by Axel Nygaard and Valdemar Andersen. Bottom left, Actress Dagmar Hansen. Bottom right, Corset of 1901

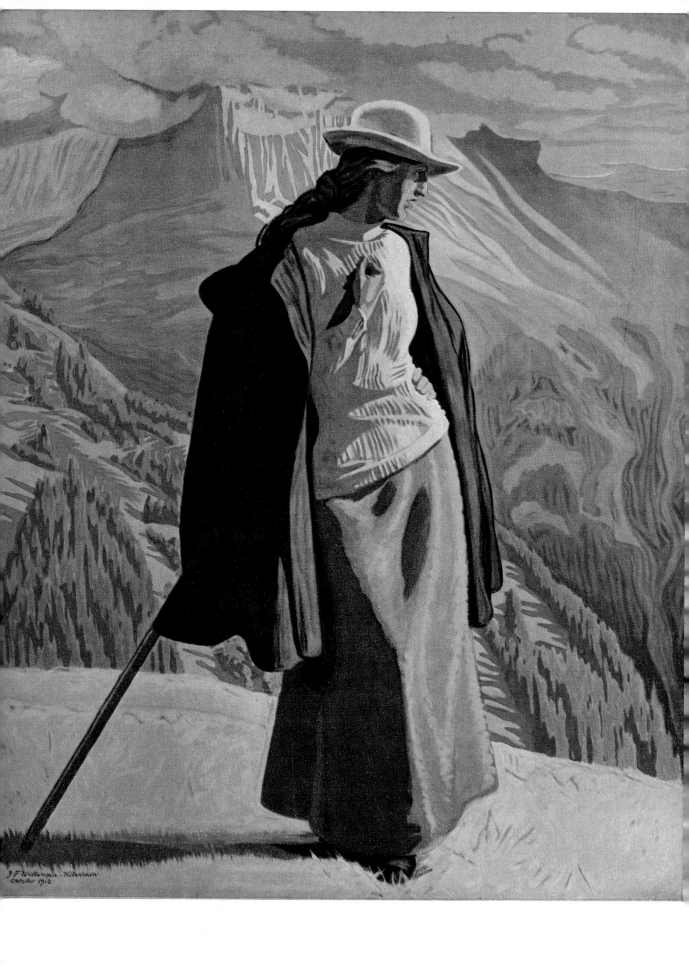

continents in thrall. Her interpretation of the barefoot dance influenced Fokine to make his Russian ballet dancers in Paris abandan their corsets. But first there was a rearguard action to be fought; the S-contour, still retaining its fascination, turned like a serpent and reversed itself, and the curved back and protruding stomach came into fashion once again. The revolution in women's dress carried through in 1910 was indeed as significant as the changes in fashion instituted at the time of the French Revolution.

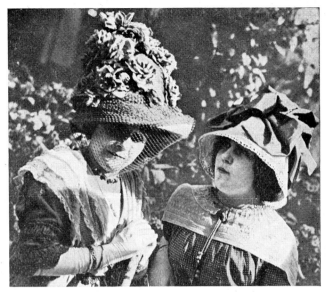
Decorated hats and lace collars on the eve of the First World War

Just as sport formed the background for English fashion, so the theatre was the main influence on French styles. The Paris dress designer, Paul Poiret, used the costumes of the Russian ballet as a basis for new French styles. Russian influence could be clearly seen in the strong colour contrasts which emerged — in the orange and lemon, bright green and indigo that took the place of the more refined and carefully harmonizing French colours.

1914

Poiret's extravagant creations were launched in an Arabian Nights atmosphere and displayed by exquisite, carefully selected mannequins. It is ironical that this dress designer who used Russian sources for one magnificent fashion after another, had no prescience of events to come. The violent reaction soon to take place in Russia itself was hardly dreamt of in the perfumed atmosphere of Poiret's villa where the *haute monde* gathered to enjoy the almost ritual presentation

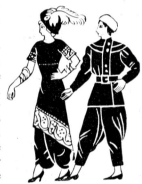
Poiret's trouser-dress of 1911 and working woman's outfit of 1917

of the latest fashions. Who indeed could have forecast that the glittering semi-oriental court of the Russian Tsar would soon be overtaken by a tidal wave forcing a passage from a quite different source? Similarly who could have guessed that the everyday dress of the working-class woman was stealthily effecting an entrance into the very salons themselves of France?

When Poiret endeavoured to introduce the trouser-dress, leaders of fashion were aghast. However, his vertical line was accepted in 1913. Poiret's narrow hooped dress had the semblance of trousers but did not, in fact, have separate legs, merely a narrow slit at the bottom which allowed the legs to move.

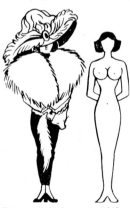
The one-legged woman, 1913

The First World War. When the First World War broke out, the initiative in fashion passed from high society to the women in the factories and elsewhere who were engaged in the war effort. When the men left their normal occupations for the Front their place was taken by the women, who carried out every kind of work. Women became factory hands, bus conductors and chauffeurs, and they also worked on the land. This meant that of necessity the long tight-fitting dresses had to be abandoned, and this was done with tremendous gusto. Poiret had previously dictated that a loose chemise dress be worn on top of the narrow skirt. All, therefore, that women had to do to suit the new conditions was simply to discard the skirt and lengthen the chemise.

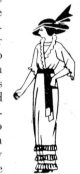
Hooped dress of 1913

When both money and materials were in short supply a 'war crinoline' that needed a lot of material became, understandably, a fashionable status symbol. Several petticoats were also needed underneath the 'crinoline' to make it stand out.

A more lasting change took place in the realm of underwear, now that the use of elastic was properly understood; coloured taffeta and crêpe de chine took the place of plain linen. Before bathrooms were widespread, white underwear was looked to as proof of personal freshness. Now this standard no longer applied and charming lightweight underwear could be found beneath working clothes, made in pretty pastel shades. The tragic background to this development was the sudden disappearance of almost an entire generation of potential husbands and this involved

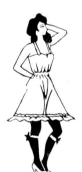
Négligé of 1916

Opposite   Copy (1912) of painting by J. F. Willumsen, 1904

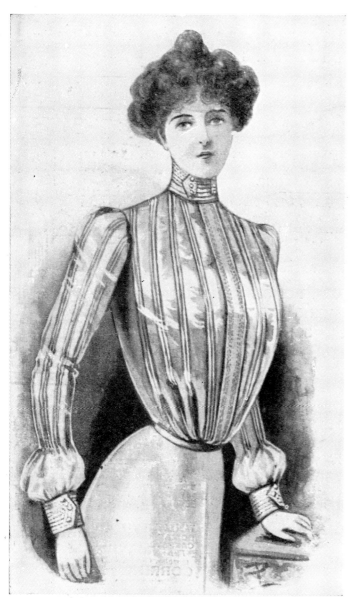

Woman wearing corset, 1901

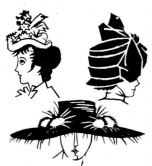

Hats in 1900, 1910 and 1919

down over the ears. In 1913, the cloche hat came into fashion, shaped to the head and adorned with all sorts of odd feathers. Several new hair styles came in at the beginning of the First World War: the hair combed back to frame the face and done up in a bun at the back, the page-boy bob, and the shingle which was first introduced by nurses and factory girls.

The khaki uniforms influenced the colour of women's clothes, as it was found to be a practical colour for working clothes.

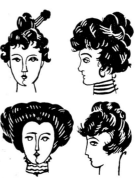

Hair styles in 1895, 1900, 1910 and 1920

Fur coats — the normal winter outfit of the Russians — became an essential item in the wardrobe of the well-dressed woman.

Cosmetics. During the war years, all sorts of cosmetics insinuated their way into society, from the lower strata up. Rouge, lipstick, mascara and face powder graduated from the brothel to the stage and thence to Bohemian society. The lady's maid might well convince her mistress of the attractions of make-up. When the men came home on leave all women made use of cosmetics to enhance their good points. From a sociological viewpoint the adoption of make-up was another milestone on the road of women's progress, indicating her assumption of an active role. Man's ancient prerogative, that of covering his body with paint, had now become the monopoly of the fair sex.

Women's Legs. It is natural that there was a similar trend in the matter of legs. The female leg was

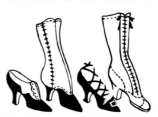

Female footwear in 1890, 1910, 1912 and 1918

exposed to the public after thousands of years of obscurity. By 1915, the hemline of the skirt had been raised to the top of the buttoned boots and the leg moved out of the reserves to the front line of attack.

women in fierce competition for those men who had survived.

Hats became smaller at this time and a peculiar relationship was to be seen between headwear and dress. Following an inverse ratio, a large hat went with a neat dress and a small hat with a bulky dress. In 1900, a small hat was worn well forward on the head. When the motor car arrived in about 1906 the hat needed to have a veil to stop it blowing off. In 1910, hats looked like generously decorated millstones or inverted churns pulled

From this time, the following procedure was observed by males, young and old alike, when eyeing the female: first the face,

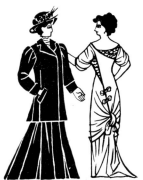

English walking costume and
evening dress, 1910

1916 and 1919

then the legs with the eye
travelling in an upward direction, and last a survey of
the whole figure.

Prostitutes could not, of
course, restrict themselves to
an occasional glimpse of the
ankle; they therefore made
use of the négligé for a better display of the eternal feminine charms. Women of
the most unassailable respectability could also employ
these blitzkrieg tactics. Short

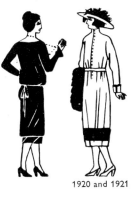

1920 and 1921

skirts and slighter boots were now the order of the
day. Shoes worn with a strap over the instep became

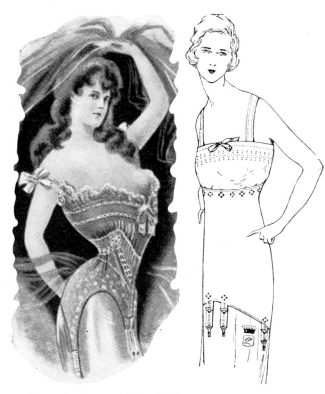

Corset advertisements, 1913 and 1924

fashionable in 1915. The strap gradually became
wider until it developed into two flaps. Eyelets and
cords were added and thus laced shoes came into
existence.

The Schoolgirl Ideal. It now became evident that
the age considered the height of women's attractiveness
had altered. At the beginning of the century, a full-
busted woman in her thirties was most admired. By
the end of the First World War the ideal was the
schoolgirl figure. In the old days little girls would
dream of the day they would wear long dresses. Now,
however, it was the older women who turned their
attention back to the short skirt, and the more flat
chested they could make themselves look the better.

During the war years men were largely confined
to each other's company and we cannot rule out the
possibility that the attraction of the boyish female
image involved a degree of homosexual feeling. The
short hair of women at that time also adds to this
general impression.

Male Defences. Men seemed to take
little interest in their appearance, and
male fashions certainly did not change
as frequently as women's fashions.
The truth is that men always have
been much more conventional in the
matter of dress. Contrary to the general impression, civilized peoples
have at least as many taboos and inhibitions as their more primitive for-
bears. Male dress became increasingly
rigorously fixed. The strait jacket effect of their clothes; the hard hat, tight
collar and sleeves finished off to look
like hand-cuffs, gave the impression of
a stultified spirit. The heavy armour
of the knight in days gone by had
conveyed a feeling of strength and a
sense of chivalry and moral responsibility. This was also true of men's
clothes in later times; substantial and
well moulded to the body, they suggested moral fibre and self-discipline.
The crisp shirt and stiff collar indicated self-control — behind a crumpled shirt-front a fickle heart must
surely beat.

The soft felt hat had replaced the
tall silk hat at the beginning of the
century and was now competing with
the bowler for popularity. Before the
First World War it was quite unthinkable for a man to be seen outdoors
without a hat.

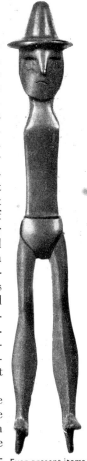

Ever-present items
of dress: Bronze
Age figure wearing
hat and pants

Ready-made Clothes. In the middle of the nineteenth century, the American clothing industry provided factory-made garments for the Negro slaves in

213

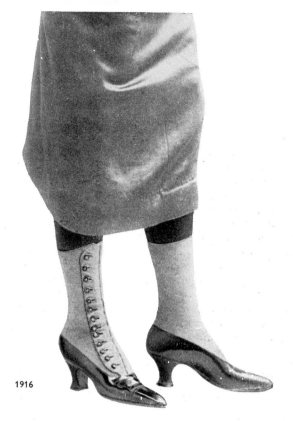

1916

strange reversal then took place. The ready-made clothing manufacturers threw themselves into a positive orgy of padding and pleating so that people would be deceived into thinking that the cheap ready-made garment was an individually tailored article. The genuine bespoke tailors moved in precisely the opposite direction in catering for the upper classes and the aristocracy. Here the aim was to produce loose-fitting, comfortable clothes which gave a casual impression and even suggested a certain degree of carelessness on the part of the wearer.

Sportsmen and Puritans. Two completely different attitudes were expressed in these two distinct styles. One reflected the old puritan outlook which regarded the body as something shameful and unpleasant. The other expressed the spirit of the athletics field, a love of life and freedom.

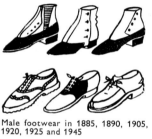

Formal wear was loth to make compromises to comfort. The stiff collar, for example, so much a symbol of correct behaviour and gravity was, at the turn of the century, still a part of formal wear. The First World War, however, brought the soft collar into fashion for everyday wear. The tie was no longer buckled at the back but was placed round the neck and tied in a knot or a bow in front. New types of cloth hats and caps were also introduced to provide an alternative to the ordinary felt hat.

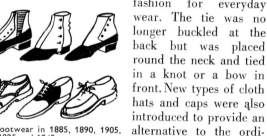

Ready-tied bow-tie and ready-knotted tie

Male footwear in 1885, 1890, 1905, 1920, 1925 and 1945

the Southern States, and at the end of the century ready-made clothes were sold to the white population. England followed America's example at the beginning of the present century, and by the First World War ready-made clothes were generally accepted in most countries, with the exception of France. They were nevertheless regarded with a good deal of suspicion. Could a suit fit properly if not cut and shaped to the individual wearer?

Men's suits were beginning to look like the suit of the present day. The jacket was cut with narrow lapels and was buttoned up to the neck. Trousers were narrow and frequently of a lighter shade than the jacket. They were kept immaculately pressed and looked as if they had just arrived from the tailor. The creases were at the front and back instead of down the sides as in 1840. The cuffs became trimmer and neater.

Men's clothing, in theory and in practice

Leisure Clothes. Men continued to wear stiff uncomfortable suits for parties and on Sundays. The individual still found it necessary to prove to the outside world that he had no need to work. When leisure clothes appeared on the scene, however, the whole attitude to clothing changed.

When it came to shooting tigers or escaping from a wounded rhinoceros, freedom of movement was essential. Jacket and trousers became looser in cut, the soft shirt replaced the starched front, and the soft felt hat came into general wear. The tailor was required to make suits which were easy and comfortable. A

214

Collars worn in 1905

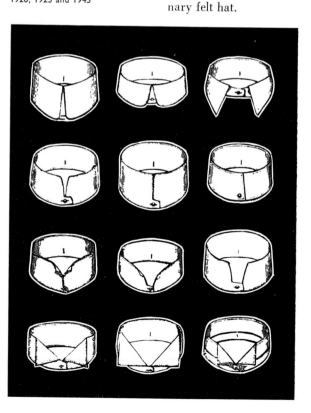

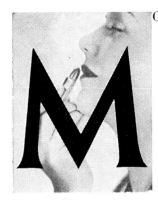

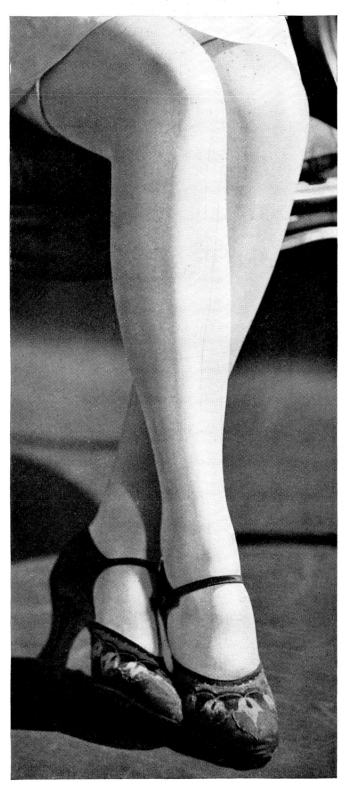

MOTOR CARS were in general use in 1920 and were also more efficient. In fact, that year marked the beginning of a new era. The aviation industry was rapidly expanding. Rutherford split the atom in 1919, and the talking pictures came into existence through the work of Marsolle, Engel and Vogt. The radio became part of most households during the twenties, television arrived in 1928 and penicillin was discovered in 1929. All these inventions had a tremendous impact. An abstract style of painting, Cubism, was introduced, which reduced natural forms to fundamental geometric shapes. Within architecture, functionalism was the dominant trend.

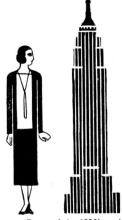

Young people saw a bright future ahead and were firmly resolved not to repeat the stupidities of the past. The First World War had provided ample proof of failure on the part of the older generation and the young people wished to disassociate themselves from this failure as completely as possible. The balance between the sexes was upset by the large number of men who had lost their lives in the war. For the first time in modern history,

Dress of the 1920's and a skyscraper

there was a surplus of women, but it was made rather less noticeable by the boyish look of so many women.

The Self-Supporting Woman. A number of new occupations opened their doors to women, and as a

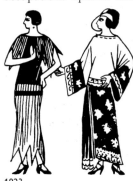

result they assumed a new place in society. The opportunity to earn their own living gave them a feeling of augmented independence. Young unmarried daughters left the bosom of their families and installed themselves in rooms or flats complete with up-to-date furniture, radiogram and all the latest records, and moreover were eager to

1923

215

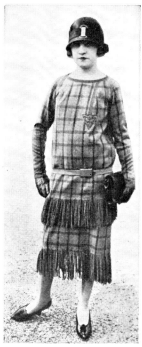

Ca. 1925

take this step. No longer was it a matter of demanding concessions but rather there was a belief in a woman's inherent right to live her own life in her own way. But, unlike their sisters of the emancipation, these women did not wish to segregate themselves from the opposite sex. The girl typical of this time was not the untouched innocent, but rather the girl who could be both work-mate and companion to the man.

Returning soldiers still sought partners even if they lacked the financial standing to start a family. The old romantic clichés were out of date and a poetic manner of speech gave way to a clipped,

Silk Stockings and Cloche Hats. The most striking aspect of these new fashions concerned the legs, which were now exposed up to the knee. Stockings were made of silk or of artificial silk which had become reasonable in price. Black or dark coloured stockings were worn up to 1924, but light colours gradually came in after that, in shades such as flesh pink and, later, beige and tan.

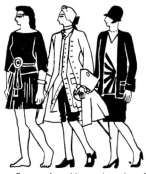

Bronze Age skirt, male attire of 1725, and female dress of 1927

As regards footwear, the curved Rococo heel gave way to an upright heel, and a low-heeled shoe with a thick sole became fashionable. A development of the rubber boot of the war years became the vogue for a short time and was known as the Russian boot. This protected the flimsy silk stockings well, but revealed all too clearly that the wearer belonged to that section of society which did not own motor cars and therefore had to walk.

Permanent waving had become less expensive. The

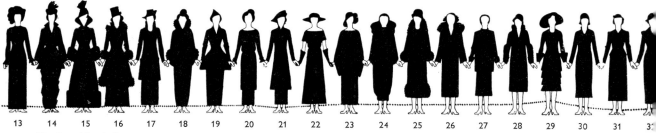

| 13 | 14 | 15 | 16 | 17 | 18 | 19 | 20 | 21 | 22 | 23 | 24 | 25 | 26 | 27 | 28 | 29 | 30 | 31 | 3 |

The dotted line indicates gross annual national product of the United States from 1913 to 1953. The silhouetted figures indicate the average length of wom... American economy alone, is a decisive factor

consciously tough diction. Young girls lectured their rather embarrassed parents on the theory that spiritual and bodily welfare went hand in hand with a sensible sex life.

Youth. The call was for youth and the young in spirit. Young men home from the war, who had sampled the pleasures of the brothels, looked for something better from their girl friends. Women became interested in diet and the newly discovered vitamins; they did exercises to keep their bodies young and in good shape.

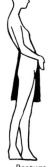

Posture of the late 1920's

The corset, which had been the basic foundation for women's dresses since 1830, was finished. In its absence, suspender belts were used to keep the stockings in position, and brassieres were worn to flatten the bust. During the mid twenties, dresses usually took the form of sleeveless open-necked tunics. The waistline disappeared in 1921, and in 1923 the belt descended to the level of the hips, a revival of a male fashion of the Middle Ages.

shingle was the most popular hair fashion after 1924, when it displaced that token of radical tendencies, the page-boy cut. Short hair was probably a legacy of the war years, when all women involved in the war effort had, for practical reasons, to wear their hair short. Nor was there any room for long hair inside the cloche, that belated imitation of the soldier's tin helmet.

Hair styles

1922	1923	1930
1935	1939	1940
1942	1944	1950

No Pretence. People of this time neither minced nor wasted their words. They took daily baths, no longer washing themselves in sections. Among this generation of high-brows, the body was found rather unsubtle from a sensual viewpoint; the old black-and-white films of the time, in which dress was little

216

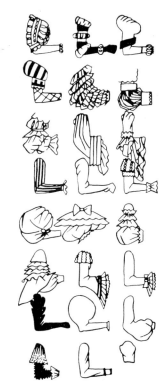

Sleeves of women's dresses

1525	1550	1577
1577	1590	1644
1660	1724	1770
1789	1800	1822
1830	1834	1838
1860	1870	1878
1890	1894	1903
1909	1920	1939

emphasized, supports this impression. Mostly we get close-ups of the heroine with her large face, big emotional eyes and straight mouth.

Beauty treatment became normal after the war. Cosmetics were used openly and to great effect, but too much deception was not approved of. A great deal of interest was, however, centred on the face as the mirror of the soul. Women no longer wished

were as scantily attired as mythical Dianas in sleeveless dresses that hung nonchalantly from the shoulders. Personal charm and attraction depended entirely on good lines, on the shape of the legs, the curve of the neck, on young slender arms, and, above all, on a vivacious and intelligent face.

Short Dresses. The cloth manufacturers were naturally concerned over the popularity of the short dress which was curtailing the demand for their products. The Parisian fashion houses co-operated with the textile factories and endeavoured to introduce styles which would require the yards of material that were needed in the good old days. One of these was an ankle-length dress made in transparent material and worn over a similar dress in heavy material. The optimistic hope was that one layer of tulle would be followed by another, but the plan was not successful.

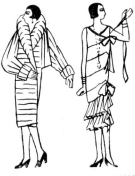

1926 and 1927

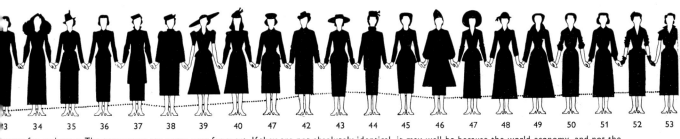

3 34 35 36 37 38 39 40 47 42 43 44 45 46 47 48 49 50 51 52 53

esses for each year. The two curves are never very far apart. If they are not absolutely identical, it may well be because the world economy, and not the

to have milk-white skins and pink cheeks to contrast with the weather-beaten workers in the fields. The new ideal was a sun-bronzed complexion as a contrast to the pale-faced workers in factories, offices and shops. Eyebrows were trimmed to a narrow line and arched with an eyebrow pencil. The shape of the mouth was altered with lipstick, which was available in colours varying from violet to orange red. Nail-polish was introduced after 1930 and red laquered nails became popular.

A high degree of freedom existed and women did exactly as they wanted. The most well brought up girl would drink and smoke in public, and the use of cars and motor cycles increased the general sense of liberty. In the ballroom partners would dance close together and 'petting', derived from America, became known. Dancers no longer swayed to the romantic music of the violin but hopped about to the sexy bleat of the saxophone. The new dances emphasized energetic bodily movement and gesture, and the Negro jazz band ousted the old gypsy orchestra.

Never before were women's clothes so straightforward and so honest. There was no deception; women

Women still wished to show their legs, and while they did accept a formal gown which came down to the ankles at the back, the front still remained knee-length, as short as ever.

The short dress remained the mode for as long as America dominated the financial world, the hemline rising and falling slightly in accordance with the economic situation. The general trend was a steady upwards movement, starting in 1918 at ankle-length and reaching the knee in 1927.

A sensation occurred in the fashion world in the autumn of 1929 when the skirts of day dresses suddenly dropped to mid calf and those of evening dresses to the ground. It may be a coincidence, but a month later saw the Wall Street crash and the collapse of the money market in America.

The athletic American girl has always been quite open about showing her legs, in contrast to French girls whose attitude is much more subtle and coquettish.

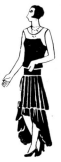

Dinner dress of 1928, short in front and long at the back

217

Dress Materials. Not only was less material used in a dress but the materials themselves had become much lighter. Heating in houses had improved and physical exercise had made people hardier and less sensitive to the cold. Women's underwear became merely a thin silk combination garment of slip and short knickers made in one, known as cami-knicks, and kept in position by shoulder-straps.

No generation approves of the fashion of the preceding generation, a principle which has held good

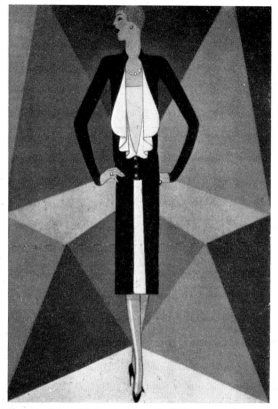

Dress made from black and white satin, 1927

throughout history. The fashions of the twenties had several notable characteristics. Simplicity was the keynote and materials were appreciated for their own intrinsic qualities. Ostentatious jewellery was com-

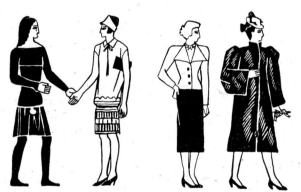

Male attire of 1350 and women's dresses in 1927, 1936 and 1938

pletely out of favour and platinum was preferred to gold. The style of this period cannot be regarded as deficient in taste. If anything, it tended in general to be over-critical.

Male Dress. Men abandoned their long underpants when women decided to expose their silk-clad legs. Short underpants were adopted that were similar to present-day underpants, except that they were kept up by tapes which fitted over the ends of the braces. While women's skirts were becoming short and slim, the men scored with the new fashion of the wide Oxford Bags.

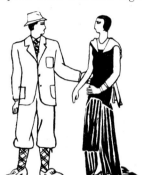

Man 1927 and woman 1924

Apart from these changes male fashion did not alter greatly. Jackets became shorter and the vent at the back was thus no longer essential. The sports jacket came into vogue; worn wih the Oxford Bags, it was usually in a checked material with a halfbelt at the back. The ready-made clothing industry was not anxious constantly to alter

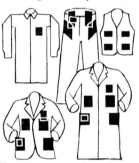

The twenty-two pockets of the man's suit, shirt and overcoat

its production system in order to meet the new styles. It was much easier to clothe men as if they were tailor's dummies. Men were expected to fit themselves into ready-made suits; as far as the man in the street was concerned the old tailor's craft of cutting and fitting was a thing of the past.

Male clothing became more and more fossilized and cluttered with out-dated items with no practical use, such as buttons, cuffs and surplus pockets. Only one of the twenty-two pockets on an average suit could be used by a gentleman of fashion, and that was the outside breast pocket, ostensibly made for a handkerchief, and not really supposed to be used. A suit was littered with unnecessary buttons; both the double-breasted jacket and the double-

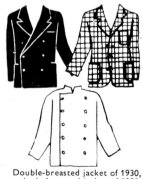

Double-breasted jacket of 1930, single-breasted jacket of 1950, and a chef's jacket today

breasted waistcoat sported double rows of buttons. Lapel buttonholes had no corresponding buttons, cuff buttons had no corresponding buttonholes. Cuff buttons have remained with us, however: a sad remind-

Opposite Chic Parisienne. Painting by H. C. Etcherry, 1928

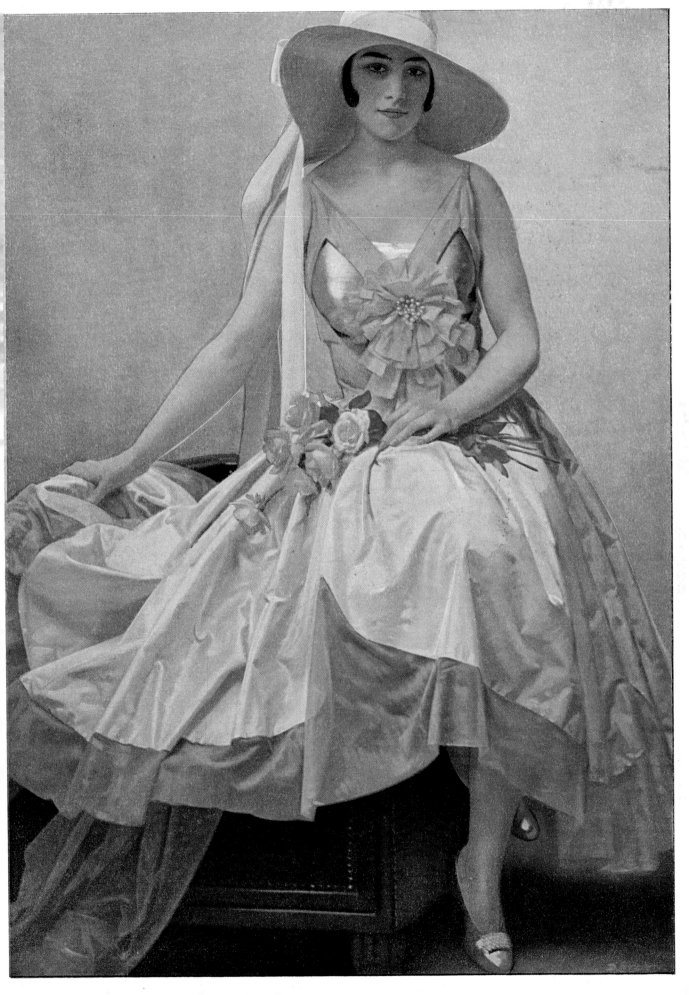

er of the handsome cuff of Rococo times.

Dark, drab colours were used for men's suits, which made the wearers look as if they were in low spirits. A man who wore informal or brightly coloured clothes would find his way barred

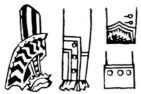

Cuffs in 1689, 1787, 1809 and 1825

to decent establishments. In some countries in Europe even the inns along the quayside of large harbour

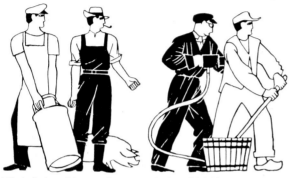

Work clothes: dairyman, farmer, mechanic and bricklayer

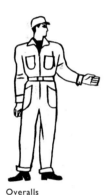

Overalls

towns carried stocks of ties for the use of tie-less patrons. Conventional evening dress is now regarded as something of a joke where it does not appear as the normal attire of waiters and diplomats.

The function of the overall was extended at this time, having been previously reserved for factory workers and mechanics. The boiler-suit copied the design of the battledress worn by soldiers during the war.

Accessories. Spats were worn by the well-dressed man between 1910 and 1920. Spectacles, which had previously drooped sadly over the nose merely as a

Spectacles in 1870, 1935 and 1945

corrective to weak eyesight, now assumed heavy frames of horn or tortoiseshell and became the aristocratic symbol of the intellectual. The walking stick was an essential part of the well-dressed gentleman's outfit during the latter part of the previous century. Now it appeared again, but in a size and shape which denied any suggestion that its user needed any assistance in walking. The pipe, however, became the most outstanding male ornament and has indeed remained so. Firmly gripped between the teeth, the pipe should convey an impression of mature and deep reflection. It can also be used to keep the hands occupied and to cover any awkward pauses in conversation. Cigarettes

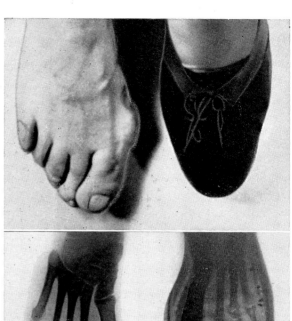

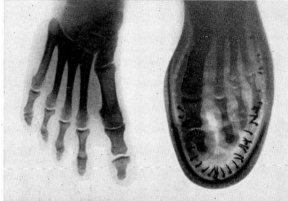

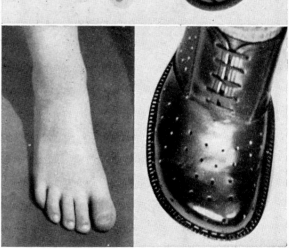

Top row, The 'normal' European foot, bent and stunted by pointed shoes. Middle row, X-ray of the feet of an Indian who has never worn shoes. His left foot has been forced into the largest shoe Copenhagen could provide. Bottom row, Scandinavian child's unspoiled foot, and a Swedish shoe healthily shaped and with vents

fulfil the same function but in a more lighthearted manner. A man without a pipe or cigarette may be compared to a woman without make-up.

In contrast to these additions, the hat, previously a token of extreme dignity, now ceased to be popular. Ceremonial occasions were the only exception when the silk top hat was taken out for an airing. Young men would sometimes wear a beret or, in cold weather, a leather cap, but usually they would go bareheaded.

Male deportment changed after the First World War. The straight-as-a-ram-rod pose became old-fashioned and a relaxed, slightly drooping posture was considered the thing. Both men and women ceased to walk with their feet turned out at right angles to each other; an angle of about thirty degrees became the accepted position.

A Look at the Thirties. The economic crisis which followed the 1929 Wall Street crash in America cast a general gloom all over Europe. New wars darkened the horizon: war in Abyssinia, war in the Far East, the Civil War in Spain and then the devastation of the Second World War.

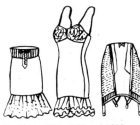

Girdles in 1920, 1930 and 1935

Political and economic development ground to a standstill. Fascism, Nazism and the Spanish Falange movement were established. Discipline and hypocrisy became the order of the day, the greatest successes being scored by propaganda.

In this atmosphere, dress could not fail to lose its simplicity and sense of freedom. Immediately after 1930, the narrow waist and high shoulders returned. A back door was opened for the re-entry of the corset by a new interest in national costumes. National costumes are basically picturesque anachronisms which are actually unsophisticated versions of Baroque court dress. Skirts grew wider at the hem and lace edging reappeared. The old conception of women returned, best described by the German expression, *Kinder, Kirche und Küche* — children, church and kitchen. The night-dress came back into general use.

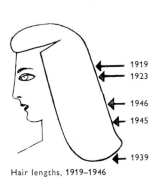

Hair lengths, 1919–1946

Boyish hair styles gave way to hair done up in a small roll at the back. Short hair became fashionable again for a while in 1933 when it was made to appear windswept. This changed to the longer style popularized by Greta Garbo. The next change occurred in 1938, just before Chamberlain

and Hitler had their Munich meeting, and called for the hair to be gathered on top of the head.

The cloche hat had had its day and great ingenuity was expended to find a suitable successor. The new hat, when it arrived, permitted a number of variations in the way it was placed on the head.

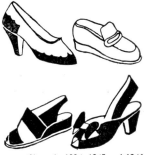

Shoes in 1934, 1945 and 1946

Sometimes it was set at a jaunty angle, at other times it was tilted well forward over the forehead. The Tyrolean hat with a feather stuck in the band became popular at about the same time as Hitler came to power in Germany. But political dictators were not the only influence on this period. Surrealism and cartoon films played their part; in 1933 Schiaparelli shocked the fashion world by producing a hat which was modelled on an old shoe.

Fashion in the 1930's. Women now started to wear shorts and slacks for sport. Young people normally went hatless. Boots ceased to be worn by women at all except for skating and ski-ing. Sandals came into everyday use and were no longer considered eccentric. Bare legs or short ankle socks became acceptable and the sandals allowed red lacquered toenails to be seen. For the first time in two thousand years, women's feet were, albeit hesitantly, exposed to view. This was surely a demonstration long overdue of the fact that feet are provided with ten toes.

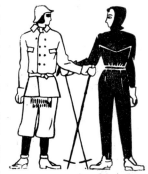

Ski clothes, 1929 and 1945

Styles of female dresses now alternated between the

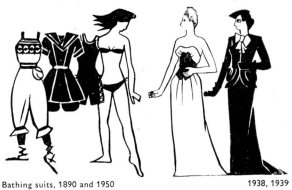

Bathing suits, 1890 and 1950   1938, 1939

old and the new. Many new materials were available and many new colours could be produced by dyes.

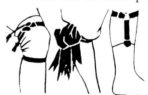
Ski-boot

The conception of the perfect woman changed from a slim young girl to a more archaic type. Sculptors searched for models who were heavy, massy-limbed, almost negroid in type. In this atmosphere, not even the spiritual intelligence of a Garbo, with her awkward figure, broad shoulders, flat chest and undistinguished legs, could have had the world at her feet. A far less perfect ideal of womanhood appeared on the scene. The traditional beauty was deposed from her seat of majesty and was metamorphosed into the pin-up girl with her soulless sex appeal.

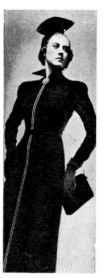
The zip arrived in 1933

The contrast between party clothes and working clothes became more marked. Evening dresses were so clinging that they looked as if they were slightly damp. Perhaps this was a democratic fashion in as much as every individual has a unique body to display. This kind of dress clung closely to the posterior and was obviously meant to be looked at from behind. The back was left completely bare and even the shoulder straps eventually disappeared. Fashion then swung sharply in the opposite direction and, by 1940, both day and evening wear had become high-necked at both front and back.

The bathing suit now turned into a two-piece garment. The first harbingers of sense made their appearance: the Swedish shoe on page 220 and the toe-stocking below.

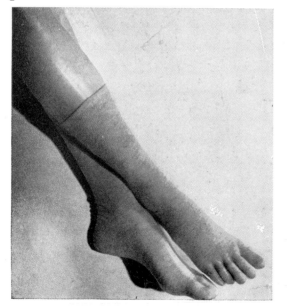

Separate Collars. Although minor changes took place, male fashions remained largely conservative. Many layers of clothing continued to be worn and the male figure to act like a thermos flask.

The human body has, as already mentioned, an immense capacity for regulating its body temperature. Experiments have proved that the body can withstand temperatures hot enough to cook a steak, provided the surrounding air is dry and evaporation can take place freely. Instead, however, of finding ways and means of ventilation, man proceeds to seal his body off from the outside atmosphere. His collar and tie interfere with the free movement of the head. This in turn restricts the use of neck and shoulder muscles, giving rise to headaches and to fibrositis.

Shirts appeared in coloured or striped materials. During the 1920's, collars were made separate from the shirt itself, but in 1930 a shirt with a front opening was introduced to which the collar was permanently attached. The shirt was buttoned all the way down the front and thus did not have to be pulled on over the head. The vest under the shirt was usually sleeveless and the underpants, or shorts, were held in

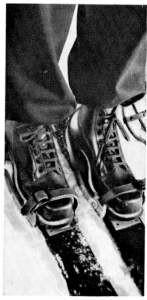

position by elastic in the waistband. Casual clothes for men gained general acceptance, and shorts became normal sportswear. Sock suspenders were seldom used and the knitted pullover went a long way towards ousting the formal waistcoat.

The garter in 1579, 1635 and 1930

Belts replaced braces except when the waist of the trousers was cut sufficiently narrow to keep the trousers up by itself.

The Vanishing Tie. When colour was introduced into shirts, socks, pullovers, pyjamas and dressing-gowns, the popularity of coloured ties began to wane. Previously the tie had been the only coloured item permitted in male attire. This restriction no longer applied, and if a tie had still to be worn with business or professional dress, its colour was usually dark. A loosely folded scarf or cravat was sometimes worn with an open-necked shirt for off-duty occasions and during the weekend. Hats for men declined further in popularity, and people started to walk with their feet pointing straight forward like soldiers.

Ski trousers

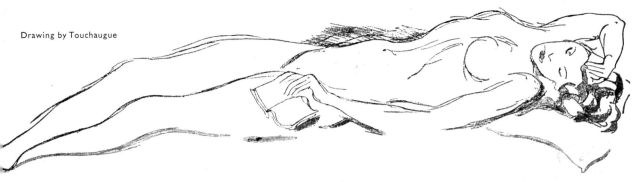

The Second World War. Many shortages existed during the Second World War, not least in the realm of clothing. Many items disappeared from the market completely, and the people of all those countries affected showed great spirit and ingenuity in doing without or in finding alternatives. Footwear was made with cork soles and wedge heels. Head scarves were used to cover the hair. Women adopted long trousers both as a countermeasure to the fuel shortage and for convenience in air-raid shelters.

The New Look. A move was made towards the return of feminine fashions as the end of the war approached. Hips became rounder, waistlines were more

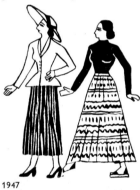

1947

clearly defined and brassieres were designed to enhance the effect of the bust. The New Look introduced these and other changes, including longer hair, but failed to eliminate the broad-shouldered effect. The corset tried to make a comeback, after being rejected by younger women who preferred the new close-fitting elastic girdle. Brassieres came into such wide use that doctors predicted serious injury if they continued to be worn so tight. The artificial support given was thought certain to weaken the natural muscles, and the overall effect was considered likely to have a harmful effect on the natural function of the breast.

Indeed, the women living on the Malabar Coast in India quite recently adopted the brassiere and already their beautifully rounded breasts are showing signs of losing their beauty.

Glamorous materials such as tulle and lace were com-

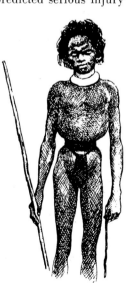

Native of New Guinea wearing a girdle

monly used for ball dresses and evening gowns but it was difficult to incorporate these materials into dresses for everyday wear.

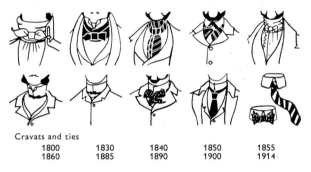

Cravats and ties

| 1800 | 1830 | 1840 | 1850 | 1855 |
| 1860 | 1885 | 1890 | 1900 | 1914 |

This was definitely a period of uncertainty in fashion. No one was deluded into thinking that the 1945 victory was a victory for humanity or that a clear road lay ahead to freedom and a better way of life. On the contrary, propaganda instilled uncertainty and fear into people's minds. The armaments race was revived and it was clear to all that stout hearts and strong muscles would still be needed. A new form of psychological warfare, connected with ideology and art and inevitably involving the world of fashion, came on the scene. It is generally accepted that a uniform standard of dress goes a long way towards achieving uniformity of outlook and action and convincing others of its existence.

The experiment of endeavouring to revive the fashions of the 1880's was given the title of the New Look, an ambiguous term capable of various interpretations.

The New Look constituted a splendid war cry for those campaigning for a return to the old

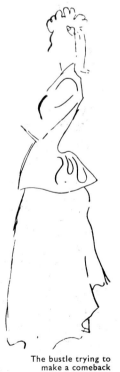

The bustle trying to make a comeback

223

styles; the very words themselves had a psychological implication. All things considered, a strong reaction against the modern fashions was to be expected, and yet how long did the New Look survive? The brassiere, of course, became even more widely used, because it gave the impression of full and well-developed breasts. Certainly high heels, which had been in fashion for a considerable time, are not seen as frequently on the street now as in the shoe shop.

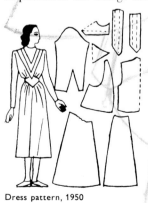

Dress pattern, 1950

Above, Christian Dior's first sketch of the New Look, 1947

The ratio between men and women in the world population was gradually changing. The male birth-rate has always been higher, but the higher mortality rate among boy babies inevitably caused a surplus of women. Moreover, statistics prove that women are married at an earlier age. This fact, too, has implications for the world of fashion.

Let us now visit the workshops behind the scenes in the theatre of world fashion.

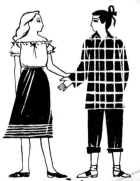

Teenagers of 1944 and 1948

Paris. It is to be expected that the leading workshops should be found in Paris. Two world wars have done no more to challenge the leadership of Paris in haute couture than the two hundred years of history which went before them. This predominance has existed ever since Versailles was the court of courts. It is true that the character of French leadership has changed since the French king decided to send dolls dressed in Paris fashions all over the world. But the fashion magazines have taken over and are no less categorical and authoritarian in their decrees.

Paris continues to be leader and dictator of the fashion world, but it is no longer Frenchmen who are the greatest creators. Ever since 1846, when the Englishman, Worth, arrived in Paris as an unemployed shop assistant to establish the first world fashion house and to launch the first mannequin parade, foreign influence has been at work. Transfusions of foreign blood have improved the circulation of the French fashion industry, and impulses from all over the world have made themselves felt in Paris. Fashion, through the influence of the cinema, television, radio and air transport has become democratic in nature and character. It is no longer confined to one particular class but is available to all. The fashion world is governed by a court where talent is the one and only qualification for gaining favour.

The artist is employed in many other industries, but fashion is the only industry which the artist has completely in his control. A vast amount of capital is involved in this industry, but the real direction lies in the hands of some thirty to forty top designers. The real capital of the big fashion houses lies not in buildings, stock or bank accounts, but in its artists and designers.

The Fashion Designer. The fashion designer is a licensed genius. It would be of no significance were he brute, buffoon or criminal. If his passions run contrary to the law of the land, arrangements will be made to keep him clear of prosecution.

Several dress designers have been homosexuals, indulging in activities outside the law of France. Perhaps the mother-worship and the woman-hatred of such people explain the distorted and yet glowing elements in fashion. The dress designer's creations come to seem ugly so quickly, while the creations of other types of artists, although at first appearing grotesque, come to reveal their beauty after time has worked its spell. It is also the fate of the designer to be destroyed by his first failure to produce a successful line. His fall is immediate and irrevocable, and all of his creations will vanish as if he had never existed.

These dress designers come from every corner of the world. They congregate and thrive in Paris, yet their world is very small. The area in which they work is bounded by Boulevard Haussmann on the north, the Seine on the south, Place Vendôme on the east and the Étoile on the west. Surrounding this area is a vast city in which around one hundred thousand

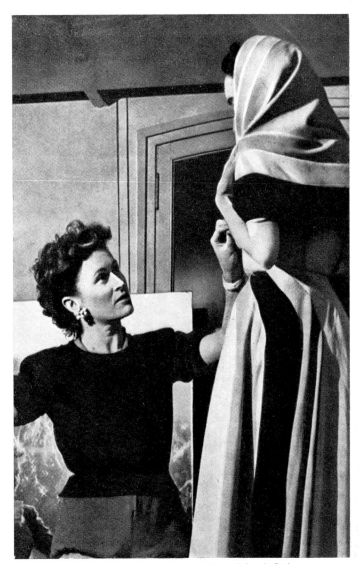

A couturier's workshop in Paris

people make their living in the fashion industry — designers, dressmakers, shoemakers, hairdressers, jewellers and artisans of every description. These people possess a specialized knowledge of all the most modern methods and techniques. Their number even includes apparent layabouts who descend from their dingy garretts with exquisite handicraft wrapped up in newspaper. These people are true artists and will not be dictated to: indeed, they are dictators in their own right. They are not impressed by money, honours, glowing compliments or any other form of psychology attempted by their social superiors, and they possess in this way the wisdom of Socrates.

Surrounding the sanctuary of the haute couture exists an aura of superficiality, moodiness and futile endeavour, and this too in the centre of a world filled with technological discovery, economic drive and strict discipline. Behind the worldly strife can be heard the sighs of billions, striving to express themselves, yearning to live in beauty.

TODAY'S FASHIONS
– AND WHAT THE FUTURE MAY BRING

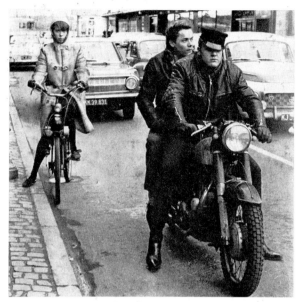

Riders in leather armour on iron horses

spicuous failure because the bosom which it was supposed to reveal simply didn't exist any longer, thanks to the pressure applied for so long by the brassiere.

Teenage girls, with their voluminous parkas and bulky Icelandic sweaters, had already reached full maturity; they did not feel the need to simulate

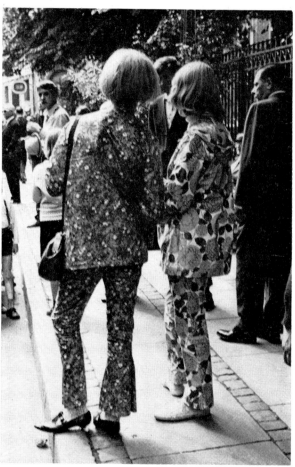

Since the end of the Second World War, the world of fashion has admittedly been in a state of flux. In marked contrast to its former air of authority and self-confidence, it has been characterized by a feeling of uncertainty and a lack of direction. The New Look, the sack dress, the trapeze line, the A-line, the H-line — all of these aimless forays into history and geography have superseded one another at an ever greater pace; but all of them have been little more than whims and fancies, and turned out almost immediately to be merely old wine in new bottles.

Today's fashions have sometimes even encouraged the aristocratic artificiality that was de rigeur in ages long past. Wigs, for instance, have been reintroduced; no woman of fashion is without at least a dozen. At other times, fashion has made an almost convulsive leap back to nature. The V-neck is a case in point. This, however, was an immediate and con-

The future that is already past

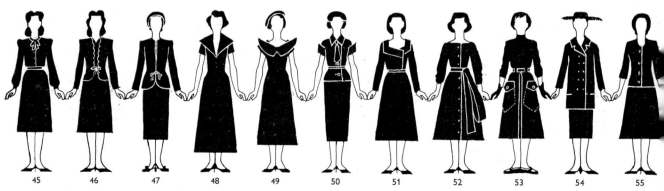

45   46   47   48   49   50   51   52   53   54   55

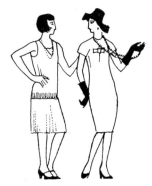

womanliness with the purchased attributes of 'war paint'. The V-neck was merely one of the many vain attempts that Paris couturiers made to break down the barrier between what was, until recently, the command centre of world fashion and the millions of youngsters of the new generation.

Women escaped from the dress in the 1920's, but in 1958 they crawled into the sack

At last, at the moment of writing, the oracles of world fashion have seen the writing on the wall and after countless evasions have given in. It would be foolish to imagine that they decreed unthinkingly hemlines which reached no further down than mid-thigh. The textile industry is losing money to the tune of millions. Present-day youth refuses to commit itself to a future of wars and armaments; women will no longer dress themselves in sackcloth and ashes and conceal the fact that they can stand on their own two feet.

Nor did the footwear industry regard the disappearance of the stiletto heel and the pointed toe with any joy. Those insane shapes brought with them an unprecedented acceleration in demand, for a shoe which does not conform to the shape and function of the foot quickly loses its attraction.

But it is possible that these changes of mind, if not heart, have come too late.

The Revolt of the Masses. The inconceivable has happened. The unchallenged rule of haute couture over dress is passing away. The time has gone when women farm-workers went about their tasks in the fields dressed in their best crinolines. But it is not the fact that something now exists called work clothes that shakes the fashion oracles so deeply and which gives rise to desperate, seemingly deranged fashions. They had written off work clothes a long time ago anyhow. Nor is it because the lustre of the Sun King's city is fading and new creations consequently are given their first showing in other cities, in Rome or in New York, rather than in Paris. What is incredible is that the small minority who do not look up to

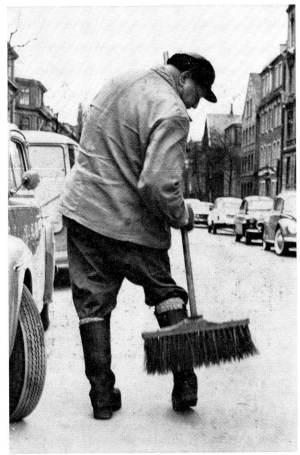

Another type of battledress

Paris, Rome and New York, but rather ridicule the entire high-heeled comedy that is the world of haute couture has grown into a great number.

Today very many young people all over the world have turned that sacred principle of the fashion industry — the one which equates newness and beauty — firmly on its head. They wash their new clothes and soak them over and over again, even scrubbing them with sandpaper and ripping them, in order to disguise the fact that they are new. Canny businessmen advertise clothes that 'look used'. Today's youth has turned its back on the pursuit of the new that the clothing industry so assiduously encouraged. For them

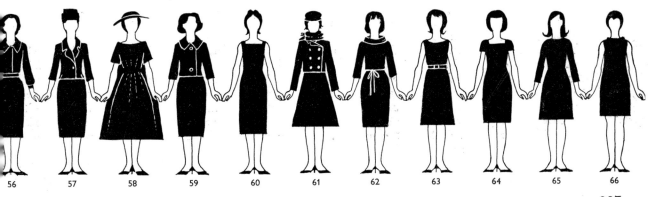

56   57   58   59   60   61   62   63   64   65   66

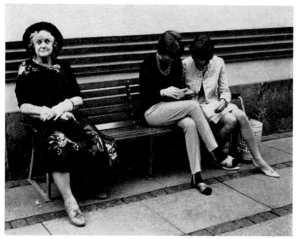

Two generations of women

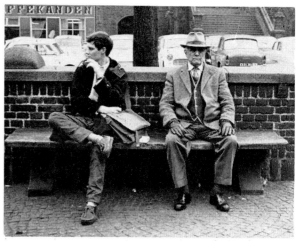

Two generations of men

new clothes are as comical and vulgar as a shiny new American car.

I admit that, for my part, I do feel an historian's reverence for the old and the used. I have often watched workers streaming out of a factory and noticed their work clothes, sometimes closely fitted and at other times arranged like Grecian draperies, rich in colour with all the nuances of blue and green, with violet shades and orange and rust-red stains. At such a time I have always been struck by the none too cheerful thought that these Homeric heroes in their sturdy battledress were going home to don carefully pressed trousers, jackets and starched shirts, in a vain attempt to exchange their square shoulders, strong muscles and broad chests for the sloping shoulders, flat chest and big behind of the bank clerk.

The distinction between the value of a man and the beauty of his clothes is now recognized by more than just a handful of painters and poets. Millions of young Europeans now are acutely aware of the distinction. Unimpressed, they see straight through the antics of advertising. Crumpled trousers are in no way an indication of worthlessness; it is the personality that should put a stamp on those garments that are privileged to clothe the human body.

Young people's dress is revolutionary in another even greater way: it can be identical for both sexes. Both can wear the same tight jeans, coloured shirts and jackets. The elimination of the difference between the two sexes' style of dress constitutes the first step towards a cure for a sickly phase in our cultural development. The abnormal concentration of European fashion during the last few centuries on minor differences suggests something was seriously wrong in sexual relationships.

A Look at the Present Day. Let us concentrate on the disappearing present and consider this creative warfare between past and future in some detail.

Those who feel that young people are behaving like morons and do not deserve to be taken seriously,

228   Helmet and mail

should remember that even such a curious feature as the stovepipe hat was once a symbol of revolution. Rather later on, the soft felt hat was taken as infallible proof of subversive political views and brought mass arrests in its wake.

Nowadays, boys as well as girls wear tight jeans or cowboy pants, and tight dress is undoubtedly militant dress. It is nothing less than the fur which a hunter has skinned from the animal and turned inside out while still wet, so that it fits like a glove. The armour of the astronauts is in the same category. There are exceptions, however, such as fringes and bell-bottomed trousers. It is noteworthy that girls' trousers also have a fly with a zip in front.

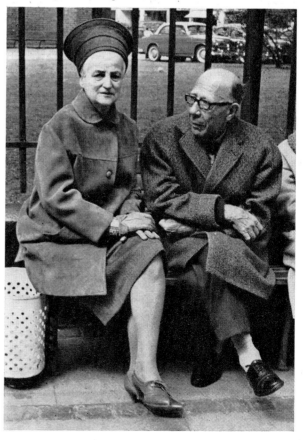

way, as the hats which form part of police and military uniform and whose stiffness remind one of Nazi Germany.

Both sexes wear their hair long, and many of the young men sport beards. There is absolutely no doubt that cutting ones hair and shaving are, in the final analysis, physical amputation and that it is more natural not to perform such operations. But equally, long hair and luxuriant beards are demonstrations of dissociation on the part of the young from the closely-shaven older generation. As those who have followed this historical account will have by now realized, it is a misconception based on nothing short of ignorance to associate feminine nature with long hair and masculine nature with short-cropped hair. Some readers will recall that in the stories about Red Indians read during their childhood, the women of the Crows and other tribes always wore their hair short, while the men wore theirs long. This is actually more or less common practice among primitive peoples living in a matriarchal society. Margaret Mead's researches into the Tchambuli of New Guinea revealed that the men spent a long time combing, plaiting and curling their hair, while the women wore their hair short.

Within our own cultural tradition, both men and women in Ancient Egypt shaved all the hair from their bodies, since it was considered hygienic in such a hot climate. But long wigs and false beards were worn. The reigning Pharaoh always wore a plaited beard of goat's hair, even if the ruler was a woman. The wigs of men and women were of equal length since the two sexes were considered equal.

The Jews of the Old Testament had long hair and the story of Samson demonstrates that they looked upon it as a sign of male strength. Samson says to his temptress: 'If I shave it off, my strength will leave me and I will become as weak as other mortals.' In

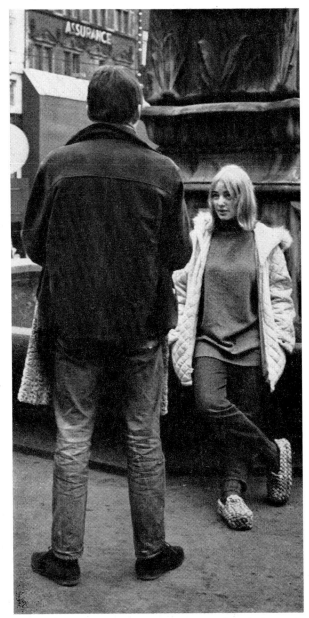

Visors are raised and eyes meet

Both sexes wear coloured shirts and jackets. Many girls' pullovers are actually men's woollen pullovers that have been dyed. Outer clothing usually consists of army surplus jackets inscribed with the names of their heroes, navy peajackets, or donkey jackets, or uniforms that belonged originally to porters, soldiers or policemen. As far as material and tailoring are concerned, both are of an inferior quality.

All young people wear shoes that acknowledge the basic shape of the foot; boys wear either suede campaign boots or sandals, while girls prefer sandals with wooden soles or Cossack boots.

Handbags, it is felt, are only permissible if they look like sacks. Caps have to have broad peaks and soft floppy crowns; they are as symbolic, in their own

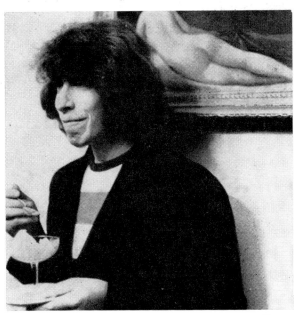

Samson

229

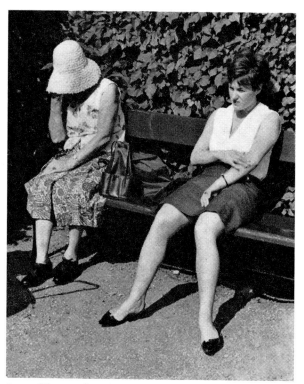

An age difference of twenty years ...

own view, again, was the one current in Tarsus in Asia Minor, where he had grown up.

Paul says, 'Does not even nature itself teach you that, if a man have long hair, it is a shame unto him? But if a woman have long hair, it is a glory to her, for her hair is given her for a covering.'

Greek men in earliest times wore their hair long. Cretan wall-paintings show men with long plaited hair, and Zeus himself, father of all the gods, was represented with long flowing locks. Later, Greek men had short hair since it was more practical for sport, while the long hair of the women showed that their place was not on the athletics field. But in Sparta all unmarried women wore short hair just like the men. The emancipated women of Rome at the time of the Empire preferred the same short style favoured by the men.

In Northern Europe, there is much evidence to support the theory that long hair was greatly valued from ancient times on; slaves, on the other hand, could be identified by their short-cropped hair. When Klodomir was captured in battle, the Burgundians realized who he was by his unusually long hair. After the year 800, long hair lost favour. Charlemagne still wore hair down to his shoulders, but his son's hair was short and his grandson was known as Charles the Bald.

About 1100, Henry I of England formally banned long hair and had his subjects' heads forcibly trimmed; his example was followed in Russia six hundred years later by Peter the Great. In Normandy, a sermon by the monk, Selo, moved Henry I to tears, so that there and then he allowed Selo to cut his hair as well as that of his entire retinue. This episode in particu-

the Second Book of Samuel we are told that no one in Israel looked so splendid as Absalom: when he shaved his head — which happened at the end of every year — he weighed the hair of his head at two hundred shekels.

Women in this society had their hair cut when they were married. The Ethiopian ruling house cites this custom as the indirect reason for its illegitimate descent from King Solomon. When the Queen of Sheba learnt that, in order for her to enter into a lawful marriage with the King, her hair would have to be cut short, she changed her mind and went back home to Ethiopia.

Despite the fact that the Old Testament became part of the Christian Bible, the attitude of Christianity towards the length of hair of the two sexes differed from that of the ancient Jews. The Christian view of hair styles, as of the relationship between men and women in general was decisively influenced by the views and teaching of St. Paul. His

230   ... And a difference of five hundred years

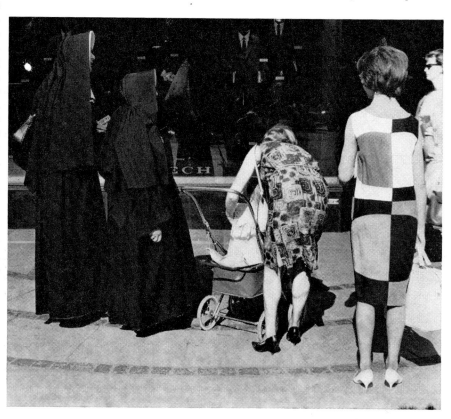

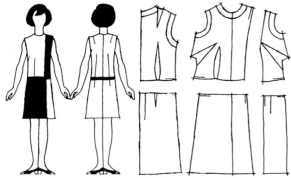
Pattern of a symmetrical op-art dress, 1966

lar would seem to indicate that it is Christian agitation which spells the end of long hair for men!

As Christianity became disseminated, women's hair went into hiding. The enjoyment of a married woman's hair was the monopoly of her husband. On her wedding night it was concealed beneath tight strips of cloth, with the result that it eventually rotted on the scalp. And so women became as bald as eggs.

Women's hair began to peep out from under their head-dresses again at the end of the sixteenth century, but it was artificial hair made by female wigmakers. These wigmakers figure largely in letters of the time exchanged between noblewomen.

Two hundred years later, the coiffures of high-born women were three feet or more in height, and no one but an expert could tell which parts were natural hair and which artificial. On top of each coiffure, flower baskets, baskets of fruit, replicas of temples or three-masted ships were set.

Women during the French Revolution wore their hair short like the men, thus returning to the styles of Antiquity. Curly locks were popular, while women wih less extreme tastes wore their hair in a Greek bun. Later, hair was massed over the forehead and built up with a hairpiece of artificial hair to which were added several artificial plaits.

Long-haired Boys, Short-haired Girls. In our own times, the old subconscious associations fostered by Christianity are fast disappearing. The revolt of the modern generation against them has a background entirely other than most outraged critics of the young realize or than most young people themselves realize.

Women's long and smouldering resentment of the Paul-inspired fear has now burst out violently. The earliest manifestation of protest occurred during the Middle Ages, when the Virgin Mary was installed as the third member of the Christian Trinity instead of the theologians' hopelessly moribund construction, the Holy Ghost.

Growing female self-confidence expressed itself in hair styles for the first time during the Renaissance, when learned and well-read women dared to reveal that they had their own or false hair just like the men. This new assertiveness opened the way that led eventually to the monstrous coiffures of Baroque and Rococo times. Then, during the French Revolution,

women suddenly discovered that they had the courage to allow hair styles to reveal the shape of the head.

Whenever fashion has dictated short hair, artists have reaffirmed their preference for the natural by letting their hair grow longer than is common among the short-cropped bourgeoisie. Their gesture in itself constitutes a criticism of the increasing standardization essential to a completely rationalized society. The long, wavy hair of a teenage boy is a comparable revolt, a joyful and successful revolt against being merely a functional cog in a sterile machine. I was recently sitting behind a young man at a meeting, when it suddenly struck me that there, in front of me, was a survival from the great age of the Valdemars. The magnificient gleaming shock of red-gold hair falling over a neck, young and slim but already muscular, recalled pictures from the Middle Ages of those men who brought about the greatest century of Denmark's history.

Those who react angrily to long hair on men should not be too convinced that determinedly male styles in hair and dress are not a device to conceal impotence and repression.

The hair we are now concerned with, be it long or short, is the person's very own. Consequently it displays countless individual variations from person to person. Soldiers, it should be noted, are not allowed to grow their hair. Throughout the ages the military ideal has been a head as closely cropped as possible; the German shorn neck is the closest that civilian society has come to this ideal. (The American author, Scott Wood, has very aptly remarked that the natural soldier can be identified by the fact that he does not have to unbutton his shirt in order to pull it over his head!)

As for girls with short hair, they are our Amazons and they take no pains to hide their aggressive intent.

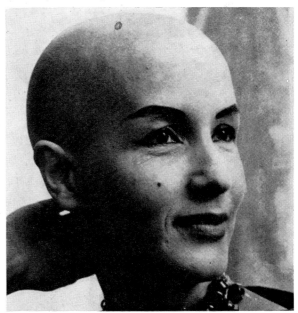
Amazon of 1966

231

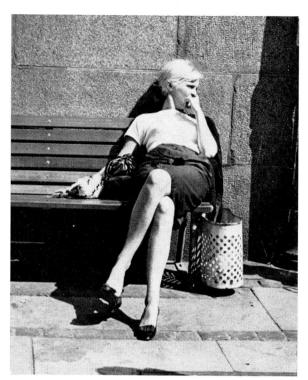

The eternal Eve

They look upon the long hair of the past as a device to conceal women and as one of the many fetters that bound them in a position of social inferiority. They have thrown off the fetters, and it is the young men who have now seized them. And that is only fair!

The sexes may continue their struggle for dominance, as they have done for thousands of years. It is not impossible, however, to conceive of a pact which could entail co-operation and mutual help. The conflict has had its periods of armistice, evidenced by the fact that mankind has not yet died out.

The Battle for Ideals. It is within the realm of possibility that one day the leather jacketted youths, with their immaculate white shirts, terylene trousers and pointed, high-heeled boots might oust the long-haired youths from Europe's main streets. Contrary to opinion, these youths are in fact idealists; the ideals they are fighting for are simple ones, as un-

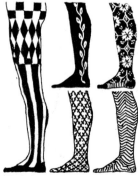

Men's hose in 1550 and women's stockings in 1968

complicated as those which drew volunteers to the Nazi cause and, as soldiers, spurred them on right up to the steppes of Russia.

Our indignation has little rational basis, for the Leather Jackets are trying hard, according to their own lights. It is no fault of theirs if society has provided little to sustain them beyond movies and comic strips and that they are at

the mercy of advertising and publicity campaigns. It shocks them deeply that so many young people scoff quite openly at the ideals and achievements of European culture. Their heroes who embody their ideals are the bull-fighters, gunmen and astronauts of today. The faith they are loyal to is the violent solution of the flick-knife.

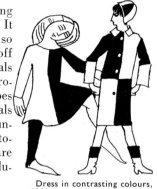

Dress in contrasting colours, 1350, and op-art dress of 1966

Their anger, no less despairing on the one hand than that of their long-haired counterparts, is, on the other, not as devoid of illusions. They accept trustingly those self-same caricatures that they are offered as the genuine article. When they attack asocial individuals who seem to them to be sneering at the consumers' great society, they are merely acting out the violent hostility felt by many respectable citizens.

Other more liberal observers believe that the clothes and hair styles affected by the long-haired young people signify the utter hopelessness induced by the threat of nuclear destruction.

What has actually happened is that our welfare state has in fact produced a thoroughly apolitical generation. Neither the Leather Jackets nor the long-haired youths are prepared to give credence to the menace of the bomb. They have no faith in any words or speeches of the older generation, whether they are threatening or reassuring. They disassociate themselves from everything connected with the parent generation that brought them up and tried to pass onto them the fruits of its experience. But for the first time in history, the older generation has not been able to teach its children the fundamental art of living in the world. The fully mechanized society into which the young have been born is an impersonal chilly one. But both their leather jackets and long hair conceal hearts as ardent as young people of all ages and all countries have always possessed.

Their attitude towards the atomic bomb differs significantly from that of their parents. They have an equal conviction that it will one day be dropped, but they have an inborn faith, that even the materialistic society in which they have come to maturity has failed to crush, that mankind will survive. Their faith in life is far more securely based than our fear of death.

If history teaches any moral, it must be that never has any opportunity for the commission of human error been passed by. But up till now, the destructive forces have always been made, ultimately, to serve a constructive purpose. One shock has, up till now, been enough to bring men to their senses and to make them realize what they are about.

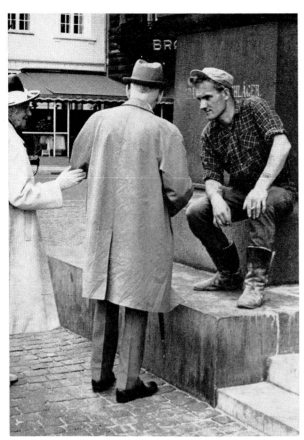

White-collar worker and manual worker

ous' metals and 'real' stones.

Since they themselves prefer old, worn clothes, they naturally feel an affinity with those peoples prevented by their poverty from sharing in the largesse of the textile industry. Since they reject the sexually differentiated Western styles of dress, they naturally tend to identify themselves with those peoples whose garments, like those of the Chinese, are similar for both sexes.

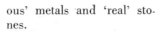
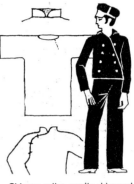

Chinese collar, coolie shirt and coat, St. Laurent model, 1966

The intense loathing that their specific situation arouses in them is expressed in antisocial behaviour that is a protest only different in degree from the Buddhists, who burn themselves to death in Vietnam.

Involvement with Others – But with whom? If politicians were not so blind, they would quake at the sight of young people's clothes today. They constitute, in effect, banners, which proclaim almost legibly that the young steadfastly refuse to assume the responsibility that has not been entrusted to them. Modern power politics and acrobatics performed in space by cosmanauts fail alike to impress them. They take note of them. They register the fact that men can travel as quickly to Vietnam today as they did to a neighbouring town a hundred years ago. And the conclusion they draw is that events in Vietnam now concern them as intimately as events in their next town.

Innumerable details of their dress convey the involvement which they feel with distant peoples and cultures: Arab kaftans, Cossack boots, Chinese collars, African jewellery made from seeds, wood and leather, instead of 'preci-

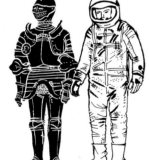

Suit of armour of 1550, and space suit of 1968

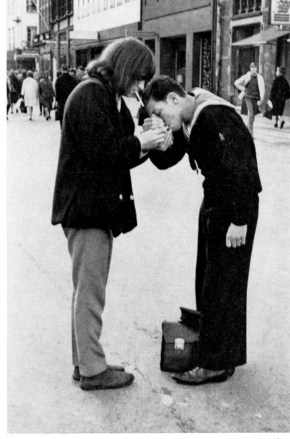

Two kinds of uniform

233

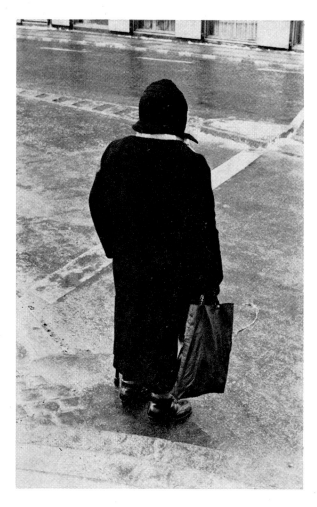

leaders in fashion and dress. Men could well take a lesson from their innovations, were they not so inhibited by their vast superiority complex. Women's clothing weighs between a half and a tenth of the weight of men's clothes and is also far more efficiently ventilated. In winter, women sensibly wear fur coats for extra warmth. Their clothes permit freedom of movement, are easier to carry and provide much greater choice in material, colour and cut. Until quite recently, artificial silks which allow ultraviolet rays to pass through them, were reserved for women's wear. However a woman dresses, she never lets her body become a mere abstract form with her face and hands looking like surrealistic appendages.

All of this ground has been won by women fighting in the shadow cast by the lords of creation. What will be the result when women occupy their own place in the sun? Many things will alter when we cease to think in terms of men and women and begin to think in terms of people.

Throughout the history of our civilization, it has been the task of women, albeit assisted on occasions by men, to establish and maintain the home as the vital centre of family life. Men can establish a state, but what state can create a home atmosphere for its children? There are many things which will be treated with greater care and respect when a world exists in which women's power and influence is equal to that of men. When this time comes, the history of dress with which this book has been concerned, will have reached the end of an epoch and a new era will commence. No longer will dress and mode of dress be a sign of class and social standing or a method of disguise. Dress will regain its old glory and will be a delight, a true adornment and means of enchantment. The meaning and the answer to Our Lord's question will then be clear to all:

'Is not the life more than meat, and the body than raiment?'

Envoy. Good democratic fashion is, to this day, a concentration of what is best in style. The state-owned factories of Soviet Russia turn out footwear with Baroque heels like our own, and China has appropriated the dignity conferred by the blocked felt hat. We may well wonder how long it will be before the developing nations which have emerged so suddenly into an industrialized world thrust the colour, passion and temperament of Asia, Africa and Indian America into the great melting pot. For some time already, brown, yellow and black bodies have haunted the dream of fashion geniuses. That most international sphere of all, the fashion world, has become aware of a world other than the white world, and the dark skin has been brought more and more into the picture. What surprises can we expect from another and even greater movement of liberation even now on its way from north, south, east and west: the march against the tyranny of male domination in sexual relationships? This is the revolution which will liberate not only nations and social classes, but the entirety of the human race. Man will no longer be master and woman will no longer be his slave.

Women long ago took the initiative in becoming

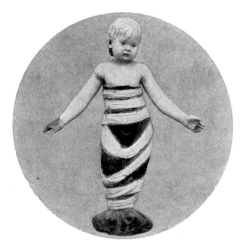

Terracotta medallion by Andrea della Robbia

EXPANDED TABLE OF CONTENTS

PRIMITIVE PEOPLES 6
The Price of Nakedness 7/ Cold
Shoulders and Empty Stomachs 7/
Flat Foreheads 11/ Plate-Shaped
Lips and Elongated Ears 11/ Self-
Mutilation and the Gods 12/ Civi-
lized Body Culture 12/ Cinderella's
Glass Slipper 13/ Colours for Iden-
tification 14/ Fear-Inspiring, Fes-
tive and Mourning Make-up 14/
Decorative Scars 15/ Moving Pic-
tures 15/ The Magic of Clothes
20/ The Mask Changes — But the
Mask Remains 21/ The Submission
of Man to Woman 23/ Mother-
Worship 23/ The Amazons 24/
Warrior versus Housewife 24/ The
Fight for Freedom 24/ The Strug-
gle for the Trousers 24/ From
Feast-Hall to Prison 25/ The Spun
Thread 27/ Female Occupations
27/

CLASSICAL DRESS 33
The Wrapped Garment 33
The Egyptian Loin-Cloth 35
The Long Dress 36/ Light Cloth-
ing 38/ The Slender Line 38/
Pharaoh's Throne 39/ Cosmetics
and Wigs 39/ Peaceful Coexist-
ence 41/
The Mesopotamian Wrap 41
Draped Clothing 42/ Heavy Wool
42/ Rich Colours 44/ Exposed
Borders — Concealing Dress 44/
Female Duties 45/
The Greek Chiton 46
The Naked Athlete 46/ Head and
Feet 46/ Greek Stances 47/ Wool
and Linen 50/ Dress and Body
50/ Democracy 51/ Status of Wo-
men 51/
The Roman Toga 52
The Toga 54/ The Tunic 56/
Beauty Culture 57/ Roman Law
58/ Pax Romana 58/
The Arab Haik 59
Abstract Sculpture in Cloth 59/
Veiled Men 60/ The Dream Wo-
men 60/ Arabian Capes 61/ Mus-
lim Dress 61/
The Indian Sari 62
Muslim and European Dress 64/

Turbans and Jewels 64/ Dance
and Sign Language 65/ Rounded
Women 65/

WORKADAY CLOTHES 67
The Armour of Antiquity 67
Armour 67/
The Goat-Skin Skirt of the Aegean 73
Nature and Culture 74/ Bathing
Trunks 74/ The Open Dress 75/
The Tailored Dress 75/ The
Naked Bosom 75/ The Bronze
Age in Nordic Countries 76/
Persian Leather Trousers 77
The Hide Dress 77/ Muslim and
Mongolian Influence 80/ Women
of the Harem 80/
The Indian Feather Poncho 83
Advanced Cultures in America 83/
Stone Age Techniques 83/ Aztecs,
Mayas and Incas 83/ Textiles
84/ Feather Mosaics 85/ Tall
Hats and Ear-rings 85/ The Pon-
cho 86/ Strength and Dignity 86/
Human Sacrifice and Flowers 86/
Spanish Central America 88/
The Mongolian Silk Kimono . . . 89
China 89/ Silk 90/ Discretion in
Dress 90/ Golden Lilies 90/ Red
Happiness — White Sorrow 93/
Family Life 96/ Technique of Love-
Making 96/ The Flat, Snow-white
Bosom 97/ Walking and Sitting
97/
The Eskimo Skin Clothes 98
The Life of the Hunter 98/ De-
corations and Patterns 98/ Pre-
paration of Hides 99/ Clothing
99/ Combinations 100/

CLOTHES AND STATUS 101
Historical Costumes 101
Robes of Byzantium 300—1100 . . 102
Ceremonial Dignity 102/ The Sinful Body 104/ Dressed in Jewellery 106/ The Dress of the Viking
Age and the Period of Great Migrations 106/ Teutons and Celts
108/ Barbarians and Byzantines
109/ Two Philosophies 110
Romanesque Shift and Monk's Cowl
800—1350 111
Knight, Cleric, Burgher 111/ The

Dawn of the Middle Ages 112/
Adam's Clothes 112/ Mantle,
Shirt, Trousers and Socks 114/
Byrnie and Helmet 117/ Silk
Shift and Head Covering 118/
Fresh Perceptions and Expressive
Bodies 119/ The Poetry of the
Troubadours 120/ The Church
and Women 120/ The Church as
Unifier 120/
Gothic Armour and Pointed Shoes
1350—1490 121
Soaring Gothic 121/ The Trium-
phant Progress of the Scissors
122/ Chaucer's Pilgrims 123/
Plate Mail 123/ The Jerkin and
the Full-Sleeved Coat 123/ Fash-
ions from Burgundy 124/ Stock-
ings become Trousers 124/ Heads
and Hair Styles 126/ Hell's Win-
dows 129/ Devil's Horn 129/
Man's Armour and Woman's Dress
130/ Differences in Male and
Female Dress 131/ Deportment
131/ Colourful Uniforms and
Black Velvet 132/ The Tailor's
Craft 132/
Renaissance Fashion 1490—1625 133
New Directions of Thought 136/
Propaganda and Expediency 136/
Venice-Madrid Axis 137/ Mobile
Men and Immobile Women 137/
The Spanish Cape and the Split
Jerkin 138/ Millstones Round the
Neck 139/ Voluminous Trousers
140/ The Codpiece 140/ Comfort-
able Shoes 142/ Hat, Hair and
Beards 142/ Décolleté 143/ Spa-
nish and French Crinolines 143/
Heads and Feet 144/ The Posi-
tion of Women 144/ Respectable
Prostitutes 145/ People of the
Renaissance 146/ Beauty Culture
146/
Baroque Lace and Footwear
1625—1710 147
Propaganda 147/ Spanish Cape
and Polish Kassak 147/ From
Ruff to Neckcloth 149/ Knee
Breeches 149/ Shoes and Stockings 149/ Hats, Hair and Wigs
151/ Military Uniform 153/ Baroque Women 153/ Puritan Dress

155/ Dressed in Silk and Lace 155/ Heels and Wigs 156/ Erotic Aspects 156/ Weak Men and Strong Women 158/

Rococo Fashion and Powdered Wigs 1710—1790 163
The Boned Skirt 163/ The Laced Bodice 163/ Négligé 164/ Hair Styles for the Crinoline 164/ Satin Shoes 165/ The Rococo Woman's Deportment 165/ Male Dress 166/ Uniforms 169/ Colours and Material 169/ Make-up 171/ Chinese Influence and Nature-Worship 171/ The Ideal Woman 172/ The Salons 173/ The World at Large 173/

CHANGING FASHIONS 175
Fashion During and After the French Revolution 1790—1830 . . 176
The Statuesque Dress 177/ The Shift 177/ The Draped Garment 177/ Long-Limbed Graces 178/ Short Hair and Small Fans 178/ Daughters of the Revolution 178/ The Return of the Crinoline 180/ Sons of the Revolution 183/ Puritans and Long Trousers 183/ Revolutionary Behaviour 184/

Fancy Waistcoats and Puritan Hats 184/ The Dress of the Commoners 184/

Crinolines and Stovepipes 1830—1870 185
The Romantic Woman 185/ Souls without Bodies 186/ The Harbingers of Emancipation 186/ Clothed in Steel 187/ Court Crinoline 187/ Restricted Muscles 188/ Décolleté and Gloves 189/ Professional Charmers 189/ New Rococo and New Revolution 190/ Red Blouses and Masculine Coats 192/ Two Varieties of Tails 192/ White Collars and Coloured Waistcoats 192/ Office Uniform 193/ Underwear 193/

Jackets and Bustles 1870—1890 . . 195
Male Accessories 195/ The Chignon and the Bustle 197/ A Curious Fashion 197/ The Rout of the Bustle 198/ The Return of the Bustle 199/ The Buxom Woman 199/ The Willowy Type 200/ The Emancipated Woman 200/

Corsetted Waist and Wing Collar 1890—1920 201
New Weapons 201/ The New Woman 202/ Sporting Dress 202/

The Turn of the Century 206/ Art Nouveau 207/ Bust and Skirts 207/ The First World War 211/ Cosmetics 212/ Women's Legs 212/ The Schoolgirl Ideal 213/ Male Defences 213/ Ready-made Clothes 213/ Leisure Clothes 214/ Sportsmen and Puritans 214/

Functional Design 1920—1950 . . 215
The Self-Supporting Woman 215/ Youth 216/ Silk Stockings and Cloche Hats 216/ No Pretence 216/ Short Dresses 217/ Dress Materials 218/ Male Dress 218/ Accessories 220/ A Look at the Thirties 221/ Fashion in the 1930's 221/ Separate Collars 222/ The Vanishing Tie 222/ The Second World War 223/ The New Look 223/ Paris 225/ The Fashion Designer 225/

Today's Fashions —
and What the Future May Bring 226
The Revolt of the Masses 227/ A Look at the Present Day 228/ Long-haired Boys, Short-haired Girls 231/ The Battle for Ideals 232/ Involvement with Others — But with whom? 233/ Envoy 234/